An Introduction to the Physiology of Hearing

An Introduction to the Physiology of Hearing

James O. Pickles

Department of Physiology,
University of Birmingham,
Birmingham, England

1982

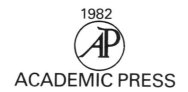

ACADEMIC PRESS

A Subsidiary of Harcourt Brace Jovanovich, Publishers
LONDON   NEW YORK
PARIS   SAN DIEGO   SAN FRANCISCO   SÃO PAULO
SYDNEY   TOKYO   TORONTO

ACADEMIC PRESS INC. (LONDON) LTD
24–28 Oval Road,
London NW1

U.S. Edition published by
ACADEMIC PRESS INC.
111 Fifth Avenue,
New York, New York 10003

British Library Cataloguing in Publication Data

Pickles, J.O.
  An introduction to the physiology of hearing.
  1. Hearing   2. Psychoacoustics
  I. Title
  612'.85   QP461

    ISBN 0-12-554750-1 Hardback
    ISBN 0-12-554752-8 Paperback
    LCCN 81-69596

Phototypesetting by Oxford Publishing Services, Oxford
Printed in Great Britain by St Edmunsbury Press, Bury St Edmunds

Preface

The last fifteen years have seen a revolution in auditory physiology, but the new ideas have been slow to gain currency outside the circle of specialists. Undoubtedly, one of the main reasons for this has been the lack of a general source for non-specialists, and it is hoped that the present book will introduce recent thinking to a much wider audience.

Whilst the book is primarily intended as a student text, it is hoped that it will be equally useful to teachers of auditory physiology. It should be particularly useful to those teaching physiology to medical students, because general texts of physiology aimed at medical students commonly contain only a small section on hearing, which is based on material that is 20 or more years out of date. The increasing concern about the extent of hearing loss in the community should increase the attention paid to auditory physiology in the medical curriculum.

The majority of the book is written at a level suitable for a degree course on the special senses or as a basis for a range of postgraduate courses. It is organized so as to be accessible to those approaching the subject at a number of levels and with a variety of backgrounds. Chapter 1 on the physics and analysis of sound contains elementary information which should be read by everyone. Those who need only a brief introduction to auditory physiology may then read only Chapter 3 on the Cochlea. Those whose interests lie in the psychophysical correlates may read Chapters 1 to 4, and then turn to Chapter 9. Those who are interested in clinical aspects may read Chapters 1 to 3, part of Chapter 4 (as indicated), and then Chapter 10. Chapter 5, which explores the newer ideas on cochlear physiology, is written at a more advanced level than the rest of the book, and if desired may be omitted without affecting the understanding of the other chapters. Chapters 6, 7, and 8, on the brainstem, cortex, and centrifugal pathways should appeal primarily to specialist physiology students, although the latter part of Chapter 7 on the cortex, and some parts of Chapter 8 on centrifugal pathways, contain much material that should be of interest to students of physiological psychology.

Only the most elementary knowledge of physiology is assumed, and even

v

such basic concepts as ionic equilibrium potentials are explained where appropriate, so that the book should be accessible to those with only a small background in physiology. The treatment is nonmathematical, and only a few very elementary algebraic equations appear. In Chapter 3, some of the reasoning behind theories of cochlear mechanics is explained verbally for the benefit of those without mathematical training. I have found that for those *with* such training, this approach makes the subject more, rather than less, confusing. I can only apologize to them, and refer them to the several excellent accounts that have already appeared at their own level (e.g. Zwislocki, 1965; Dallos, 1973a; Schroeder, 1975; Geisler, 1976; Steele, 1976; and Dallos, 1978).

I should like to express my thanks to colleagues who read and commented on sections of an earlier version of the manuscript, and in particular to G. R. Bock, S. D. Comis, J. L. Cranford, L. U. E. Kohllöffel, O. Lowenstein, B. C. J. Moore, G. F. Pick, H. F. Ross, I. J. Russell, R. L. Smith, and G. K. Yates. I am also grateful to D. Robertson for supplying the micrographs of Fig. 3.4, and to T. L. Hayward for help with the illustrations. The book was written while I was a member of the Neurocommunications Research Unit at Birmingham University, and I am grateful to my colleagues in the Unit, S. D. Comis and H. F. Ross, for many helpful discussions, and to everyone, in this university and elsewhere, who dealt patiently with a continual series of small queries.

July 1981   J. O. Pickles
                                                                              Birmingham

Contents

To Charlotte

Some of the basic concepts of the physics and analysis of sound, which are necessary for the understanding of the later chapters, are presented here. The relations between the pressure, displacement and velocity of a medium produced by a sound wave are first described, followed by the decibel scale of sound level, and the notion of impedance. Fourier analysis and the idea of linearity are then described.

A. The Nature of Sound

In order to understand the physiology of hearing, a few facts about the physics of sound, and its analysis, are necessary. As an example, Fig. 1.1 shows a tuning fork sending out a sound wave, and shows the distribution of the sound wave at one point in time, plotted over space, and at one point in space, plotted over time. The tuning fork sends out a travelling pressure wave, which is accompanied by a wave of displacement of the air molecules making them vibrate around their mean positions. There are two important variables in such a sound wave. One is its frequency, which is the number of waves to pass any one point in a second, measured in cycles per second, or hertz (Hz). This has the subjective correlate of pitch, sounds of high frequency having high pitch. The other important attribute of the wave is its amplitude or intensity, which is related to the magnitude of the movements produced. This has the subjective correlate of loudness.

If the sound wave is in a free medium, the pressure and velocity of the air vary exactly together, and are said to be in phase. The displacement however lags by a quarter of a cycle. It is important to understand that the pressure variations are around the mean atmospheric pressure. The varia-

1

tions are in fact a very small proportion of the total atmospheric pressure — even a level as high as 140 dB SPL (defined on p. 4), as intense as anything likely to be encountered in everyday life, makes the pressure vary by only 0.6%. The displacement is also about the mean position, and the sound wave does not cause a net flow of molecules.

The different parameters of the sound wave can easily be related to each

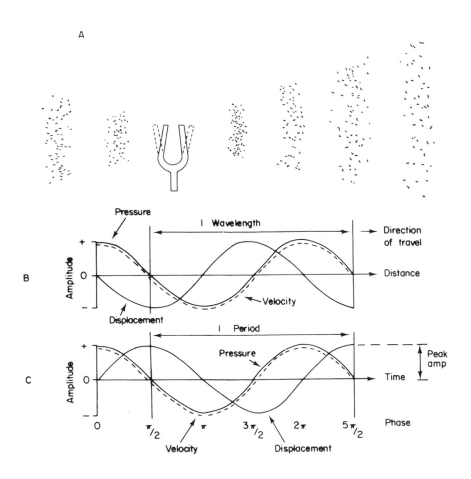

Fig. 1.1 A. A tuning fork sending out a sound wave.
B. The variation of the pressure, velocity, and displacement of the air molecules in a sinusoidal sound wave are seen at one moment in time. The variations are plotted as a function of distance. The pressure and velocity vary together, and the displacement lags by a quarter of a cycle.
C. The same variation is plotted as a function of time, as measured at one point. Because times further in the past are plotted to the right of the figure, the curve of displacement is here plotted to the *right*, not to the left as in part B, of the pressure curve. The phase increases by 2π (or 360°) in one cycle. The sound wave is defined by its peak amplitude and its frequency.

other. The peak pressure above atmospheric (P) and the peak velocity of the sinusoid (V) are related by:

$$P = RV \qquad \text{(Equation 1)}$$

where R is a constant of proportionality, called the *impedance*. It is a function of the medium in which the sound is travelling, and will be dealt with later.

The intensity of the sound wave is the amount of power transmitted through a unit area of space. It is a function of the *square* of the peak pressure, and, by equation 1, also of the square of the peak velocity. It in addition depends on the impedance; for a sine wave,

$$\text{Intensity } I = P^2/2R = RV^2/2 \qquad \text{(Equation 2)}$$

In other words, if the intensity of a sound wave is constant, the peak pressure and the peak velocity are constant. They are also independent of the frequency of the sound wave. It is for these reasons that the pressure and velocity will be of most use later.

Unlike the above parameters, the peak *displacement* of the air molecules does vary with frequency, even when the intensity is constant. For constant sound intensity, the peak displacement is inversely proportional to the frequency:

$$D = \frac{1}{2\pi f} \sqrt{\frac{2I}{R}} \qquad \text{(Equation 3)}$$

where D is the peak displacement, and f is the frequency. So for sounds of constant intensity, the displacement of the air particles gets smaller as the frequency increases. We can see correlates of this when we see a loud-speaker cone moving. At low frequencies the movement can be seen easily, but at high frequencies the movement is imperceptible, even though the intensities may be comparable.

B. The Decibel Scale

We can measure the intensity of a sound wave by specifying the peak excess pressure in normal physical quantities, e.g. newtons/metre^2, sometimes called pascals. In fact it is often more useful to record the RMS pressure, meaning the square Root of the Mean of the Squared pressure, because such a quantity is related to the energy (actually to the square root of the energy) in the sound wave over all shapes of waveform. For a sinusoidal waveform the RMS pressure is $1/\sqrt{2}$ of the peak pressure. While it is perfectly possible to use a scale of RMS pressure in terms of N/m^2, for the purposes of physiology and psychophysics it turns out to be much more convenient to use an intensity scale in which equal increments roughly correspond to equal increments in sensation, and in which the very large range of intensity used is represented by a rather narrower range of numbers. Such a scale is made by taking the ratio of the sound intensity to a certain reference intensity, and then taking the logarithm of the ratio. If logarithms to the base 10 are taken, the units in the resulting scale, called Bels, are rather large, so the scale is expressed in units 1/10th the size, called decibels, or dB.

$$\text{Number of dB} = 10 \log_{10} \left(\frac{\text{Sound intensity}}{\text{Reference intensity}} \right)$$

Because the intensity varies as the square of the pressure, the scale in dB is 10 times the logarithm of the *square* of the pressure ratio, or 20 times the logarithm of the pressure ratio:

$$\text{Number of dB} = 20 \log_{10} \left(\frac{\text{Sound pressure}}{\text{Reference pressure}} \right)$$

It only now remains to choose a convenient reference pressure. In physiological experiments the investigator commonly takes any reference he finds convenient, such as that, for instance, given by the maximum signal in his sound stimulating system. However, one scale is general use has a reference close to the lowest sound pressure that can be commonly detected by man, namely, 2×10^{-5} N/m^2 RMS, or 20 μpascals RMS. In air under standard conditions this corresponds to a power of 10^{-12} watts/m^2. Intensity levels referred to this are known as dB SPL.

$$\text{Intensity level in dB SPL} = 20 \log_{10} \left(\frac{\text{RMS Sound Pressure}}{2 \times 10^{-5} \text{N/m}^2} \right)$$

We are then left with a scale with generally positive values, in which equal intervals have approximately equal physiological significance in all parts of the scale, and in which we rarely have to consider step sizes less than one unit. While we often have to use only positive values, negative values are perfectly possible. They represent sound pressures less than 2×10^{-5} N/m^2, for which the pressure ratio is less than one.

C. Impedance

Materials differ in their response to sound; in a tenuous, compressible medium such as air a certain sound pressure will produce greater velocities of movement than in a dense, incompressible medium such as water. The relation between the sound pressure and particle velocity is a property of the medium and was given in equation 1 by Impedance $R = P/V$. For plane waves in an effectively infinite medium the impedance is a characteristic of the medium alone. It is then called the *specific impedance*. In the SI system, R is measured in $(N/m^2)/(m/sec)$, or $N\ sec/m^3$. If R is large, as for a dense, incompressible medium such as water, relatively high pressures are needed to achieve a certain velocity of the molecules. The pressure will be higher than is needed for a medium of low specific impedance, such as air.

The impedance will concern us when we consider the transmission of sounds from the air to the cochlea. Air has a much lower impedance than the cochlear fluids. Let us take, as an example, the transmission of sound from air into a large body of water, such as a lake. The specific impedance of air is about $400\ N\ sec/m^3$, and that of water $1.5 \times 10^6\ N\ sec/m^3$, a ratio of 3750 times. In other words, when a sound wave meets a water surface at normal incidence, the pressure variation in the wave is only large enough to displace the water at the boundary by 1/3750 of the displacement of the air near the boundary. However, continuity requires that the displacements of the molecules immediately on both sides of the boundary must be equal. What happens is that much of the incident sound wave is reflected; the pressure at the boundary stays high, but because the reflected wave is travelling in the opposite direction to the incident wave it produces movement of the molecules in the opposite direction. The movements due to the incident and reflected waves therefore substantially cancel, and the net velocity of the air molecules will be small. This leaves a net ratio of pressure to velocity in the air near the boundary which is the same as that of water.

One result of the impedance jump is that much of the incident power is reflected. Where R_1 and R_2 are the specific impedances of the two media, the proportion of the incident power transmitted is $4\ R_1\ R_2/(R_1 + R_2)^2$. At the air–water interface this means that only about 0.1% of the incident power is transmitted, corresponding to an attenuation of 30 dB. In a later section (p. 15) we shall see how the middle ear converts a similar attenuation in the ear to the near-perfect transmission estimated as occurring at some frequencies.

Finally, in analysing complex acoustic circuits, it is convenient to use analogies with electrical circuits, for which the analysis is well known. Impedance in an electrical circuit relates the voltage to the rate of movement of charge, and if we are to make an analogy we need a measure of impedance which relates to the amount of medium moved per second. We can therefore define a different acoustic impedance, known as acoustic ohms, which is the pressure to move a unit *volume* of the medium per second. Acoustic ohms will not be used in this book, and where necessary, values will be converted from the literature, which is done by multiplying the number of acoustic ohms by the cross-sectional area of the structure in question.

D. The Analysis of Sound

Figure 1.2 shows a small portion of the pressure waveform of a complex acoustic signal. There is a regularly repeating pattern with two peaks per cycle. The pattern can be approximated by adding together the two sinusoids shown, one at 150 Hz, and the other at 300 Hz. Such an analysis of a

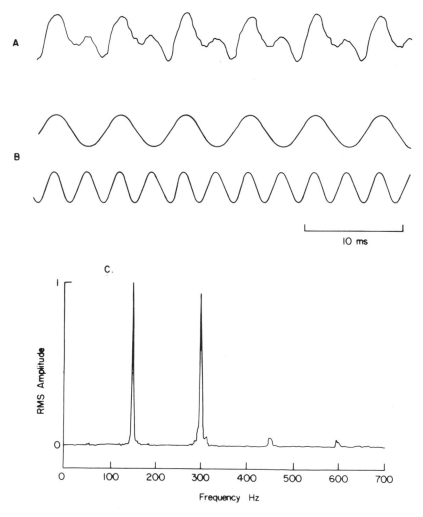

Fig. 1.2 A. A portion of a complex acoustic waveform.
B. The waveform can be closely approximated by adding together two sine waves.
C. A Fourier analysis of the waveform in *A* shows that in addition to the main components, there are other smaller ones at higher frequencies. Components at still higher frequencies, responsible for the small high frequency ripple on the waveform in *A*, lie outside the frequency range of the analysis, and are not shown.

complex signal into component sinusoids is known as Fourier analysis, and forms one of the conceptual cornerstones of auditory physiology. The result of a Fourier transformation is to produce the *spectrum* of the sound wave (Fig. 1.2C). The spectrum shows here that in addition to the main components, there are also smaller components, at 1/15th of the amplitude or less, at 450 Hz and 600 Hz. Such a spectrum tells us the amplitude of each frequency component, and so the energy in each frequency region.

Why do we analyse sound waves into sinusoids rather than into other elementary waveforms? One reason is that it is mathematically convenient to do so. Another reason is that sinusoids represent the oscillations of a very broad class of physical systems, so that examples are likely to be found in nature. However, the most compelling reason from our point of view is that the auditory system itself seems to perform a Fourier transform, like that of Fig. 1.2C, although with a more limited resolution. Therefore sinusoids are not only simple physically, but are simple physiologically. This has a correlate in our own sensations, and a sinusoidal sound wave has a particularly pure timbre. In understanding the physiology of the lower stages of the auditory system, one of our concerns will be with the way in which the system analyses sound into sine waves, and how it handles the frequency and intensity information in them.

Figure 1.3 shows some common Fourier transforms. In the most elementary case, a simple sinusoid, which lasts for an infinite time, has a Fourier transform represented by a single line, corresponding to the frequency of the sinusoid (Fig. 1.3A). A wave such as a square wave, similarly lasting for an infinite time, has a spectrum consisting of a series of lines (Fig. 1.3B). But physical signals do not of course last for an infinite time, and the result of shortening the duration of the signal is to broaden each spectral line into a band (Fig. 1.3C). The width of each band turns out to be inversely proportional to the duration of the waveform, and the exact shape of each band is a function of the way the wave is turned on and off. If for instance the waveform is turned on and off abruptly, sidelobes appear around each spectral band (Fig. 1.3D).

In the most extreme case, the wave can be turned on for an infinitesimal time, in which case we have a click. The spread of the spectrum will be in inverse proportion to the duration, and so, in the limit, will be infinite. The spectrum of a click therefore covers all frequencies equally. In practice, a click will of course last for a finite time, and this is associated with an upper frequency limit to the spectrum (Fig. 1.3E). Another quite different signal, namely white noise, also contains all frequencies equally (Fig. 1.3F). Although the spectrum determined over short periods shows considerable random variability, the spectrum determined over a long period is flat. It differs from a click in the relative phases of the frequency components, which for white noise are random.

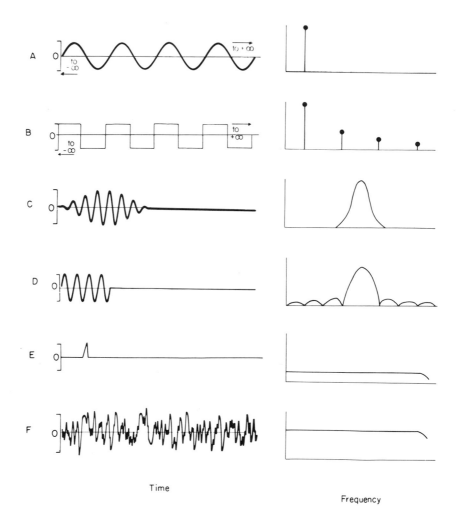

Fig. 1.3 Some waveforms (left) and their Fourier analyses (right).
A. Sine wave. B. Square wave (in these cases the stimuli last an infinite time, and have line spectra, the components of which are harmonically related). C. Ramped sine wave. D. Gated sine wave. E. Click. F. White noise.

E. Linearity

One concept which we shall meet many times, is that of a *linear* system. In such a system, if the input is changed by a certain factor k, the output is also changed by the same factor k, but is otherwise unaltered. In addition linear systems satisfy a second criterion, which is that the output to two or more inputs applied at the same time, is the sum of the outputs that would have been obtained if the inputs had both been applied separately.

We can therefore identify a linear system as one in which the amplitude of the output varies in proportion to the amplitude of the input. A linear system also has other properties. For instance, the only Fourier frequency components in the output signal are those contained in the input signal. A linear system never generates new frequency components. Thus it is distinguished from a non-linear system. In a non-linear system, new frequency components are introduced. If a single sinusoid is presented, the new components will be harmonics of the input signal. If two sinusoids are presented, there will, in addition to the harmonics, be intermodulation products produced; that is, Fourier components whose frequency depends on *both* of the input frequencies.

In the auditory system, we shall be concerned with whether certain of the stages act as linear or non-linear systems. The tests used will be based on the properties described above.

F. Summary

1. A sound wave produces compression and rarefaction of the air, the molecules of which vibrate around their mean positions. The extent of the pressure variation has a subjective correlate in loudness. The frequency, or number of waves passing a point in a second, has a subjective correlate in pitch. Frequency is measured in cycles per second, known as hertz (Hz).

2. The particle velocities produced by a pressure variation depend on the impedance of the medium. If the impedance is high, high pressures are needed to produce a certain velocity.

3. When a sound pressure wave meets a boundary between two media of different impedance, some of the sound energy is reflected.

4. Complex sounds can be analysed by Fourier analysis, that is, by splitting the waveforms into component sine waves of different frequencies. The cochlea seems to do this too, to a certain extent.

5. In a linear system, the output to two inputs together, is the sum of the outputs that would have been obtained if the two inputs had been presented separately. Moreover, in a linear system, the only Fourier frequency components that are present in the output are those that were present in the input. Neither is true for a non-linear system.

II. The Outer and Middle Ears

The outer ear modifies the sound wave in transferring the acoustic vibrations to the eardrum. Firstly, the resonances of the external ear increase the sound pressure at the eardrum, particularly in the range of frequencies (in man) of 2 to 7 kHz. Secondly, the change in pressure depends on the direction of the sound. This is an important cue for sound localization, enabling us to distinguish above from below, and in front from behind. The middle ear apparatus then transfers the sound vibrations from the eardrum to the cochlea. It acts as an impedance transformer, coupling sound energy from the low impedance air to the higher impedance cochlear fluids, substantially reducing the transmission loss that would otherwise be expected. The factors allowing this will be described, and the extent to which the middle ear apparatus acts as an ideal impedance transformer will be discussed. Transmission through the middle ear can be modified by the middle ear muscles, and their action, and possible hypotheses for their role in hearing, will be described.

A. The Outer Ear

The outer ear consists of a partially cartilaginous flange called the pinna, which includes a resonant cavity called the concha, together with the ear canal or external auditory meatus leading to the eardrum or tympanic membrane (Fig. 2.1). The effect of the outer ear on the incoming sound has been analysed from two approaches. One is the influence of the resonances of the outer ear on the sound pressure at the tympanic membrane. The other is the extent to which the outer ear provides directionality cues for help in sound localization.

10

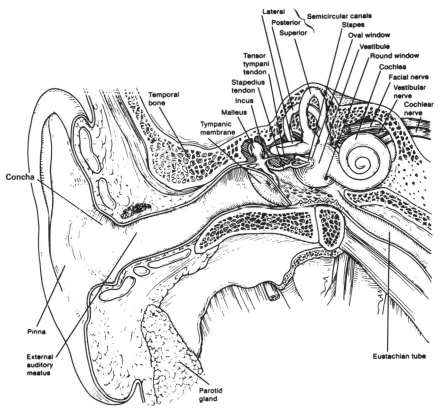

Fig. 2.1 The external, middle, and inner ears in man. From *Tissues and Organs: A Text-Atlas of Scanning Electron Microscopy*, by R. G. Kessel and R. H. Kardon. W. H. Freeman and Company. Copyright © 1979.

1. The Pressure Gain of the Outer Ear

The concha, meatus and tympanic membrane provide the main elements of a complex acoustic cavity, such a cavity being expected to increase and decrease the sound pressure at the tympanic membrane at different frequencies. The data of Wiener and Ross (1946) in man showed a broad peak of 15–20 dB at 2.5 kHz in the sound pressure gain at the tympanic membrane. A recent synthesis of the available data by Shaw (1974) shows very much the same effect (Fig. 2.2). Shaw studied the contributions of the different elements of the external ear by adding the different components sequentially in a model. The results of such an analysis are shown in Fig. 2.3. The 2.5 kHz peak is provided by a resonance of the combination of the meatus and concha. The 5.5 kHz peak is due to a resonance in the concha

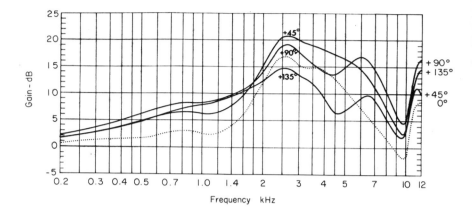

Fig. 2.2 The average pressure gain of the external ear in man. The gain in pressure at the eardrum over that in the free field is plotted as a function of frequency, for different orientations of the source in the horizontal plane ipsilateral to the ear. Zero degrees is straight ahead. From Shaw (1974), Fig. 5.

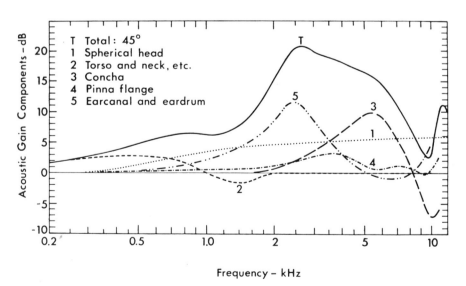

Fig. 2.3 The average pressure gain contributed by the different components of the outer ear in man. The analysis assumes that the components are added in the order shown: e.g. curve 5 is the change produced when the ear canal and eardrum are added to the other components listed. Stimulus in the horizontal plane, 45° from straight ahead. From Shaw (1974), Fig. 11.

alone. It appears that the main pressure gains are complementary, increasing the sound pressure relatively uniformly over the range from 2 to 7 kHz. In increasing the pressure in this way the external ear does not of course provide any actual *power* amplification of the incoming sound wave, because it consists of entirely passive elements which are unable to introduce any extra energy.

2. The Outer Ear as an Aid to Sound Localization

The most important cues for sound localization in man are the intensity and timing differences in the sound waves at the two ears. The sound wave from a source on the right will strike the right ear before the left and will be more intense in the right ear. However this does not account for our ability to distinguish in front from behind, or above from below. The information for such localization comes from the pinna and concha.

When the wavelength is short compared with the dimensions of the pinna, the pinna will show a directional selectivity in the reception of sound. We expect the pinna to be useful in this way only in the high kHz range of frequencies. Some bats, which use frequencies of many tens of kHz for echolocation, have pinnae with a high degree of directional selectively. They may have fantastically developed pinnae, sometimes resembling microwave radio horns. Such directional selectivity for sound is commonly associated with mobile pinnae. For instance the echolocating horseshoe bat *Rhinolopus Ferrumequinum* can change the shape of its pinnae, and rotate them independently through wide angles, the movements accompanying the emitted echolocating pulses (Griffin *et al.*, 1962).

The frequency range of man is too low for the pinnae to be of much use in producing a similar degree of directional selectivity. Nevertheless the pinna does provide useful directional cues. When a sound is behind the ear, the wave transmitted directly interferes with the wave scattered off the edge of the pinna, reducing the response in the 3–6 kHz region (Shaw, 1974). It is in this region that there are the greatest intensity changes as a sound source is moved in the horizontal plane (Fig. 2.2). The obvious dip at 10 kHz is due to out-of-phase reflections off the back wall of the concha. The low frequency cut-off frequency of the dip is raised when the sound source is elevated, and there is psychophysical evidence that such information is used to judge the elevation of sound sources (Hebrank and Wright, 1974).

The external ear therefore produces a spectral modulation of the incoming sound. In using such a coloration to make directional judgements, we are obviously able to make subtle judgements about the modulation of the spectra of perhaps unknown sound sources.

B. The Middle Ear

1. Introduction

The middle ear couples sound energy from the external auditory meatus to the cochlea, and by its transformer action matches the impedance of the auditory meatus to the much higher impedance of the cochlear fluids. In the absence of a transformer mechanism, much of the sound would be reflected.

The sound is transmitted from the tympanic membrane to the cochlea by three small bones, known as the *ossicles*. They are called the malleus, the incus, and the stapes (Figs 2.1 and 2.4). The first two bones are joined comparatively rigidly so that when the tip of the malleus is pushed by the tympanic membrane, the bones rotate together and transfer the force to the stapes. The stapes is attached to a flexible window in the wall of the cochlea, known as the oval window (Fig. 2.4).

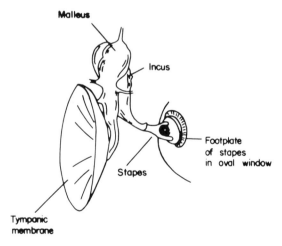

Fig. 2.4 The three ossicles, called the malleus, incus, and stapes, transmit the sound vibrations from the tympanic membrane (eardrum) to the oval window of the cochlea.

A second function of the ossicles is to apply force to one window only of the cochlea. If the ossicles were missing, and the pressure of the incoming sound wave were applied to both windows equally, there would be no net flow of cochlear fluids. Nevertheless, in many species the other window of the cochlea, the round window, is shielded from the incoming sound wave by a bony ridge. In these cases, if the ossicles are missing, the sound pressure is still primarily applied to one window of the cochlea, and some hearing, although without the benefit of the impedance matching, is still possible.

2. The Middle Ear as an Impedance Transformer

(a) The nature of the problem

The middle ear transfers the incoming vibration from the comparatively large, low impedance, tympanic membrane to the much smaller, higher impedance, oval window. As was explained above in Chapter 1 (p. 5), when a sound wave meets a higher impedance medium, much of the sound energy is normally reflected. The middle ear apparatus, by acting as an acoustic impedance transformer, reduces this attenuation substantially.

As a first approximation, Wever and Lawrence (1954) said that the cochlear fluids would have an impedance approximately equal to that of sea-water, namely 1.5×10^6 N sec/m^3, and this led to the calculation, detailed above (p. 5), that if the sound met the oval window directly, only 0.1% of the incident energy would be transmitted. As pointed out by Schubert (1978), although the numerical result is approximately correct, the physical reasoning behind it is not. Specific impedances are defined for progressive acoustic waves in an effectively infinite medium. In the range of audible frequencies, the cochlea is far smaller than a wavelength of sound in water, and so cannot develop such waves. The actual cochlear impedance is determined entirely by the fact that cochlear fluid flows from one flexible window, the oval window, to another, the round window, and the cochlear impedance depends on the way the fluids flow, and on the distensibility of the cochlear membranes. The input impedance of the cochlea has been determined either theoretically, for instance by Zwislocki (1965), or experimentally, for instance by Khanna and Tonndorf (1971). Khanna and Tonndorf's direct measurements in the cat suggest a cochlear impedance of about 2×10^5 N sec/m^3 at 1 kHz,[*] much lower than expected from Wever and Lawrence's approximation.

(b) The mechanism of the impedance transformer

In matching the impedance of the tympanic membrane to the much higher impedance of the cochlea, the middle ear uses three principles.

(i)   The area of the tympanic membrane is larger than that of the stapes footplate on the cochlea. The forces collected over the tympanic membrane are therefore concentrated on a smaller area, so increasing the pressure at the oval window. The pressure is increased by the ratio of the two areas (Fig. 2.5A). This is the most important factor in achieving the impedance transformation.

(ii)   The second principle is the lever action of the middle ear bones. The

---

[*]This is derived from their measurement of 1.7×10^6 c.g.s. acoustic ohms, by multiplying by a stapes footplate area of 1.2×10^{-2} cm^2 to get a specific impedance, and converting to SI units by multiplying by 10.

arm of the incus is shorter than that of the malleus, and this produces a lever action that increases the force and decreases the velocity at the stapes (Fig. 2.5B). This is a comparatively small factor in the impedance match.

(iii)   The third factor is more subtle, and depends on the conical shape of the tympanic membrane. As the membrane moves in and out it buckles, so that the arm of the malleus moves less than the surface of the membrane (Fig. 2.5C). This again increases the force and decreases the velocity (Khanna and Tonndorf, 1972). It also is a comparatively small factor.

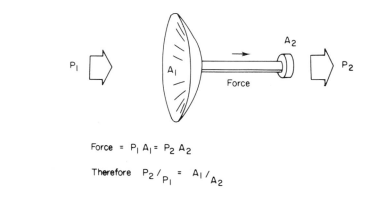

Force $= P_1 A_1 = P_2 A_2$

Therefore $P_2 / P_1 = A_1 / A_2$

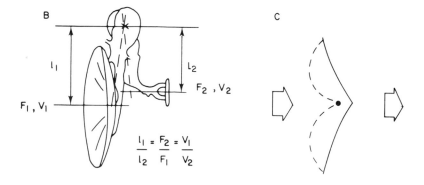

Fig. 2.5 The three mechanisms of the middle ear acoustic impedance transformer.

A. The main factor is the ratio of the areas of the tympanic membrane and oval window. The middle ear bones are here represented by a piston.

B. The lever action increases the force and decreases the velocity.

C. A buckling motion of the tympanic membrane also increases the force and decreases the velocity. A: area, F: force, L: length, P: pressure, V: velocity.

(c) Calculation of the transformer ratio

It might be thought that determining the transformer ratio would be a matter of comparatively simple anatomy, and would have been settled in an uncontroversial way a long time ago. This is not so; the actual transformer ratio depends on the exact way the structures vibrate in response to sound. As the movements are microscopic or submicroscopic, and probably depend on the physiological state of the animal, the determination of the transformer ratio is a rather complex measurement. For instance, Khanna and Tonndorf (1972) had to use a method such as holography to determine the movement of the middle ear structures in the cat. It is their results that will be used here.

The most important factor is the ratio of the areas of the tympanic membrane and the oval window. In the cat, the tympanic membrane has an area of 0.42 cm^2, and the stapes footplate about 0.021 cm^2. The *pressure* on the stapes footplate is therefore increased by $0.42/0.012 = 35$ times.

The effective length of the malleus is about 1.15 times that of the incus, and so the lever action multiplies the force 1.15 times. However the velocity is *decreased* 1.15 times. The lever action therefore increases the impedance ratio (being the pressure/velocity ratio) $1.15^2 = 1.32$ times.

The buckling factor was assessed to decrease the velocity two-fold and increase the force two-fold. The impedance ratio is therefore changed four-fold.

The final transformer ratio, calculated here as an impedance ratio, can be obtained by multiplying all these factors together. The ratio was assessed as $35 \times 1.32 \times 4 = 185.$*

Does this theoretical transformation ratio give the ideal transformation required to match the air to the cochlea? Unfortunately, to answer this we need to know the input impedance of the cochlea, a measurement which has been subject to some variability. In the cat, Khanna and Tonndorf (1971) applied known pressures to the oval window, and measured the displacement of the window indirectly, by measuring the equivalent displacement of the other window in the cochlea, the round window. They found the impedance of the cochlea at 1 kHz to be about 2×10^5 N sec/m^3. The impedance transformer of the middle ear will make this appear to be $2 \times 10^5/185 = 1100$ N sec/m^3 at the tympanic membrane. This is significantly higher than the impedance of air, which is 430 N sec/m^3. The middle ear transformer ratio is not therefore adequate for perfect transmission.

Such a value, which was determined indirectly, can be compared to direct

---

*The reader may be puzzled to see very different numbers in the literature. This may be for two reasons. Firstly, the impedances will probably be defined in acoustic ohms (see p. 5). Secondly, the transformer ratio is often quoted as the *square root* of the impedance ratio in acoustic ohms. Such a ratio is also equal to the pressure transformation ratio. The latter is calculated below on p. 20.

measurements of the input impedance of the middle ear as seen at the tympanic membrane. At 1 kHz, Møller (1965) measured the input impedance to be 1680 N sec/m³ in the cat. As not all of the impedance seen at the tympanic membrane will be due to the cochlea, but will also depend on losses in the middle ear, this agreement does not seem unreasonable. Møller's value leads us to expect that at 1 kHz, 65% of the stimulus power will be absorbed.

Such derivations of the middle ear transformer ratio have been a matter of disagreement over the years. For instance, von Békésy (1960) showed that the eardrum in man was hinged on one side, so that it flapped like a door rather than moving in and out like a piston. Obviously, a point near the hinge will contribute less to the total force transmitted than a point near the free edge, and this has led to the use of an 'effective area' for the tympanic membrane which is less than the real area. Similarly, the way the tympanic membrane moves will affect the effective lever ratio of the middle ear bones, and Wever and Lawrence (1954) for this reason took a lever ratio of 2.5, rather than the 1.15 of Khanna and Tonndorf.

The transformer ratio was calculated for one species, the cat, and applies in one frequency range, around 1 kHz. It seems that at other frequencies, additional factors affect the movement. For instance, above 2 kHz the buckling motion of the tympanic membrane breaks up into separate zones, and as the frequency is raised further the effective area of the tympanic membrane becomes progressively reduced, until it becomes equal to the area of the arm of the malleus. This will reduce transmission (Khanna and Tonndorf, 1972). Transmission through the middle ear is also affected by factors such as elasticity and friction in the middle ear bones and their attachments, particularly at low frequencies. The inertia of the middle ear bones and their imperfect coupling, in addition to acoustic resonances in the middle ear cavity, will also affect transmission. If we wish to determine the way in which the middle ear affects the transmission of sound over a range of frequencies, it is therefore necessary to measure the transmission experimentally. This can be done by measuring the *transfer function*, that is, the ratio of the output to the input, as a function of frequency.

(d) The transfer function of the middle ear

The middle ear transforms the sound pressure variations of the ear canal into a sound pressure variation in the scala vestibuli of the cochlea. The transfer function can be shown by plotting the ratio of the two pressures, at different stimulus frequencies.

Nedzelnitsky (1980) measured the pressure in the cochlear duct of the cat, just behind the oval window, for constant sound pressures at the tympanic membrane. Figure 2.6 shows the pressure gain as a function of frequency.

The curve has a bandpass characteristic, greatest transmission being seen around 1 kHz. There, the sound pressure variations are 30 dB greater than those at the tympanic membrane. The response shows an irregularity around 4 kHz, but otherwise declines smoothly towards low and high frequencies.

We can attempt to identify some of the factors governing this bandpass characteristic. One factor, which attenuates the response at low frequencies, is an *elastic stiffness*. This has variously been ascribed to an elasticity in the tympanic membrane and the ligaments of the middle ear bones, and to a compression and expansion of air in the middle ear cavity. For instance, as the tympanic membrane moves in and out, air in the middle ear cavity is compressed and expanded, so reducing the movement of the tympanic membrane. The importance of this factor can be shown experimentally, because when the middle ear cavity is vented to the atmosphere, transmission is increased at low frequencies but not at high (Guinan and Peake, 1967). But why should elastic stiffness be particularly important at low frequencies? This follows simply from the mathematical relation between the pressure of the sound wave and the displacement of the air, and so of the tympanic membrane. Recall from equation 3 (p. 3), that for a constant sound pressure level, the displacement of the air varies inversely with the frequency. At low frequencies, a constant sound pressure will produce a comparatively large displacement of the tympanic membrane and middle ear structures. The forces to overcome an elasticity depend on displacement, and so the forces will increase as the frequency drops. This explains why transmission is reduced at low frequencies.

The drop at high frequencies is affected by many factors, and their relative importance is not known. For instance, Khanna and Tonndorf (1972) showed that at high frequencies the vibration pattern of the tympanic

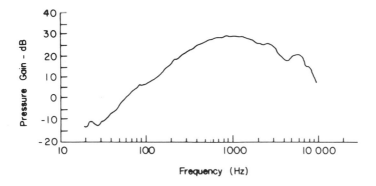

Fig. 2.6 The transfer function of the middle ear, according to Nedzelnitsky (1980). The gain of pressure in the cochlea (the scala vestibuli, basal turn) over that at the tympanic membrane, is shown as a function of frequency. From Nedzelnitsky (1980), Fig. 7.

membrane broke up into separate zones, reducing the effectiveness of the transmission. We would also expect the mass of the middle ear bones to have a significant effect at high frequencies. Constant sound pressure level corresponds to a constant velocity. The accelerations, and so the forces on the structures involved, therefore increase in proportion to frequency. Further, the ossicular chains begins to flex at high frequencies, also reducing transmission (Guinan and Peake, 1967).

The position is in addition complicated by acoustic resonances in the middle ear cavity, responsible for the peak and dip in the transfer function near 4 kHz. The middle ear cavities of many small animals are enlarged by a bony bulge, called the bulla, extending below the skull (incidentally, this probably serves to increase the low frequency response of the middle ear, because it will reduce the low frequency stiffness of the system). In many animals the bulla is divided into two by a bony wall, called the septum. The septum has a small hole, and the two cavities with a small intercommunicating hole form coupled acoustic resonators.

In the midfrequency range, around 1 kHz, many of the factors affecting transmission at lower and higher frequencies will be small. Møller (1965) showed that in this frequency region it was the input impedance of the cochlea itself that was the main factor governing transmission. He disconnected the cochlea by disarticulating the joint between the incus and stapes, and showed that the input impedance at the tympanic membrane fell by 90%. It is in this frequency region that the theoretical calculation of the transformer ratio, described above, will be most nearly accurate; the transfer here will be least affected by factors other than the input impedance of the cochlea. Therefore we can see here whether the actual pressure gain observed by Nedzelnitsky (1980) agrees with the value expected from Khanna and Tonndorf's transformer ratio, calculated from the displacements of the middle ear structures. Khanna and Tonndorf would lead us to expect the area ratio to increase the pressure by 35 times, the lever ratio to increase it by 1.15 times, and the buckling factor to increase it by two times. The product is 80.5 times, or 38 dB. This is in the same range as, although rather greater than, the 30 dB increase in pressure observed in the same species, and at the same frequency, by Nedzelnitsky. The disagreement, unless due to inter-animal variation, may be a result of transmission losses.

Consideration of transmission through the middle ear is not complete without a description of the linearity of the response (see p. 8). Guinan and Peake (1967) found that the stapes movement increased in proportion to the input up to 130 dB SPL below 2 kHz, and up to 140–150 dB above. This suggests that the movements are linear up to these intensities. It also suggests that there are unlikely to be significant harmonics or intermodulation products at much lower intensities. Guinan and Peake were not able to see any harmonics, although their method only allowed them to detect 10–20% of odd harmonics. In view of these measurements, it is likely that the middle ear is linear in the usual range of physiological and psychophysical measurements.

3. The Middle Ear Muscles

Transmission through the middle ear can be controlled by means of the middle ear muscles. They are two small striated muscles attached to the ossicles. The *tensor tympani* is attached to the malleus near the tympanic membrane, and is innervated by the trigeminal (fifth) cranial nerve. The other muscle, the *stapedius muscle*, is attached to the stapes and is innervated by the facial (seventh) cranial nerve.

Contraction of the muscles increases the stiffness of the ossicular chain. As was explained above (p. 19), below 1–2 kHz transmission through the middle ear is stiffness-controlled. The stiffness arises from the elasticity of the tympanic membrane and the ligaments of the ossicles, as well as from the compression and expansion of air in the middle ear cavity. The stiffness reduces the transmission of sounds of low frequency. When it is augmented by a stiffening of the ossicular chain, the low frequency response is attenuated still further. On the other hand, at high frequencies, above 1–2 kHz, where transmission is not stiffness-controlled, the response is hardly affected by the middle ear muscles (Møller, 1965). Although this seems to be the main mechanism of middle ear muscle action, the real position is more complicated, because in the cat the position of the notch in the transfer function around 4 kHz, arising from resonances in the bulla, is changed as well (Simmons, 1964).

Contraction of the middle ear muscles can be elicited by loud sound (more than 75 dB above absolute threshold), or by vocalization, or by general bodily movement (Carmel and Starr, 1963). In some cases, the middle ear muscles can be contracted voluntarily without any other discernable movement.

Several functions have been suggested for the middle ear muscles.

(i)   The contraction to loud sound suggests that the reflex might be of use in protecting the inner ear from noise damage. This indeed seems to be the case. For instance, Zakrisson and Borg (1974) showed that in patients with unilateral Bell's palsy, where the stapedius muscle is paralyzed, low frequency noise produced greater temporary threshold shifts in the abnormal than in the normal ear. A temporary threshold shift, which may continue for minutes or hours after an auditory stimulus, is a sign that fatigue, and hence potential damage, has been produced in the auditory system. But the reflex is too slow to protect the ear against impulsive noises.

(ii)   The fact that the muscles contract with vocalization or bodily movement suggests that they may also reduce the perception of self-produced sound.

(iii)   It has been suggested that the middle ear muscles may be able to keep intense low frequency stimuli near a lower part of the intensity range. Wever and Vernon (1955) showed that the reflex maintained the intensity of the input to the cochlea relatively constant when the intensity of the stimulus was varied. This near-perfect automatic gain control functioned for a range of 20 dB above the reflex threshold, and, of course, only applied to low frequency stimuli.

(iv)   The middle ear muscles may also have a beneficial effect on the frequency response of the middle ear. As mentioned above, the transmission characteristic shows a sharp dip near 4 kHz, due to resonances in the bulla. Simmons (1964) showed that the middle ear muscles could shift the frequency of the dip slightly. In cats which were awake and had intact middle ear muscles, the dip was not apparent, suggesting that the continually fluctuating tone in the muscles had averaged it out.

(v)   At high intensities, low frequency stimuli can mask higher frequency stimuli over a wide range of frequencies. Selective attenuation of low frequencies by the middle ear muscles can therefore be expected to affect the perception of complex stimuli with low frequency components, such as speech, at high intensities.

C. Summary

1. The outer ear has two roles in transmitting sound to the tympanic membrane or eardrum. It aids sound localization by altering the spectrum of the sound, depending on the direction of the source. It also, by resonances, increases the sound pressure at the tympanic membrane.

2. The middle ear apparatus couples sound energy from the tympanic membrane to the oval window of the cochlea. The sound is transmitted by three small bones, the ossicles, called the malleus, incus, and stapes. The middle ear acts as an acoustic impedance transformer, coupling energy from the low impedance air to the higher impedance cochlear fluids, so reducing the reflection of sound energy which would otherwise occur.

3. The middle ear transformer uses three principles. The area of the oval window is smaller than that of the tympanic membrane, increasing the pressure. The lever action of the ossicles increases the force, and decreases the velocity. The buckling motion of the tympanic membrane does likewise.

4. Transmission through the middle ear depends on the frequency of the stimulus. Greatest transmission is produced (in the cat) in the range around 1–2 kHz. Below that frequency, transmission is reduced by the stiffness of the middle ear structures and by compression and expansion of air in the middle ear cavity. Above that frequency, many factors, including the mass of the ossicles, and less efficient modes of vibration of the structures, reduce transmission. There are also dips in the response arising from acoustic resonances in the middle ear cavity.

5. Transmission through the middle ear is affected by the middle ear muscles, which reduce the transmission of low-frequency sounds. They may serve to protect the ear to some extent from noise damage, reduce the effect of self-produced sounds, act as an automatic gain control for low frequency stimuli over a narrow range of intensities, reduce the perturbing effects of middle ear resonances, and reduce the masking of stimuli that are higher in frequency.

D. Further Reading

The outer ear has been comprehensively discussed by Shaw (1974).

The middle ear has been described by Dallos (1973), Chapter 3, pp. 83–126, and parts of Chapter 7, pp. 465–501, and by Møller (1974), and Zwislocki (1975).

III. The Cochlea

The chapter on the cochlea is a key one, and forms the foundation for much of the rest of this book. The anatomy of the cochlea will be described first. This is followed by a description of cochlear mechanics, including von Békésy's pioneering observations, then a non-mathematical description of some theories of cochlear mechanics, and the recent measurements of basilar membrane vibration. The electrophysiology of the cochlea, starting with the standing potentials and the grossly recordable sound evoked potentials, and ending with hair cell potentials, will then be discussed. The transduction process will be provisionally interpreted in terms of Davis's (1958, 1965) battery and resistance modulation theory. Davis suggested that the standing potentials of the cochlea drove current through variable resistances in the apical membrane of the hair cells. The resistances were varied by the mechanical vibration of the cochlear partition, and this led to the recordable cochlear potentials and activation of the synapse at the base of the hair cells. The theory is still controversial, and recent ideas will be discussed in Chapter 5.

A. Anatomy

1. General Anatomy

Figure 2.1 shows the position of the human cochlea in relation to the other structures of the ear. It is embedded deep in the temporal bone. Overall, the cochlea stands about 1 cm wide and 5 mm from base to apex in man, and contains a coiled basilar membrane about 35 mm long. Figure 3.1A shows the turns of the cochlea in more detail, and in particular the longitudinal division into three scalae. The scalae spiral together along the length of the cochlea, keeping their corresponding spatial relations throughout the turns. The osseous spiral lamina divides the scala vestibuli from the scala tympani on the side near the modiolus (Fig. 3.1B). The scala media is separated from the scala vestibuli above by Reissner's membrane, and from the scala tympani below by the basilar membrane. The two outer scalae, the scala vestibuli and scala tympani, are joined at the apex of the cochlea by an opening known as the helicotrema (Figs 3.1A and C). The two outer scalae contain perilymph, a fluid which is similar to extracellular fluid in its ionic composition. The scala media forms an inner compartment which does not communicate directly with the other two. It contains endolymph, which is similar to intracellular fluid in its ionic composition.

The vibrations of the stapes are transmitted to the oval window, a membraneous window opening onto the scala vestibuli. Fluid in the cochlea is displaced to a second window, the round window, opening onto the scala tympani. The flow causes a wave-like displacement of the basilar membrane and the structures attached to it (Fig. 3.1C). It is this that is thought to be responsible for the stimulation of the hair cells, and the first stage of the analysis of the incoming sound is performed by the spatial distribution of the resulting displacements.

The basilar membrane undergoes an important gradation in dimensions up the cochlea; although the cochlear duct is broad near the base and narrow towards the apex, the basilar membrane tapers in the opposite direction, the difference being filled by the spiral lamina.

The organ of Corti on the basilar membrane constitutes the auditory transducer and it is here that the nerve supply ends (Figs 3.1B and D). The nerve supply and the blood vessels of the cochlea enter the organ of Corti by way of the central cavity of the cochlea, the *modiolus*, the spiral structure of the cochlea imparting a corresponding twist to the nerve and blood vessels during development.

2. The Organ of Corti

The highly specialized structure of the organ of Corti contains the hair cells, which are the receptor cells, together with their nerve endings and supporting cells. The hair cells consist of one row of inner hair cells on the modiolar side of the arch of Corti, and between three and, towards the apex, five rows of outer hair cells. There are about 25 000 hair cells in man (Guild, 1932) and 12 500 in the cat (Schuknecht, 1960).

The organ of Corti itself sits on the basilar membrane, a fibrous structure dividing the scala media from the scala tympani. Often, though misleadingly, the whole complex is referred to as 'the basilar membrane'.

The organ of Corti is given rigidity by an arch of rods or pillar cells along its length, the upper ends of the rods ending in the *reticular lamina* which forms the true chemical division between the ions in the fluids of the scala media and those of the scala tympani (Fig. 3.1D). The arch is surrounded by phalangeal cells; that is, by cells with processes which end in a plate in the

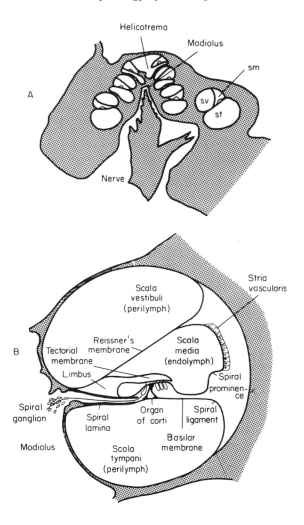

Fig. 3.1 A. In a transverse section of the whole cochlea, the cochlear duct is cut across several times as it coils round and round. Abbreviations: sv: scala vestibuli; sm: scala media; st: scala tympani.
B. The three scalae and associated structures are shown in a magnified view of a cross-section of the cochlear duct.

reticular lamina. The inner phalangeal cells completely surround the inner hair cells. The outer phalangeal cells, which are also known as Deiters' cells, form cups holding the basal ends of the outer hair cells. The outer phalangeal cells send fine processes up to the reticular lamina, leaving spaces between the outer hair cells. External to the outer hair cells there is a row of supporting cells known as Hensen's cells, and on the modiolar side of the

C

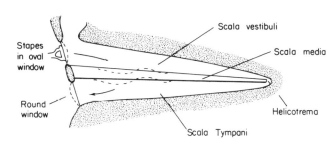

D

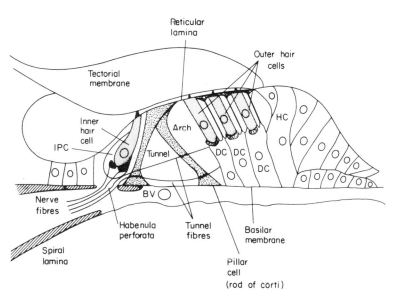

C. The path of vibrations in the cochlea are shown in a schematic diagram in which the cochlear duct is depicted as unrolled.
D. A cross-section of the organ of Corti, as it appears in the basal turn. BV: blood vessel; DC: Deiters' cells; HC: Hensen's cells; IPC: inner phalangeal cell.

organ of Corti there is a further row of supporting cells. The distribution of the supporting cells changes in the different turns of the cochlea (Fig. 3.2).

The organ of Corti is covered by a gelatinous and fibrous flap, the tectorial membrane. The tectorial membrane is fixed only on its inner edge, where it is attached to the limbus, although some investigators believe it to make contact with the reticular lamina on its outer edge (Kronester-Frei, 1979). The longer of the hairs on the outer hair cells have been reported to be shallowly but firmly embedded in the under-surface of the tectorial mem-

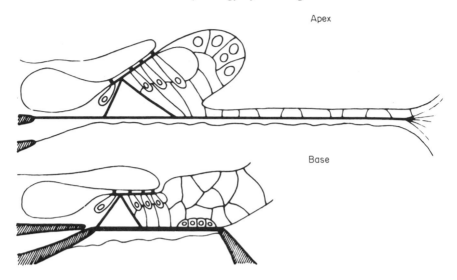

Fig. 3.2 The organ of Corti shows morphological differences along the length of the cochlea. Moreover, near the apex the basilar membrane is wide, and near the base it is narrow. From Spoendlin (1972), Fig. 1.

brane (Engström and Engström, 1978). The hairs of the inner hair cells are probably not embedded and may well be only loosely attached to the under-surface of the gelatinous covering. The tectorial membrane is attached only on one side and is raised above the basilar membrane. Therefore when the basilar membrane moves up and down a shear or relative movement will occur between the tectorial membrane and the organ of Corti, with the result that the hairs will be bent (Fig. 3.3). The arch of the pillar cells (the arch of Corti) would seem well suited to maintaining the rigidity of the organ of Corti during such a movement.

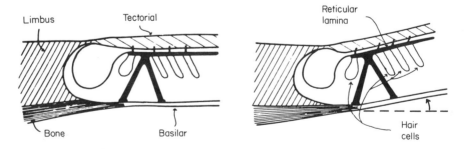

Fig. 3.3 In Davis's hypothesis for the lever action of the cochlea, the stereocilia on the hair cells are deflected as a result of vertical displacements of the basilar membrane. From Davis (1958), Fig. 8.

Figure 3.4 shows views of the upper surface of the organ of Corti once the tectorial membrane has been removed. The hairs or stereocilia of the hair cells are seen projecting through the reticular lamina. On each inner hair cell the hairs are arranged in two closely spaced rows, the rows being slightly curved, whereas on the outer hair cells there are three or four closely spaced rows, with the rows making a V or W shape. The geometric patterns on the reticular lamina between the hair cells reveal the pattern of the supporting cells making up the lamina. The pattern is formed by small microvilli, which cover the apical surfaces of the supporting cells, bunching more thickly around their edges.

An inner hair cell is shown in Fig. 3.5A. It is about 35 μm in length, and about 10 μm in diameter at the widest point (chinchilla: Smith, 1968). The shape is commonly likened to that of a flask. The cuticular plate, in the reticular lamina, is set at an angle to the axis of the cell. The nucleus is central, the mitochondria are scattered, though denser above the nucleus, and the cellular organelles are most prevalent at the apex, near the cuticular plate. The nerve endings are situated near the base of the cell. These terminals are associated with the afferent fibres of the auditory nerve, conveying information from the cochlea to the brain stem. The synapse is often marked by small dense synaptic bars or invaginations at right angles to the cell wall, or rounded synaptic bodies, together with a few vesicles (Ades and Engstrom, 1974).

The outer hair cells are approximately 25 μm long in the basal turn and 45 μm long in the apical turn, and 6–7 μm in diameter (chinchilla: Smith, 1968). The nucleus is located basally (Fig. 3.5B). The mitochondria are primarily situated at the base below the nucleus, and at the apex below the cuticular plate. The afferent terminals are faced with short synaptic bars, but not round synaptic bodies (Ades and Engstrom, 1974).

The stereocilia, or hairs, are 6–7 μm long and 0.3 μm wide on the outermost of the closely-spaced multiple rows on each hair cell, tapering almost to zero on those of the rows on each hair cell that are nearer the modiolus. The hairs are joined by bridges of very fine fibrils so that all the hairs on one cell tend to move together when the longest ones are pushed (Flock, 1977). The hairs are similar to the sterocilia seen generally on hair cells of the acousticolateral system, although many of the other acoustico-lateral hair cells have an additional hair of different appearance known as the kinocilium. The kinocilium is present in the embryonic cochlear hair cells, but gradually disappears to leave a stub known as the basal body. The hairs themselves have a membrane which is continuous with the hair cell surface membrane. The centre of each hair is filled with fine filaments which continue down into the cuticular plate (Fig. 3.5C). The hairs appear to consist of actin in a paracrystalline array, which probably accounts for their mechanical rigidity (DeRosier *et al.*, 1980). They also contain myosin

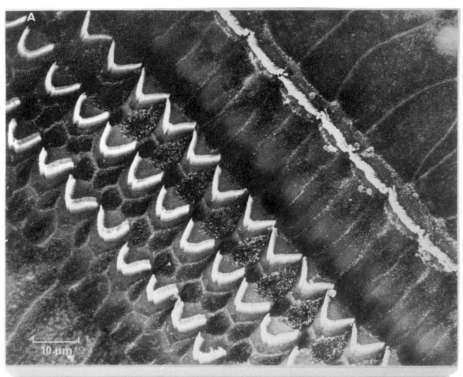

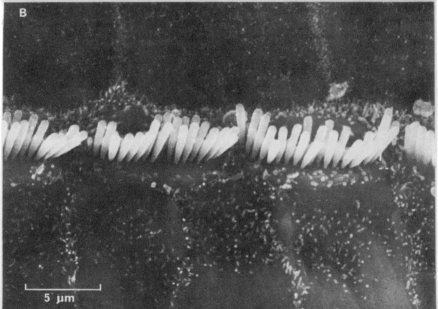

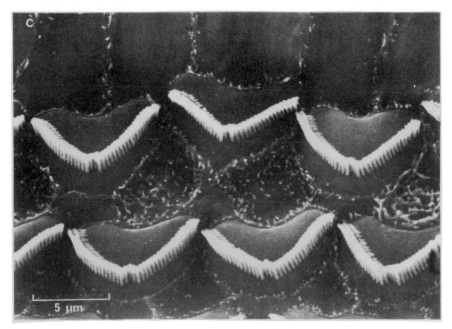

Fig. 3.4 A. A scanning electron micrograph of the upper surface of the organ of Corti, when the tectorial membrane has been removed, shows three rows of outer hair cells and one row of inner hair cells.
B. The stereocilia on inner hair cells form a nearly straight row.
C. The stereocilia on outer hair cells are smaller and the rows form a V or W.
Guinea-pig. Photographs by courtesy of D. Robertson.

(Macartney *et al.*, 1980). The presence of actin and myosin suggests that the hairs may be able to actively change their mechanical properties, or may even be motile.

3. The Innervation of the Organ of Corti

The cochlea is innervated by about 50 000 sensory neurones in the cat, and about 30 000 in Man (Spoendlin, 1972). There are also about 1 800 'efferent' or centrifugal neurones, by means of which the central nervous system is able to influence the cochlea (shown in the cat; Warr, 1978).

The afferent fibres, which convey auditory information from the cochlea to the central nervous system, have their cell bodies in the spiral ganglion in the modiolus on the inner wall of the spiral lamina (Fig. 3.1B). The cells are bipolar, with one process projecting to the hair cells and the other to the cells of the cochlear nucleus in the brain stem. The axons project into the cochlear duct through openings in the bony shelf of the spiral lamina, known as the habenula perforata. About 90–95% (90% in the guinea-pig; Morrison *et al.*,

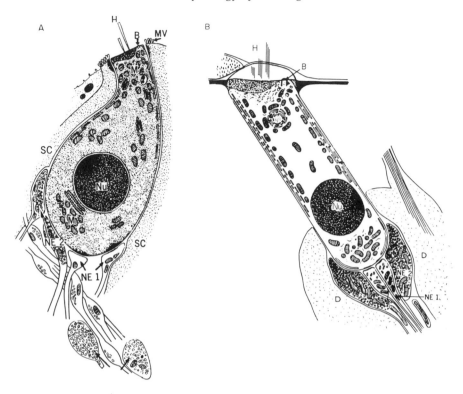

Fig. 3.5 A and B. Inner hair cells are shaped like a flask (A), and outer hair cells are shaped like a cylinder (B). B: basal body; H: hairs or stereocilia; M: mitochondria; D: Deiters' cell; MV: microvilli, NE 1: type 1 endings (afferent); NE 2: type 2 endings (efferent); Nu: nucleus; SC: supporting cell. From Engström *et al*. (1965), Figs 8 and 13.

1975; 95% in the cat; Spoendlin, 1972) of the afferent fibres connect directly with the inner hair cells (Fig. 3.6). Each inner hair cell receives about 20 fibres. The remaining 5–10% go to the much more numerous outer hair cells. Whereas the axons to the inner hair cells contact the cell directly opposite their habenular opening, those to the outer hair cells take a much more oblique course. They turn basally for five hair cells or so, and cross the tunnel of Corti on the basilar membrane where they are known as basilar or lower tunnel fibres. They then run towards the base of the cochlea for some 0.6 mm, first running along the outer edge of the tunnel of Corti, where they are known as the fibres of the outer spiral bundle. They then spiral outwards among the rows of the outer hair cells, synapsing with about 10 hair cells on the way (Fig. 3.6). However each outer hair cell also has synapses from several other afferent fibres. The innervation of the two types of hair cell is therefore completely different, that of the inner hair cells showing a great

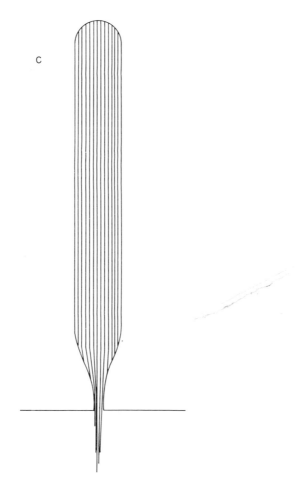

C. Stereocilia are composed of actin filaments, some of which extend into the rootlet in the cuticular plate.

deal of divergence, and that of the outer hair cells showing both convergence and divergence.

The efferent or centrifugal axons arise in the superior olivary complex of the brain stem, and will be discussed in detail later (Chapter 8). Warr (1978) has established in the kitten that there are about 800 centrifugal fibres to the outer hair cells, and about 1000 to the region of the inner hair cells. The fibres to the region of the inner hair cells do not generally contact the inner hair cells directly, but rather terminate on the dendrites of the afferent fibres under the inner hair cells. The fibres to the outer hair cells cross the tunnel half-way up the tunnel of Corti, where they are known as the upper tunnel fibres, and then ramify outwards among the outer hair cells, showing considerable branching. Near the base of the cochlea, each hair cell receives six to eight efferent terminals, and near the apex, rather fewer. The efferent terminals are large and vesiculated, and tend to envelope the base of the cell and its afferent terminals.

The cochlea also receives an adrenergic, sympathetic, innervation (Spoendlin and Lichtensteiger, 1966; Densert and Flock, 1974; Pickles, 1979b). Some of the fibres appear to end on blood vessels in the spiral lamina. Others appear to terminate near the afferent nerve fibres as they pass through the habenula perforata.

B. The Mechanics of the Cochlea

1. The Travelling Wave

When a sound impinges on the eardrum, the vibrations are transmitted to the oval window by the middle ear bones. The vibrations then cause a movement of the cochlear fluids and the cochlear partitions, displacing fluid to the round window (Fig. 3.1C). This initiates a wave of displacement on the basilar membrane, which then travels apically in the cochlea. The wave is a very important stage in the analysis of sound by the auditory system,

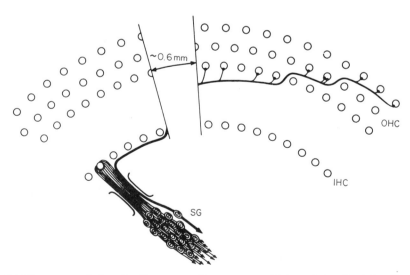

Fig. 3.6 The great majority of auditory nerve fibres connect with inner hair cells. A few fibres pass to outer hair cells, after running basally for about 0.6 mm. IHC: Inner hair cells; OHC: Outer hair cells; SG: Spiral ganglion. From Spoendlin (1978), Fig. 8.

because the *pattern* of movement of the basilar membrane depends on the frequency of the stimulus. The way this happens depends on the mechanics of the basilar membrane and the cochlear fluids. Much of our knowledge of the mechanics of the system depends on the work of the pioneer in the field, G. von Békésy, and the more recent results will be discussed in relation to his work.

Von Békésy in a long series of experiments, described in a collected form by von Békésy (1960), examined the movement of the cochlear partition in human and animal cadavers. Temporal bones were rapidly dissected soon after death, and were immersed in saline solution. Rubber windows were substituted for the round and oval windows, and a mechanical vibrator was attached to one of them. The cochlear wall was opened under water for observation of the partitions within. By microscopic and stroboscopic observation of silver particles scattered on Reissner's membrane, von Békésy was able to plot out the now-classic travelling-wave pattern of Fig. 3.7. He presumed that this was similar to the movement of the membrane carrying the transducers themselves, namely the basilar membrane. For a stimulus of fixed frequency the cochlear partition vibrated with a wave that grew in amplitude as it moved up the cochlea from the stapes, reached a maximum, and then rapidly declined. The wave of displacement moved more and more slowly as it passed up the cochlea, so the phase changed with distance at an accelerating rate, and the apparent wavelength of the vibration decreased. However, the frequency of vibration at any point was, of course, the same as that of the input.

Von Békésy's plots were made in two ways. By opening a length of

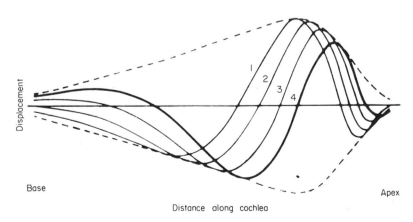

Fig. 3.7 Travelling waves in the cochlea were first shown by von Békésy. The full lines show the pattern of the deflection of the cochlear partition at successive instants, as numbered. The waves are contained within an envelope, which is static (dotted lines). Stimulus frequency: 200 Hz. From von Békésy (1960), Fig. 12–17.

cochlea it was possible to see the pattern of movement distributed along the membrane, and so plot the waveforms and their envelopes for sounds of different frequencies. The vibration envelopes found by von Békésy are shown in Fig. 3.8. They show the important point that as the frequency of the stimulus was increased, the position of the vibration maximum moved towards the base of the cochlea. Thus high frequency tones produced a vibration pattern confined to the base of the cochlea. Low frequency tones, in contrast, produced most vibration at the apex of the cochlea, although, because of the long tail of the vibration envelope, there was some response near the base as well.

A second way in which von Békésy measured the vibration pattern is indicated by Fig. 3.9. He opened the cochlea at certain points, and measured the vibration at those points as the frequency was varied. Figure 3.9 shows his results for six points on the membrane, the peak-to-peak stapes displacement being kept constant as he varied the frequency at each point. Note that, as before, it is the most basal point that responds best to the highest frequencies. In going from the space axis of Fig. 3.8 to the frequency axis of Fig. 3.9 the direction of variation of the parameters marked on the curves and the abscissa have to be reversed, although the positions of the steep and shallow slopes are the same.

There is no doubt that high frequencies peak near the base of the cochlea, and that low frequencies activate most of the cochlea and peak near the apex. However the curves of Fig. 3.9 are misleading because they might appear to suggest that for a constant *sound pressure level* (SPL) the response

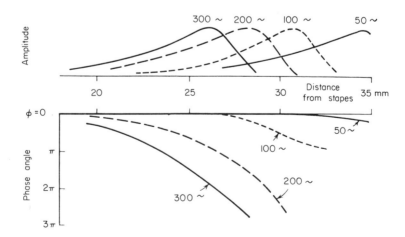

Fig. 3.8 Displacement envelopes on the cochlear partition are shown for tones of different frequency. The lower plot shows the relative phase angle of the displacement. From von Békésy (1960), Fig. 11–58.

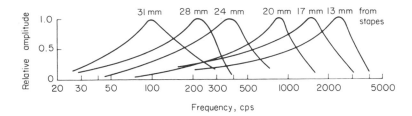

Fig. 3.9 Frequency responses are shown for six different points on the cochlear partition. The amplitude of the travelling wave envelope was measured as the stimulus frequency was varied with constant peak stapes displacements. The position of the point of observation is marked on each curve. From von Békésy (1960), Fig. 11–49.

at any one point of the cochlea peaks at one frequency, and that the response is smaller for lower frequencies. In contrast, it must be emphasized that each of the plots of Fig. 3.9 was made for constant peak *stapes displacements* and that *different displacements were used for each point on the cochlear partition*. As was shown in Chapter 1, Section A, for a constant sound pressure level it is the peak *velocity* of the air particles that stays constant, whereas the displacement goes down in inverse proportion to frequency. Figure 3.10A shows the curves of Fig. 3.9 redrawn to give the displacement for a constant peak stapes velocity, which with certain assumptions (Eldredge, 1974) would be a better indication of an input of constant SPL at the tympanic membrane. It shows that the displacement is now approximately constant up to a certain frequency, at which point it drops sharply. With this knowledge, it is possible to redraw vibration envelopes, such as appear in Fig. 3.8, to show the pattern of basilar membrane movements as a function of distance along the basilar membrane for different frequencies (Fig. 3.10B). Thus at constant SPL, high frequencies produce small maximal vibrations which are confined to the base. As the frequency is lowered, the amplitude of vibration at the base stays constant, but the envelope of the vibration grows towards the apex.

The results of von Békésy can be summarized as follows: vibration of the stapes gives rise to a travelling wave of displacement on the basilar membrane. For a vibration of a particular frequency, the vibration on the basilar membrane grows in amplitude as the wave travels towards the apex, and then, beyond a certain point, dies out rapidly. The wave travels more and more slowly as it travels up the cochlea. Low frequency sounds peak a long way along the membrane, near the apex, and high frequency sounds only a short way along, near the base. At constant SPL, any one point on the basilar membrane has an almost constant response at low frequencies. As the frequency is raised, a certain cutoff frequency is reached at which the response drops sharply. The membrane therefore acts as a low-pass filter.

2. Theories of Cochlear Mechanics

The vibration of the cochlear partition has been investigated theoretically, first by means of models by von Békésy and others, and more recently mathematically. Von Békésy (1960) showed the following:

(i) the vibration of the cochlear partition does not depend on a simple resonance analogous to that of a simple mass-and-spring resonator. In an analogy of such a system, we can think of playing a note into the body

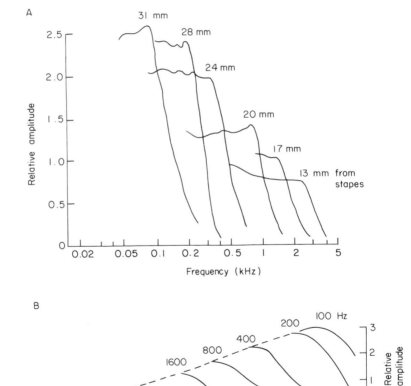

Fig. 3.10 A. When the frequency responses of Fig. 3.9 are recalculated for constant peak stapes velocity, the basilar membrane is seen to have a low-pass, rather than a bandpass, characteristic. Points of observation marked as mm from stapes. From Eldredge (1974), Fig. 3. B. Calculated envelope of displacement of the cochlear partition, for stimuli of constant peak stapes velocity (frequency marked on each curve). From Eldredge (1974), Fig. 4.

of a piano so that any string tuned to the input frequency will vibrate in sympathy. This was the resonance theory of Helmholtz (1863). The theory in its simple form is untenable because the phase changes observed along the basilar membrane were much greater than 180° (or π). It is known that in a simple resonant system, such as a stretched string, the phase differences between the input and the output cannot be greater than 180°. Moveover there are no suitable structures which could act as resonators: in view of the degree of damping in the fluid-filled cochlea, any such resonators would have to be stiffer and denser than is reasonable.

(ii) The observed travelling wave depends on an interaction between the fluid flow along the cochlea and the displacement of the cochlear partition, and is dependent on the increasing compliance of the basilar membrane towards the apex.

(iii) The travelling wave does not depend on longitudinal coupling along the basilar membrane, of the sort that would be seen if it were a stretched elastic sheet. Rather it depends on its stiffness to deflection, as though it were made of stiff bars at right angles to the long axis of the cochlea. The longitudinal coupling is provided by the fluid flow.

(iv) The direction of propagation of the wave is always from the point of highest stiffness to the point of lowest stiffness, and does not depend on the way that the vibrations are introduced. For instance, vibration of the stapes, or vibration of the bony walls of the cochlea as in bone conduction, produce the same travelling wave. And in birds, the vibrations are introduced into the 'roof' of the cochlea, rather than at one end. The introduced pressure, which initiates the travelling wave, travels almost instantaneously along the cochlea, taking very much less time than the 5 ms or so taken by the travelling wave.

Two theoretical approaches have been used in understanding the mechanics of the basilar membrane. In the analysis of Zwislocki, the inertia of the fluid flow at right angles to the basilar membrane can be neglected, and this leads to an analysis analogous to 'shallow water' or 'long' waves (Zwislocki, 1965). Von Ranke (1950) did not make this assumption and developed an analysis analogous to 'deep water' or 'short' waves. The various mathematical treatments and the relations between them have been summarized by Geisler (1976). The simpler arguments based on those of Zwislocki will be presented. This is not the place to present the mathematics, of which a particularly clear account will be found in Zwislocki (1965), and it is hoped that some understanding will be conveyed by verbal arguments. The cochlea is taken as straight, narrow compared with the wavelength of the travelling wave, and divided into only two scalae. The cochlear fluids are taken as incompressible.

It is convenient to use three stages in considering the travelling wave.

(i)   According to the direct measurements of von Békésy (1960) the cochlear partition near the base is stiff and becomes more compliant by a
factor of over 100 towards the apex. The movement of the partition in
response to a pressure difference between the two scalae will be partly
affected by the stiffness of the partition. But as the partition moves, it
displaces fluid along the cochlea, and if the forces due to the inertia of
the fluid are great compared to those due to the stiffness, it will be the
mass of the fluid that limits the movement. It is known that when mass
limits movement, the displacement lags behind the driving force. On the
other hand, where the stiffness is dominant, as it is near the base, the lag
is smaller. If therefore, the pressure in one of the two scalae is suddenly
increased, the stiffness-dominated membrane near the base will be the
first to move, followed by the membrane towards the apex. A wave of
displacement will travel from base to apex, the direction depending only
on the gradation of compliance, and not on *how* the pressure increase is
introduced.
(ii) Fluid displaced along the cochlea after a deflection of the partition will,
with a phase lag, deflect adjacent portions of the membrane. Thus
potential energy is handed along the membrane by the kinetic energy of
the fluids, and an associated wave, consisting of a pressure difference
across the cochlear partition, will travel up the cochlea with a monotonically decreasing amplitude. But because the stiffness of the membrane decreases still faster, the amplitude of the associated deflection
grows.
(iii) Because there is viscosity in the fluids and friction in the membrane,
these large movements are associated with heavy damping, and the
movements die out. Thus the wave reaches a maximum and then declines rapidly. The effects of friction are greater at high frequencies, and
so the wave dies out sooner.

Zwislocki's model predicts a pattern of movement which is similar to that
found by von Békésy. However it does not predict the greater degree of
frequency selectivity found by recent investigators (see next section).
An analysis by Peterson and Bogert (1950) and Bogert (1951), in
which mass plays more of a role and damping less of a role, produces sharper
peaks. In this model, the motion of the membrane is dominated by the
stiffness of the membrane on the basal side of the resonant point, and by the
mass of the membrane and fluid on the apical side. At some point in
between, the system resonates.
If there were no damping in the system, the oscillation would be infinite at
resonance. By choosing a suitable amount of damping, the magnitude of the
oscillation at resonance, and the sharpness of the tuning, can be varied at
will. In this analysis, therefore, very sharp peaks can be produced by making

the damping small. It differs from the analysis of Zwislocki, because the presence of the peak in the travelling wave is produced by an interaction of stiffness and mass, rather than of stiffness and damping. The difficulty of the model is that when the parameters in the equation are derived from measured quantities, resonant peaks cannot be predicted over the whole of the observed frequency range (Geisler, 1976)*.

One difficulty with both of these models is that mechanical models have shown some fluid flow at right angles to the basilar membrane, so that the assumption of shallow-water, or long, waves is not necessarily justified (von Békésy, 1960; Tonndorf, 1973). Moreover, near the peak of the travelling wave the wavelength on the basilar membrane is comparable to the diameter of the cochlear duct, also meaning that shallow water waves are not applicable (Kim and Molnar, 1975). Analyses not making such an assumption are discussed by Geisler (1976) and Steele (1976).

3. Current Status of the Travelling Wave

Von Békésy's observations have been questioned on two grounds. Visual observations meant that the vibrations had to be at least of the order of the wavelength of light, and the high intensities (130 dB SPL) necessary, may make extrapolation to a more physiological range unjustified. Secondly, his measurements were performed on cadavers, and it is now known that the properties of the basilar membrane change after death (Kohlloffel, 1972a). Indeed, it is now suspected that any physiological deterioration of the cochlea from its normal state due, for instance, to anoxia, will affect its mechanical properties. Recent experiments have tried to rectify these points, and extend the observations to a wider frequency range.

Since von Békésy, only Kohlloffel (1972 a,b) has measured the movements of the basilar membrane as a pattern distributed over space. He used a laser method, which depends on the speckled appearance of a surface in laser light. When the surface moves the speckles shift and this allows movements down to one sixth of a wavelength of light to be detected. His intensity range could be lower than that of von Békésy, going down to 100 dB SPL. Measurements were made in the 5–10 kHz region of the guinea-pig cochlea. However, the extensive dissection needed to expose a length of basilar membrane meant that the spatial distributions could be measured only in cadavers. Kohlloffel saw a travelling wave similar to that of

---

*A perspicatious reader may ask, how does this model differ from the resonance model of Helmholtz, which was discounted on the grounds that it could not predict large enough phase lags? The difference is that in Helmholtz's model the introduced sound was coupled directly to each resonant element. In the model discussed here, the force on one resonant element is supplied via the fluid flow resulting from the movement of the adjacent parts of the basilar membrane. Therefore the model is still a travelling wave model, and large phase delays can be accumulated along the basilar membrane.

von Békésy, which grew to a peak along the cochlea and then died out rapidly. Observations were also made at single points near the basal (high frequency) end of the living guinea-pig's cochlea; unlike von Békésy he showed a broad bandpass characteristic, with a low frequency slope of 10 dB/octave for a constant SPL input. The high frequency slope at 100 dB/octave was rather steeper than that of von Békésy (Fig. 3.11A).

Wilson and J. R. Johnstone (1975) measured the movement of the living guinea-pig's basilar membrane in the 20 kHz region by means of a capacitive probe. In this technique, an electrode was brought near the basilar membrane and the capacitance between the electrode and the membrane was measured by the impedance to an applied radio-frequency current. The capacitance is a function of the separation between the two structures. Wilson and Johnstone plotted the response of different points along the basilar membrane as a function of frequency. For a constant SPL at the tympanic membrane they found a frequency response with a slope of 5 dB/octave on the low frequency side, a flat top, and a mean slope of 130 dB/octave on the high frequency side, thus giving an asymmetric bandpass characteristic (Fig. 3.11B). The intensities used were between 40 and 140 dB SPL, so for the first time we have mechanical measurements in the range of many psychophysical and neurophysiological measurements. Wilson and Johnstone found complete linearity at the peak of the basilar membrane response, although there was some nonlinearity on the high frequency slope. If the same findings on linearity can be applied to von Békésy's results, it would be possible to extrapolate his measurements to the lower intensities of the physiological range.

B. M. Johnstone *et al.* (1970) used the Mössbauer technique to measure the movement of the basal end of the living guinea-pig's cochlea. The Mössbauer technique involved the placing of a small piece of stainless steel enriched with ^{57}Co on the basilar membrane. The ^{57}Co decays to ^{57}Fe in an excited state, and the ^{57}Fe decays emitting a γ-ray. If the emitted radiation has exactly the right frequency, it will be absorbed by a piece of ^{57}Fe-enriched foil nearby. If the source frequency is changed by a Doppler shift due to movement of the source, a smaller proportion of the radiation will be absorbed, and the increase in transmitted radiation can be detected. The spectral lines are so incredibly narrow that velocity disparities of 0.2 mm/sec can be detected; because it is a *velocity* detection, the technique does not require very rigid stabilization of the preparation, and is most sensitive at high frequencies. The frequency response is shown for an 18 kHz point in the guinea-pig in Fig. 3.11C. The curves were sharper than those found by von Békésy at much lower frequencies, and were in agreement with those of Kohllöffel in the same frequency region, giving for constant SPL 7 dB/octave on the low frequency side, and about 100 dB/octave on the high frequency side. The measurements were made down to 70 dB SPL.

Rhode (1971) used the Mössbauer technique in the 7 kHz region of the squirrel monkey's cochlea, thus filling in the frequency gap between the results of von Békésy, and those of the others. His measurements were made down to 65 dB SPL and are shown for both constant malleus displacement in Fig. 3.11D and constant SPL at the tympanic membrane in Fig. 3.11E. The results are unlike the others in that they showed a clear nonlinearity at the peak — that is, the peak was relatively sharper at low intensities (Fig. 3.11D). At constant SPL, the low frequency response was very nearly flat, increasing to 18 dB/octave just below the peak. The mean maximum high frequency slope was 100 dB/octave.

How do the results for the five different groups of workers agree?. In making comparisons we have to be sure that we are comparing responses at either constant SPL, or constant velocities or displacements of the middle ear bones. Responses at constant SPL will in addition be affected by the middle ear characteristics. With this proviso, all the results show an envelope for the travelling wave with a relatively shallow low frequency cutoff, and a much sharper high frequency cutoff. All the low frequency cutoffs when referred to constant stapes velocity are flat below 3.5 kHz, increasing to 4–6 dB/octave at higher frequencies below the cutoff (Wilson, 1974). Rhode showed still steeper slopes just below the cutoff. Only Rhode in the squirrel monkey showed a sharp peak at the tip of the response curve, and only Rhode showed a clear nonlinearity at the tip. However all the recent measurements agree in showing mean high frequency cutoffs of the order of 100–150 dB/octave. The phase data agree in showing a progressive increase in the phase of the travelling wave along the basilar membrane, although there is disagreement as to the actual values, Rhode having shown greater increases in phase than the others.

The experiments described hitherto, have measured the response to a sine wave, a stimulus that, conceptually at least, has no frequency spread and lasts for an infinite time. We can also measure the response to the complementary stimulus, a click, which consists of a wide band of frequencies and which lasts for a very short time. The response to a click is known as the impulse response, and if the system is linear it is a simple matter to calculate by means of Fourier transforms the frequency response from the impulse response and vice versa. A sine wave can, after all, be thought of as the sum of a large number of impulses, all of the right amplitude and polarity. There will for a linear system also be a simple relation between the impulse response and the frequency response. If the frequency response has a bandpass characteristic the system will 'ring' after a stimulus, and the ringing will go on for longer as the bandwidth of the system decreases (showing the complementary relations of the Fourier transform pairs of Fig. 1.3). Some basilar membrane impulse responses are shown in Fig. 3.12. That of Wilson and Johnstone (1975), appropriate for the wide bandwidth of their fre-

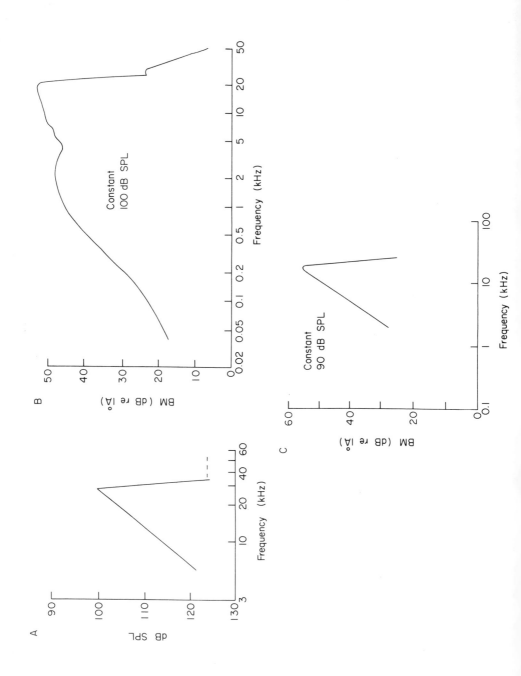

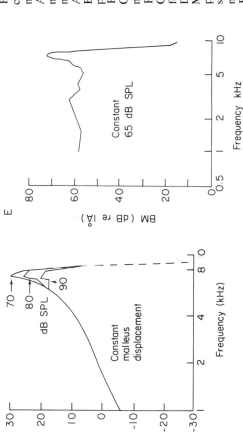

Fig. 3.11 Envelopes of vibration of the cochlear partition, according to recent measures.

A. Guinea-pig, measured by laser. The SPL necessary to give a constant amplitude of movement of the basilar membrane is shown. Adapted from Kohllöffel (1972b).

B. Guinea-pig, measured by capacitive probe. From Wilson and Johnstone (1975), Fig. 7.

C. Guinea-pig, measured by Mössbauer technique. From Johnstone and Boyle (1967), Fig. 1.

Copyright 1967, by the American Association for the Advancement of Science.

D. and E. Squirrel monkey measured by Mössbauer technique. Note that the sharp peak appears only at the lowest sound pressure levels (65–70 dB SPL). D is for constant malleus displacement, E for constant SPL. From Rhode (1971), Fig. 6, and Rhode, (1978), Fig. 7.

quency response, rang for only a few cycles, whereas that measured by the Mössbauer technique in the squirrel monkey rang for many cycles. However it must be remembered that the basilar membrane response measured by Rhode in the squirrel monkey was not linear. Just as the tuning curves appear to saturate at high intensities, so did the early parts of the impulse response (this is quite apart from a peak clipping which can be produced by the measurement technique). This makes it appear that the motion after an impulse is decaying more slowly than would be expected from a linear transformation of the basilar membrane frequency response; the later cycles, being of a lower amplitude, become relatively larger.

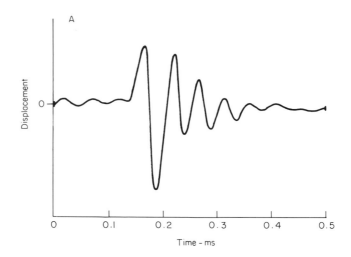

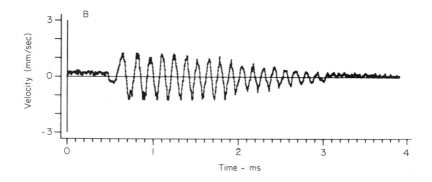

Fig. 3.12 Impulse responses of the basilar membrane show ringing.
A. Guinea-pig, measured by capacitive probe, at the 23 kHz point on the membrane. From Wilson and Johnstone (1975), Fig. 18.
B. Squirrel monkey, *velocity* of the impulse response, measured by the Mössbauer technique. From Rhode *et al.* (1976). Fig. 5.

The basilar membrane shows considerably less frequency selectivity than do either the inner hair cells of the cochlea, or the single fibres of the auditory nerve. In this regard, the data of Rhode (1971) have attracted most interest because they appear to indicate that the apparently poor tuning shown by the basilar membrane could be a result of the high sound pressures needed for the measurements. Auditory nerve fibres show their best frequency selectivity only at low intensities, and this has led to the opinion that, were it possible to measure the mechanics at still lower intensities, the peak of the basilar membrane responses of Fig. 3.11D would become still sharper and the neural and the mechanical responses would match. However, the whole question of the sharpness of the tuning and the linearity of the basilar membrane at medium and low intensities, and indeed at high intensities, is at the moment controversial. We do not for instance know whether the techniques provide an accurate picture of the movement of the membrane, or whether the surgical intervention necessary for the measurements alters the motion. The notion of nonlinearity is for instance contradicted by measurements of Wilson and Johnstone (1975), who showed linearity over the range from 40–140 dB SPL. In contrast, evidence from distortion products and from the evoked mechanical cochlear response, to be discussed in Chapter 5, suggests that there may be a nonlinearity even at the very lowest intensities. (See important note on p. 70.)

In spite of the broad agreement of the results, there is therefore some disagreement between the different investigators in the degree of linearity of the response, and in the sharpness of the tuning. When there is disagreement it is natural to suspect the validity of the methods. The Mössbauer technique involves loading the basilar membrane with a metal source, and although the mass (0.1 μg) is small, it could conceivably affect the movements. Both Johnstone and Boyle (1967) and Rhode (1971) checked this by doubling the mass of the source, and found no change. This of course does not necessarily mean that there would have been no difference if the mass had been *halved* instead. On the other hand, the capacitive probe measurements necessitate partially draining scala tympani so as to bring the probe close to the basilar membrane. However, Evans and Wilson (1975) performed the difficult feat of concurrently recording basilar membrane movements and auditory nerve fibre responses in the cat; they were able to obtain normal sensitivity and frequency selectivity in auditory nerve fibres, suggesting that the movements were in fact normal, while the cochlea was partially drained for the basilar membrane measurements. There is evidence that the differences are unlikely to be due to differences in technique, since both B. M. Johnstone *et al.* (1970) using the Mössbauer technique, and Wilson and J. R. Johnstone (1975) using the capacitive probe agreed in their findings in the 20 kHz regions of the guinea-pig. Rhode (1978) has also found similar results in the same region of the guinea-pig with the Mössbauer technique. The differences may well be due to differences in the frequency regions. Rhode (1978) suggested that for some reason the 20 kHz region may be more susceptible to damage, and that damage destroys the nonlinearity. He repeated his measuremements in the squirrel monkey in this frequency region and, like the others with other species, found complete linearity.

C. The Electrophysiology of the Cochlea

1. The Potentials of the Cochlea

In the transformation from the mechanical acoustic wave to neural activity, a fundamental role is played by the cochlear potentials. With gross electrodes (i.e. electrodes not expected to penetrate single cells, and often having tip sizes of 50 μm or more) it is possible to record both resting and sound evoked potentials in the cochlea. The main resting potential is the endocochlear potential, a positive d.c. potential of some 80 mV which can be recorded from the endolymph. In addition, other d.c. resting potentials have been recorded with gross electrodes, although their status is obscure and they will be dealt with only briefly. When a sound is presented, both a.c. and d.c. responses can be recorded. The a.c. change, which can best be recorded across the cochlear partition, follows the waveform of the acoustic stimulus and is known as the cochlear microphonic (CM). There is an accompanying shift in the endocochlear potential, which is known as the summating potential, and which appears as either positive or negative in the endolymph, depending on the stimulus parameters. The standing endolymphatic potential and the evoked cochlear microphonic and summating potentials are thought to be closely related to the transducer process in the cochlea, although the degree of closeness and the exact position in the chain of events is at the moment a matter of controversy. Definitely later in the chain, are the neural action potentials of the cochlea, recordable with gross electrodes as a massed action potential with two phases known as N_1 and N_2. The gross response is the result of synchronized action potentials in the auditory nerve fibres; it is therefore best seen to a stimulus with a rapid onset. An example of the gross potentials evoked by a tone burst is shown in Fig. 3.13.

Microelectrodes with tips of diameter 0.3μm or less can record the responses of individual cells, either intracellularly or just extracellularly. Recently, the responses of hair cells of the cochlea have been measured (Russell and Sellick, 1978; Crawford and Fettiplace, 1980). The responses of single fibres of the auditory nerve can be measured much more easily; the latter are dealt with in Chapter 4.

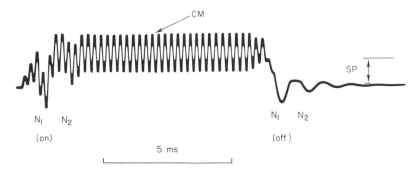

Fig. 3.13 Diagram of the response to a tone burst, recorded with gross electrodes, shows the cochlear microphonic (CM), N_1 and N_2 phases of the gross action potential to both the beginning and the end of the stimulus, and, in the d.c. shift of the microphonic from the baseline, the summating potential (SP).

2. The Standing Potentials: the Endocochlear Potential

(a) The endolymph: its composition and electrical potential

The labyrinthine cavity is composed of two separate compartments. The larger, outer, compartment, formed by the scala vestibuli and scala tympani, runs the length of the system, and is filled with perilymph. There is a smaller inner compartment also extending the entire length of the system, which is formed by the scala media and is filled with endolymph. In the cochlea itself the inner, endolymphatic space, is bounded above by Reissner's membrane, laterally by the stria vascularis, and below by the reticular lamina on the upper surface of the organ of Corti. The space is therefore nearly coextensive with the scala media, but not quite, because the structures of the organ of Corti standing on the basilar membrane are included in the scala media, but are outside the endolymph. Nevertheless, electrical responses are often stated as being recorded from the scala media; the endolymphatic space is then generally assumed. The ionic composition of the endolymph is very different from that of the perilymph; in accordance with this, the endolymphatic space is bounded on all sides by occluding tight junctions, known to inhibit the movement of ions (e.g. Smith, 1978).

The perilymph is recognized as being high in Na^+ (140 mM) and low in K^+ (7 mM; e.g. Bosher and Warren, 1968), and is therefore similar to extracellular fluid or cerebrospinal fluid. Smith *et al.* (1954) first measured the ionic content of the cochlear endolymph by microsampling. In contrast, they found high levels of K^+ (150 mM) and low levels of Na^+ (40 mM); however, their figure for Na^+ has been thought to be too high, due to contamination by the surrounding perilymph. Johnstone and Sellick (1972) suggest that

2 mM, as found with ion selective electrodes, is more accurate. The endolymph therefore has an ionic composition similar to that found intracellularly, and is unique among extracellular fluids of the body for this reason.

Von Békésy (1952) explored the fluids of the cochlea with microelectrodes. His results showed that the scala vestibuli in the guinea-pig was 5 mV positive with respect to the scala tympani, itself near the potential of the surrounding bone, and that the scala media was some 80 mV positive. The values in the scala media declined from 80–120 mV near the base of the cochlea to 50–80 mV in the higher turns. Values around 100 mV have been found in the cat (Peake *et al.*, 1969). Both the chemical and electrical properties of the endolymph therefore point to its having a special role in the cochlea, and many investigations of its functions have been undertaken. The evidence points to the endolymphatic potential as the battery driving the transduction process.

(b) The origin of the endocochlear potential

Although the endolymph has an ionic composition similar to that found inside cells, its electric potential, unlike that found intracellularly, is strongly positive. This immediately suggests that the endocochlear potential is not a K^+ diffusion potential such as is found inside nerve cells; that is, it is *not* due to K^+ ions diffusing passively down their concentration gradient taking positive charge with them and leaving a net negative charge behind. Nor does it seem to be a Na^+ diffusion potential, although the Na^+ concentration difference is in the right direction. Johnstone and Sellick (1972) increased the Na^+ concentration in scala media by perfusing with 20 mM Na^+ Ringer's solution. They found that the endocochlear potential actually increased; if it were a Na^+ diffusion potential it should have decreased, because the Na^+ concentrations in the endolymph and perilymph had become more equal.

The positive endocochlear potential is, in contrast, generally thought to be directly dependent on energy consuming, ion pumping processes in the stria vascularis. Anoxia, which of course inhibits the energy consuming processes rapidly, causes the endocochlear potential to decay to zero within one or two minutes (Johnstone and Sellick, 1972). However, a diffusion potential should be maintained even during anoxia as long as the ionic concentration differences do not decay. In fact, after a few minutes of anoxia when the presumed oxidative processes have disappeared, the positive endocochlear potential is replaced by a negative potential which can take several hours to disappear, as the ions equilibrate. This negative potential is thought to be a diffusion potential, arising from the high K^+ concentration in the endolymph (Johnstone *et al.*, 1966). Evidence that the stria vascularis is the source of the endocochlear potential comes from several sources:

(i)   Tasaki and Spyropoulos (1959) destroyed Reissner's membrane so that the endolymph and perilymph could mix. The stria vascularis was the only site from which positive potentials could then be recorded. That any potentials at all could be recorded is evidence that the endocochlear potential is not a diffusion potential, because the ionic gradient will have been destroyed.

(ii) The stria vascularis is a site of high metabolic activity. Kuijpers and Bonting (1969) analysed Na^+-K^+ linked ATPase in several structures of the cochlea, and found that its activity was some 12 times higher in the stria vascularis than in any other cochlear structure. The ATPase was inhibited by ouabain, a specific inhibitor of Na^+-K^+ linked ATPase, and showed a concentration function for its effect on the ATPase similar to that for its effect on the endocochlear potential (Kuijpers and Bonting, 1970).

(iii) Some ototoxic agents such as ethacrynic acid which have a preferential effect on the stria vascularis also reduce the endocochlear potential.

Correspondingly, it was shown by Tasaki and Spyropoulos (1959) that the organ of Corti was not the site of production of the endocochlear potential, because the endocochlear potential is present in a strain of mice known as waltzing mice, in which the organ of Corti is congenitally absent.

It appears that the stria vascularis contains an electrogenic Na^+-K^+ pump; the potential, partly at least, arises because more K^+ is pumped into the endolymph than Na^+ out. Because the pump moves both ions up their concentration gradients, energy is required, and this is supplied by the ATP (e.g. Johnstone and Sellick, 1972; Dallos, 1973a). The observed final potential will be the net result of substracting the negative K^+ diffusion potential, always expected where the ions can move down their concentration gradients, from the positive electrogenically-produced potential. The origin of the potential is further discussed by Johnstone and Sellick (1972).

3. Other Standing Potentials

Von Békésy, while exploring the cochlea with microelectrodes, found a negative potential of up to -40 mV in the organ of Corti (von Békésy, 1952). The history of the potential is one of controversy, and it has since been suggested that the potential is an injury potential recorded from the cells of the organ of Corti, rather than a potential associated with the fluid in the spaces between the cells (e.g. Dallos, 1973a; Flex, 1974; Johnstone and Sellick, 1972). In accordance with this view, Ilberg and Vosteen (1969) found that the ionic composition of the extracellular fluid in the organ of Corti was similar to that of perilymph. Engström (1960) coined the name 'cortilymph' for the fluid surrounding the organ of Corti. Cortilymph therefore seems similar to perilymph, although there is a suggestion that its protein content may be higher (Ryan *et al.*, 1980).

4. The Evoked Potentials: the Cochlear Microphonic

Wever and Bray (1930) placed a wire electrode in the auditory nerve, connected it to an amplifier in a room 16 m away, and from there to a loudspeaker. As they reported,

> "the action currents, after amplification, were audible in the receiver as sounds which, so far as the observer could determine, were identical with the original stimulus. Speech was transmitted with great fidelity. Simple sounds, commands, and the like were easily received. Indeed, under good conditions the system was employed as a means of communication between operating and sound-proof rooms."

They thought that they were recording the massed action potentials of the auditory nerve, but Adrian (1931) suggested that they were in fact recording potentials evoked earlier in the transducer chain, and called them the cochlear microphonics. Ironically, having left us with the name for the effect, he later that year decided that Wever and Bray's first interpretation was correct after all (Adrian *et al.*, 1931). It now appears that Adrian was right first time, and that the deflection of the basilar membrane in response to a sound produces a microphonic potential, which follows the movement of the basilar membrane, and occurs in the chain of events before any action potentials. Again, the closeness of the relation between the recorded microphonic and either the movement of the basilar membrane or the excitation of the auditory nerve is controversial, and the recorded microphonic has been called everything from a receptor potential (Davis, 1965) to an epiphenomenon.

(a) Generation

Tasaki *et al.* (1954) presented clear evidence as to the site of production of the cochlear microphonic. They advanced a microelectrode from the scala tympani, through the basilar membrane and the organ of Corti, into the endolymphatic space and the scala media. Their results are shown in Fig. 3.14. The d.c. record shows that as the electrode was advanced, intermittent negative potentials were recorded in the organ of Corti — the so-called organ of Corti potential — followed by a jump to a positive potential — the endocochlear potential — as the electrode penetrated the reticular lamina. The a.c. records show that at the same point as the positive potential appeared, the cochlear microphonic reversed polarity. This fixes the site of generation of the cochlear microphonic as the reticular lamina at the upper surface of the hair cells, or at least a structure, such as the hair cells

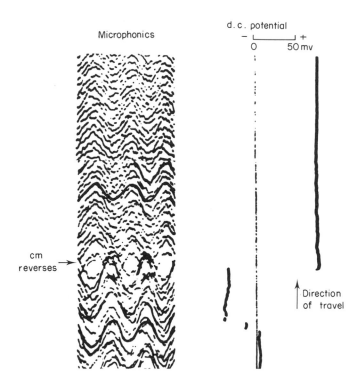

Fig. 3.14 In the classic experiment of Tasaki *et al.* an electrode was advanced through the organ of Corti. The a.c. response to a continuous tone is shown on the left, and the d.c. record on the right. The cochlear microphonic reversed polarity at the same time as the positive endocochlear potential appeared. From Tasaki *et al.* (1954), Fig. 2.

themselves, in close electrical contact with this layer. We shall see in the next section that with very fine microelectrodes it is possible to record particularly large and sharply tuned microphonics in, or very close to, the hair cells (Russell and Sellick, 1978). These lines of evidence show beyond reasonable doubt that the hair cells, if not directly responsible for, are at least closely associated with, the production of the cochlear microphonic. Dallos (1973b) selectively damaged the outer hair cells with the ototoxic drug kanamycin. This drug in the right doses can destroy the outer hair cells while leaving the inner hair cells intact, at least as judged under the light microscope. Dallos found that the cochlear microphonic dropped to 1/30th of its normal size, suggesting that, if the inner hair cells were indeed unaffected, it is the *outer* hair cells that contribute practically all the microphonics recordable in the normal animal.

The production of the cochlear microphonic is most clearly understood in terms of Davis's battery and resistance hypothesis (Davis, 1965, 1968).

According to this theory, the endocochlear potential drives current through the high resistance layer of the reticular lamina at the upper end of the hair cells. The hair cells act as variable resistances, allowing more current through when the hairs are deflected (Fig. 3.15). The travelling wave therefore modulates the current, in a way that follows the waveform of the travelling wave at that point. This produces potential changes in both the scala media and the scala tympani, of opposite phases on either side of the reticular lamina, so giving the cochlear microphonic. While this theory accounts for many experimental results in a straightforward way, it must be emphasized that there is little really direct evidence for its details, all of which have been, or still are being, questioned. Nevertheless, it seems an appropriate framework within which to interpret experimental results; the later chapter on transducer mechanisms will discuss its validity in relation to recent data.

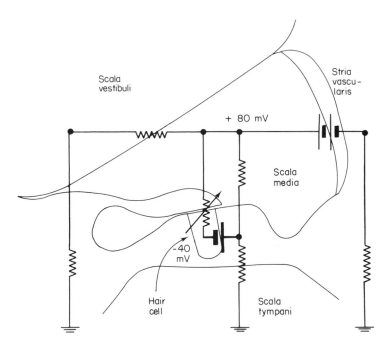

Fig. 3.15 In Davis's battery theory, the membrane at the apex of the hair cell acts as a variable resistance, modulating the current driven through the cell by the positive endocochlear potential and the negative intracellular potential. Adapted from Davis (1965).

(b) Input-output relations

Figure 3.16 shows the amplitude of the microphonic to a 1 kHz tone, recorded from the round window. The intensity function shows an increase

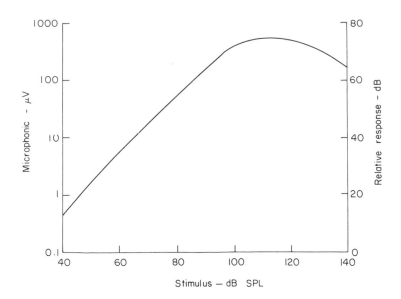

Fig. 3.16 A typical intensity function for the cochlear microphonic, recorded from the round window in response to a 1 kHz tone, shows a linear increase to 80–90 dB SPL, a maximum, and a decline at very high intensities.

proportional to the stimulus intensity up to 80–90 dB SPL, a flattening at 100–120 dB SPL, and then a downturn at 130–140 dB SPL. The actual limit of proportionality, the maximum output voltage, often between 100 and 1000 μV, and the degree of downturn, are dependent on the stimulus parameters and the recording site. As will be pointed out later, there are severe difficulties in projecting from grossly recorded responses to events at the hair cell level; nevertheless, it appears that the saturation of the microphonic has a correlate in the hair cell responses, which also saturate at similar intensities (Russell and Sellick, 1978). The limit of linearity can also be associated with an increase in the amount of distortion in the microphonic, as would be expected if the response became clipped (Wever and Lawrence, 1954), although it will also be pointed out later that the recorded distortion may be no guide to the distortion at the generator.

The mechanism of the downturn at high intensities is not known. The intensity at which it occurs depends on the stimulation conditions, the recording site, and is affected by drug damage to the cochlea.

(c) Spatial localization

As might be expected from Davis's (1965) theory, the cochlear microphonic is spatially localized in the same way as the mechanical travelling wave. Low frequencies give the greatest response near the apex, and high frequencies near the base. The records in Fig. 3.17 show this distribution clearly, especially at low intensities. In fact, the position of the peak of the response at low intensity compares well with the position of the peak of the travelling wave envelope (Eldredge, 1974, p. 568). In contrast, as the intensity is raised, the peak of the response moves towards the base of the cochlea. The detailed mechanism of this is not known, although auditory nerve fibres in some frequency ranges show an analogous shift in best frequency as the intensity is raised, and this suggests that in some cases at least it may be a product of the transducer mechanism. It is also possible to explain the shift as a result of saturation of the intensity function together with the action of spatial filtering.

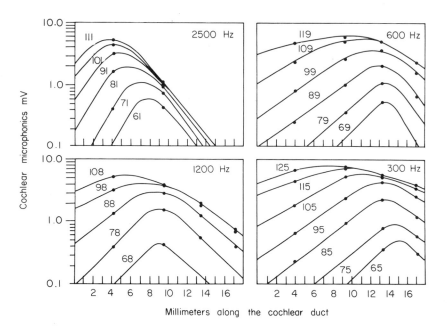

Fig. 3.17 The spatial distribution of the cochlear microphonic was estimated from four electrodes in the scala media, placed at different distances along the cochlea. Each panel shows results for a different stimulus frequency. The stimulus intensity in dB SPL is shown by the parameters marked on the curves. From Honrubia and Ward (1968), Fig. 6.

(d) Spatial filtering

Usually, the cochlear microphonic is recorded from electrodes inserted into the scala vestibuli or the scala tympani, or from an electrode placed on the round window or even more remote sites such as the surrounding bone.

Such electrodes see a spatially integrated average of the activity in their vicinity, and the relations between the recorded potentials and the activity at the generator sites can become very complicated indeed. Even if records are made between differential electrodes in the scala vestibuli and the scala tympani, so straddling the generator sites, appreciable spatial integration occurs. Many of the complexities of the grossly recorded microphonic can be understood with the concept of 'spatial filtering' introduced as a result of the analysis of Whitfield and Ross (1965).

Whitfield and Ross (1965) pointed out that an electrode integrating activity over a length of cochlea could not record the full amplitude of the potential changes if there were substantial phase changes over the distance seen by the electrode. In that case, the positive and negative phases of the microphonic would tend to cancel, with the result that the net recorded voltage would tend to be too small. The effect will be most important when the wavelength of the travelling wave is shortest, and so the effects of spatial filtering are likely to be most important at high frequencies and on the apical slope of the travelling wave envelope, for it is then that the phase changes most sharply. Figure 3.18 shows that while the envelope of the travelling wave at very low frequencies may be more-or-less faithfully recorded, when the frequency is raised and the wavelengths on the basilar membrane become shorter, the recorded envelope of the microphonic gets smaller and seems to shift basally with respect to the peak of the amplitude envelope. The recorded envelope also becomes broader. The functions in Fig. 3.17 therefore give little evidence for the degree of spatial localization of the travelling wave. Estimation from the gross microphonic to events at the generator site should be made only with the utmost caution.

Spatial filtering therefore results in the selective attenuation of high frequencies in the microphonic through the spatial integration of currents in the cochlea. We can explain other properties of the gross cochlear microphonic in terms of spatial filtering. At low intensities, for instance, the activity near the peak of the travelling wave will dominate the response. As the intensity is increased the response near the peak will limit, and the contribution from the long basal tail of the travelling wave will become relatively larger. Here, the rate of change of phase along the basilar membrane is less than near the peak, and the mutual cancellation of the generators will be relatively smaller. The peak of the distribution of the cochlear microphonic therefore moves basally (Fig. 3.17).

Spatial filtering will also reduce the amount of distortion in the recorded microphonic. High harmonics in the generator waveforms are associated with rapid spatial transitions of generator potential on the basilar membrane. These may occur over distances which are short compared with the distances seen by a recording electrode. Therefore, if in response to a sinusoid, the generators can be thought of as peak clipping and producing a

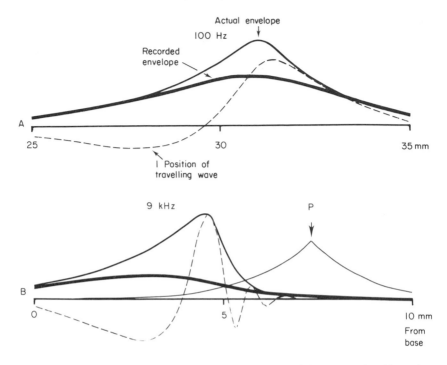

Fig. 3.18 The influence of spatial filtering on the distribution of the measured cochlear micro-phonic is shown for a low frequency stimulus, recorded near the apex of the cochlea (A), and for a high frequency stimulus, recorded near the base (B). "P" shows the potential distribution of a point source as seen by the recording electrode (decay of potentials by 6 dB/mm). Travelling wave data in A from von Békésy (1960) in man, and in B from Kohllöffel (1972a) in the guinea-pig.

square wave of activity travelling along the basilar membrane, spatial filter-ing will round the corners off, so that the recorded microphonic becomes more nearly sinusoidal.

5. The Evoked Potentials: the Summating Potential

The d.c. change produced in the cochlea in response to a sound is known as the summating potential (SP), and is visible as a base-line shift in the recorded signal of Fig. 3.13. Depending on the circumstances, it is recorded as a sustained positive or negative potential shift of the scala media during acoustic stimulation. The phenomenon is complex and the mechanism is not known precisely; nevertheless we can provisionally attempt to interpret the potential in terms of Davis's battery hypothesis. When the travelling wave reduces the resistance of the hair cells, the endocochlear potential drives current through the hair cells, producing a potential shift. Indeed Russell and Sellick (1978) found that inner hair cells were depolarized, that is, became less negative inside, in response to sound. We would therefore expect structures *below* the reticular lamina, for instance the scala tympani, to become relatively more positive, and, because the endocochlear potential is to some extent being short-circuited, we would expect structures above the reticular lamina to become more negative. The summating potential should reverse the sign around the reticular lamina. Konishi and Yasuno (1963) advanced an electrode through the organ of Corti and indeed found just such a reversal of the summating potential, at the same time as the endocochlear potential appeared and the microphonic reversed phase. Unfortunately, because there seem many different components to the summating potential, we do not know if this observation is valid for all components.

As an extension of the above hypothesis, it has been suggested that the d.c. change is produced as a distortion component of the local alternating potential. Russell and Sellick (1978) suggest that their observed intracellular d.c. change may be produced by a rectification of the a.c. driving currents. Engerbretson and Eldredge (1968) and Eldredge (1974) suggest that the summating potential is the result of asymmetric distortion in the microphonic waveform, although the evidence to be presented below suggests that the position is really more complicated.

(a) Multiple origins

In spite of the potentially simple explanation of the summating potential, there appear to be many components in its origin. As was described above, we would expect the scala media to become relatively more negative when a sound is presented. However, apparently paradoxically, the scala media can under certain circumstances become relatively more *positive* with respect to the scala tympani. In this case, contrast to the direction expected on the above hypothesis, the endocochlear potential actually *increases*. It is only at high intensities that the expected negative shift of the scala media comes to dominate the whole pattern (Dallos, 1973a). Other multiple components can be seen in the temporal responses. Honrubia and Ward (1969) showed that the summating potential had a slow component that grew for several seconds during presentation of the stimulus even though the microphonic was constant, and that this was superimposed on a component that grew instantaneously with the microphonic when the stimulus was turned on. We may expect that some of the changes were due to slow electrical changes in the neurones of the auditory nerve, and to changes in the endocochlear driving potential and maybe in the supporting cells, perhaps of metabolic origin.

For these reasons, hypotheses which explain the summating potential in terms of a distortion in the microphonic waveform, either due to mechanical nonlinearities, or to nonlinearities in the mechanoelectrical transducer, can never explain all the phenomena, although they may explain some components of the potential. However, explanations in terms of nonlinearities carry the implication that the summating potential is an epiphenomenon. In contrast, it appears that an intracellularly positive summating potential is the receptor potential for the inner hair cells, and is associated with the activation of the fibres of the auditory nerve (Russell and Sellick, 1978).

(b) Spatial distribution

Honrubia and Ward (1969) measured the position of the peak of negativity in the scala media for different frequencies (Fig. 3.19). As expected from the travelling wave, the responses to high frequencies peaked basally, and those to low frequencies apically. (It can also be seen that the low frequency tones made the scala media relatively more positive in the lower turns.) These measurements were made with monopolar electrodes, which are poor at determining the site of the potential generators, because the results can easily be influenced by current from remote sources. Dallos *et al.*

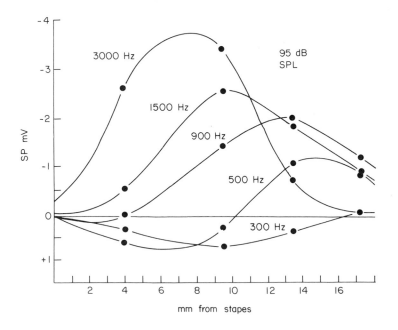

Fig. 3.19 The spatial distribution of the summating potential was estimated from four electrodes in the scala media, placed at different distances along the cochlea. High frequencies produced the greatest negativity near the base, low frequencies towards the apex. From Honrubia and Ward (1969), Fig. 2.

(1972) used bipolar recording, straddling the recording site with one electrode in the scala vestibuli and one in the scala tympani, reducing this
difficulty. Measuring at medium intensities (50 dB SPL), they showed that
the scala vestibuli, and hence the scala media, could be made more positive
by the generators on the peak, and on the low frequency slope of the
travelling wave (Fig. 3.20). It was only beyond the high frequency slope that
the generators made the scala vestibuli, and hence the scala media, more
negative. As the intensity was raised the area of negativity in the scala media
increased, and so came to dominate the whole response. The component
leading to the increased positivity of the scala media at medium intensities
can tentatively be ascribed to the outer hair cells. Kanamycin as we have
seen is thought to selectively affect outer hair cells, and Dallos and Wang
(1974) showed that, while kanamycin reduced the negative component by
26 dB, the positive component was completely abolished and replaced by a
negativity. This suggests the possibility that the positive component is

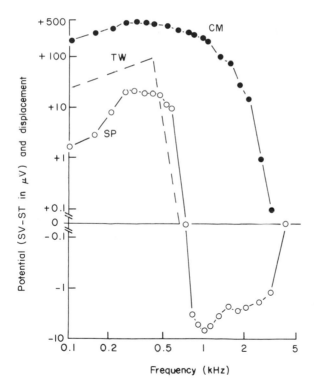

Fig. 3.20 The frequency response of the cochlear microphonic (CM), of the travelling wave on
the basilar membrane (TW), and of the summating potential, recorded across the cochlear
partition (SP), for one point in the cochlea. The plotted potentials are the potential in the scala
vestibuli minus the potential in the scala tympani. From Dallos *et al.* (1972), Fig. 21.

produced entirely by outer hair cells, and that the negative component receives contributions from both inner and outer hair cells.

The origin of the summating potential is further discussed by Johnstone and Sellick (1972), Dallos (1973a, 1975), Fex (1974) and Eldredge (1974).

6. Responses from Hair Cells

Recently, a landmark in the progress of auditory physiology has been reached with the intracellular recording of responses from individual hair cells of the mammalian cochlea by Russell and Sellick (1978) and Tanaka *et al.* (1980), and the reptilian cochlea by Crawford and Fettiplace (1980) and Weiss *et al.* (1974).

Russell and Sellick (1978) aimed fine, high impedance microelectrodes at the organ of Corti in the basal turn of the guinea-pig cochlea. They were able to dye-mark the cells penetrated, and show that they could record intra-cellularly from inner hair cells. Outer hair cells were not reliably penetrated. The cells had resting potentials of −25 to −45 mV (cf. −60 to −70 mV for nerve cells). Sound produced both a.c. and d.c. changes. The d.c. change was an intracellular depolarization: that is, the inside of the cell became relatively more positive. This is the direction expected on the basis of Davis's battery hypothesis if the sound wave reduced the resistance at the apex of the hair cells, and the changes can be provisionally understood, as can the corresponding gross potentials, in terms of the hypothesis. The d.c. depolarizations can be thought of as a correlate of the component of the summating potential that makes the scala media more negative. The maximum d.c. changes that could be recorded were some 30 mV, as against 4 mV or less for the grossly recorded extracellular summating potential. The a.c. changes followed the waveform of the stimulus, and can be thought of as an intracellular correlate of the cochlear microphonic. Near the cell's most sensitive frequency the a.c. potential changes were smaller than the d.c. potential changes, having a maximum amplitide of about 0.6 mV.

Russell and Sellick plotted the magnitude of the hair cells' responses as a function of the intensity and frequency of the stimulus in two different ways. In the first way, they held the frequency at fixed values, and plotted the magnitude of the a.c. and d.c. responses as a function of stimulus intensity. Curves plotted in this way are called intensity functions, and the curves of Fig. 3.21 show such functions for one cell for different frequencies of stimulation. In the second method, the sound intensity necessary to evoke a certain criterion magnitude of electrical response was plotted as a function of frequency; such curves are known as iso-response plots, iso-amplitude functions, or tuning curves, and are shown for another cell in Fig. 3.22.

At low intensities the intensity functions all show approximately linear increases in potential with sound level (that is, the potential increases 20 dB or 10 fold for 20 dB increases in SPL), followed by a saturation at higher levels. At one frequency, the 'best' or 'characteristic' frequency, the cell starts giving its response at the lowest intensity and saturates soonest. At frequencies lower and higher than this, the response appears first only at higher intensities. The iso-response curves (Fig. 3.22) clearly show the tuning characteristics of the cell; the cell is very sensitive at one frequency, and the responsiveness drops rapidly as the frequency is shifted by small amounts, although measurable responses still exist to frequencies well below the characteristic frequency. These curves can be directly compared with the basilar membrane tuning curves of Fig. 3.11. It is apparent that they show sharper tuning, for instance sharper than those of Wilson and Johnstone (1975) in the same frequency and intensity range in the same species, the guinea-pig, and sharper than those of Rhode (1971) at the lower levels in

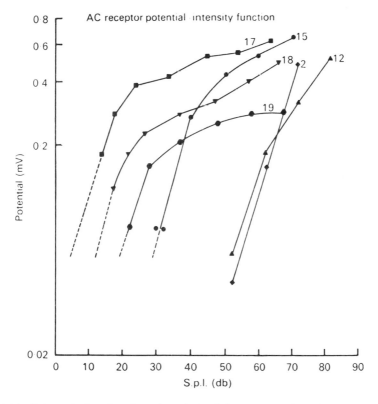

Fig. 3.21 A. C. intensity functions for an inner hair cell show an approximately linear increase in potential at the lowest intensities at each frequency, followed by a saturation. The parameter marked on each curve shows the frequency of stimulation in kHz; this cell was most sensitive at 17 kHz. From Russell and Sellick (1978), Fig. 3.

the squirrel monkey, which are the sharpest basilar membrane tuning curves that have been measured. The mechanism behind this difference is not known and will be discussed later. The selectivity is in fact comparable to that of single fibres of the auditory nerve. This may not necessarily be surprising, since 90–95% of the auditory nerve fibres synapse directly with the inner hair cells (Morrison *et al.*, 1975; Spoendlin, 1972).

The amplitude of the intracellular a.c. response, as already noted, was many times smaller than the amplitude of the d.c. response. Accurate comparison was difficult, because the high impedance electrodes attenuated the high frequency signals severely. Nevertheless, the calculated alternating voltage fell by 6–9 dB/octave, and Russell and Sellick suggested that this occurred because at high frequencies the alternating currents through the cells were short-circuited by the capacitance of the cell walls. The likely size

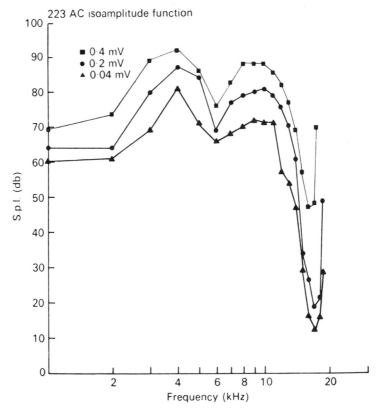

Fig. 3.22 Tuning curves for an inner hair cell show the sound pressure level to produce a constant amplitude of the electrical response, as a function of frequency. From Russell and Sellick (1978), Fig. 6.

of the effect can be calculated from the resistance and capacitance of the cells. These were assessed from the amplitude and phase of the voltage changes induced by current pulses injected into the cells. Once the resistance and capacitance had been compensated for, it was shown that the intracellular a.c. and d.c. potentials varied in a parallel fashion over the whole frequency range. On the other hand, the extracellular a.c. response was not affected by the capacitance of the cells, and showed a frequency selectivity and amplitude response similar to that of the extracellular d.c. voltage. With suitable placement, the extracellular response recorded with these fine microelectrodes was similar in frequency selectivity to the intracellular response. The maximum extracellular a.c. and d.c. response was 3 mV.

The direct measurements of resistance showed that the resistance of the cell fell when it was depolarized by sound (Fig. 3.23). The drop in resistance agrees with Davis's theory; the relation will be discussed in more detail in Chapter 5.

Outer hair cells seem much more difficult to record from than inner hair cells. Tanaka *et al.* (1980), who succeeded in recording from and dye-marking outer hair cells, report irregularly fluctuating intracellular resting potentials, with values in the range of -5 to -30 mV. In response to sound, the cells showed a.c. potential changes of a few mV peak-to-peak with a stimulus of 70 dB SPL, and negligible d.c. responses. Tanaka *et al.* were not able to measure tuning curves. It is probably too early to use such data for analysing the role of the outer hair cells in hearing. We would expect, as with inner hair cells, that over most of the frequency range a great proportion of the alternating current entering the apical membrane of the cell would pass through the capacitance of the membrane at the base. This would substantially attenuate the intracellular a.c. potential. The cells therefore seem to show neither large a.c. nor large d.c. responses intracellularly, and would seem to act merely as current shunts. In shunting current, they would be able to make a substantial contribution to the cochlear microphonic as recorded by gross electrodes.

Crawford and Fettiplace (1980) have made intracellular recordings from the turtle's homologue of the organ of Corti, the basilar papilla. They also showed sharp tuning of the alternating potentials, as sharp as, if not sharper than, that of mammalian auditory nerve fibres in the same frequency range. However they did not find similar sustained depolarizations. Their work is important because they presented evidence that the sharp tuning arises from electrical resonators in the hair cell membranes themselves. The work will be discussed later under transducer mechanisms (Chapter 5).

To what extent is it possible to explain the grossly recorded responses in terms of the individual hair cell responses? Certainly the a.c. responses are an approximation to the cochlear microphonic, and the sustained depola-

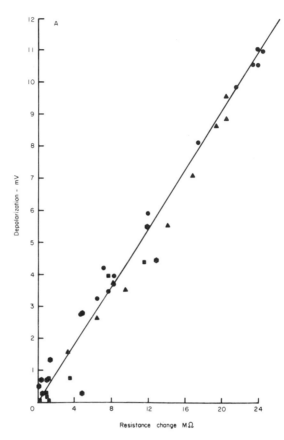

Fig. 3.23 A. Inner hair cells depolarize in proportion to the decrease in membrane resistance. The results shown here are for one cell, for different intensities and frequencies of stimulation (indicated by different symbols).

rizations of inner hair cells are an approximation to one component of the summating potential. The localization of the responses agrees with the evidence localizing the potentials to the reticular lamina. However it appears from the kanamycin studies of Dallos (1973b) and Dallos and Wang (1974) that practically all the grossly recordable cochlear microphonic is produced by the outer hair cells (p. 53), whereas it was the inner hair cells that were recorded from by Russell and Sellick (1978). We would not necessarily therefore expect the two to have the same frequency or phase response. The outer hair cells may well be broadly tuned on the low fre- quency side, and this could explain some of the broad tuning of the grossly recorded cochlear microphonic. However, we have so little evidence on outer hair cells that it is not at the moment possible to say how completely their

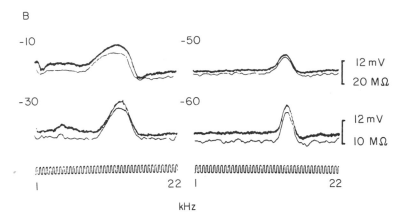

B shows that the depolarization and resistance change have the same frequency dependence. From Russell and Sellick (1978), Fig. 9.

responses account for the grossly recorded cochlear microphonic.

The negative summating potential (negative in the scala media) has a correlate in the positive intracellular depolarization of the inner hair cells, because an increase in positivity below the reticular lamina would be expected to be associated with an increase in negativity above.

As was suggested by Dallos and Wang (1974), it is the negative summating potential that is dependent on the inner hair cells, although the recorded potentials do not suggest how the inner hair cells could also contribute to the positive summating potential (positive in the scala media) as indicated by their data. Also unexplained is the finding of Dallos *et al.* (1972), shown in Fig. 3.20, that the negative summating potential was localized apically to the peak of the mechanical travelling wave, whereas the maximum hair cell depolarization seems to occur at the peak of the mechanical travelling wave (Russell and Sellick, 1978). It may be that the positive and negative contributions of different sets of hair cells show different patterns of dominance in the different parts of the travelling wave.

7. The Gross Neural Action Potential

Electrodes that are too large to record from single neural elements can nevertheless record summed neural activity produced by the simultaneous activation of many neurones. An electrode in or near to the cochlea will record a gross neural response of the cochlea to a tone onset, as in Fig. 3.13.

The two dominant waves of the gross neural response are known as N_1 and N_2, the first coming about 1 ms after the start of the microphonic, and the second about 1 ms after that. As the intensity is raised from low levels, N_1 is the first to appear, followed shortly after by N_2. At high intensities the response becomes more complex, with the appearance of other components of different latency (e.g. Antoli-Candela *et al.*, 1978). The gross potential is interpreted as the summed effect of massed action potentials travelling in a volley down the auditory nerve. Detailed experiments have supported this conclusion, although there is still doubt as to which fibres contribute most to the different phases of the gross potential, and as to the site along the auditory nerve at which the action potentials are seen by the electrode. An analysis of the mechanisms behind this potential is useful because it is this potential, rather than of course the activity of single fibres of the auditory nerve, that can be recorded clinically.

Antoli-Candela and Kiang (1978) sampled the activity of a large number of auditory nerve fibres in response to a click, and showed that it was only fibres whose best (or characteristic) frequencies were in the high frequency region, that is, above 4 kHz, whose firing was synchronized to the N_1 and N_2 phases of the gross neural action potential. We can understand how this result arises, because it is only neural action potentials that are substantially in synchrony that will add together to give a gross potential. The travelling wave travels most rapidly over the basal part of the cochlea, and more and more slowly thereafter. Therefore it is only the fibres from the high frequency, basal, region that will be activated in synchrony.

D. Summary

1. The cochlea is a coiled tube, divided lengthways into three scalae. The three divisions are known as the scala vestibuli, the scala media, and the scala tympani. The two outer scalae, the scala vestibuli and scala tympani, contain perilymph which is like normal extracellular fluid in composition and is at or near ground potential. The scala media contains endolymph which is more like intracellular fluid, and has a positive potential. The positive potential arises partly at least from an electrogenic Na^+-K^+ linked pump in the stria vascularis.

2. The auditory transducer is the organ of Corti which sits on the basilar membrane dividing the scala media from the scala tympani. The cells performing the transduction are called *hair cells*. Hair cells are of two types, known as *inner* and *outer* hair cells. They have many hairs, or stereocilia, projecting from their apical surface. It is probably deflection of these hairs that initiates transduction.

3. Deflection of the hairs is caused by deflection of the basilar membrane. The latter occurs as a result of a sound-induced displacement of the cochlear fluids interacting with the stiffness of the basilar membrane, to

produce a progressive travelling wave on the basilar membrane, which passes from base to apex.

4. Travelling waves produced by sounds of high frequency do not travel far up the cochlea, and high frequency sounds are transduced near the base of the cochlea. The travelling wave produced by low frequency sounds travels further up the cochlea, and low frequency sounds are transduced near the apex.

5. The sharpness of tuning of the peaks of the travelling wave is at the moment controversial. Some investigators show that the basilar membrane acts only as a low-pass filter, while others show a sharp resonance at the peak. (See important note on p. 70.)

6. Flexion of the stereocilia by the travelling waves probably alters the electrical resistance of the apical membrane of the hair cells, allowing the endocochlear potential to drive current through the hair cells. This produces potential changes that can be measured both in the hair cells with fine microelectrodes, and grossly in the cochlea with larger electrodes.

7. One sound induced potential that can be measured with gross electrodes is the cochlear microphonic. It is an alternating potential that follows the waveform of the stimulus. It is generated predominantly by outer hair cells. A second potential, a d.c. change, is known as the summating potential. Depending on the conditions of stimulation, it drives the scala media either more positive or more negative. The summating potential has multiple origins, with contributions from both inner and outer hair cells.

8. Inner hair cells show both an a.c. potential and a steady depolarization in response to sound. Unlike the potentials that are recorded with gross electrodes, the intracellular potentials are very sharply tuned, with low thresholds only in one frequency region. Outer hair cells are difficult to record from. They seem to show a.c. responses but not d.c. responses. It is likely that hair cell sound-induced potentials will be able to account for many of the responses found with gross electrodes.

9. The massed activity of auditory nerve fibres can be recorded with gross electrodes in response to stimulus onsets. Fibres with best frequencies of 4 kHz and above seem to make most contribution.

E. Further Reading

Aspects of cochlear anatomy have been reviewed by Ades and Engström (1974), Smith (1975), Engström and Engström (1978) and Lim (1980).

Cochlear mechanics have been reviewed by Dallos (1973a), Chapter 4, pp. 127–217, Schroeder (1975), Geisler (1976) and Dallos (1978). Measurements of basilar membrane motion have been reviewed by Rhode (1978, 1980).

Cochlear potentials and their relation to cochlear mechanics have been reviewed by Johnstone and Sellick (1972), Dallos (1973a) Chapter 5, pp. 218–390, Eldredge (1974), Dallos (1975), Dallos (1978), and Dallos (1981).

Mechanisms of transduction are further dealt with in Chapter 5 of the present work.

Note Added in Proof

Khanna and Leonard have just shown that the basilar membrane can show very sharp tuning, as sharp as that of auditory nerve fibres.

Khanna, S. M. and Leonard, D. G. B. (1982) Basilar membrane tuning in the cat cochlea. *Science* **215**, 305–306.

IV. The Auditory Nerve

We have now a comprehensive description of the responses of auditory nerve fibres to a variety of stimuli in normal, albeit anaesthetized, animals. We are also beginning to understand some of the changes that occur in auditory nerve activity during cochlear pathology. The responses of auditory nerve fibres underly the responses of the later stages of the auditory system, and perhaps even match the psychophysical capabilities of the intact organism. For these reasons, a knowledge of the material presented in this chapter is essential for the understanding of the later chapters on the central auditory system (Chapters 6–8), on the psychophysical correlates of auditory physiology (Chapter 9), and on sensorineural hearing loss (Chapter 10). Those whose later interest is primarily in Chapter 10 need here only read up to and including Section B.2 (ending on p. 85).

A. Anatomy

Auditory nerve fibres, with their cell bodies in the spiral ganglion, provide a direct synaptic connection between the hair cells of the cochlea and the cochlear nucleus. There are about 50 000 fibres in the cat and 30 000 in man (Harrison and Howe, 1974a). It was once thought that a substantial proportion of auditory nerve fibres were directed to the outer hair cells, which are of course the more numerous of the hair cells (e.g. Fernandez, 1951). Now however it is recognized that only about 5–10% of the spiral ganglion cells are connected to the outer hair cells, the majority connecting directly and exclusively to the inner hair cells (Spoendlin, 1972; Morrison *et al.*, 1975). A diagram summarizing Spoendlin's scheme is shown in Fig. 3.6. The reader is reminded that the fibres innervating the inner hair cells innervate the hair cells nearest their point of entry into the cochlea, whereas those innervating the outer hair cells run basally for about 0.6 mm before terminating. About 20 fibres innervate each inner hair cell, whereas about six fibres innervate each outer hair cell. Each fibre to the inner hair cells connects with one and only one hair cell, whereas those to the outer hair cells branch and innervate about 10 hair cells. There is evidence that the differentiation in the targets is associated with a morphological differentiation in the cell bodies and axons. About 95% (in the cat) of spiral ganglion cells are bipolar, and have myelinated cell bodies and axons, and have been called Type I cells (Spoendlin, 1978). The remainder are monopolar and are not myelinated and have been called Type II cells. It has been suggested from their differential degeneration behaviour that the myelinated Type I cells project to the inner hair cells, and Type II cells to outer hair cells. Both Type I cell bodies and the fibres in the organ of Corti which run to the inner hair cells degenerate after central section of the auditory nerve. In contrast, the Type II cells and the fibres running to the outer hair cells are preserved after the lesion (Spoendlin, 1978). There is even the suggestion that the Type II axons do not reach the central end of the auditory nerve, because of the way the cell bodies are preserved after lesions of the central end of the nerve, and because practically no unmyelinated axons are found in the central end (Spoendlin, 1978). That view is however rather controversial. These studies are nevertheless apposite, because recordings made from the central end of the auditory nerve have not so far been able to demonstrate two groups of fibres corresponding to those innervating the inner and outer hair cells.

B. Physiology

We must assume, provisionally at least, that all, or substantially all, the auditory nerve fibres recorded from in the central end of the auditory nerve innervate the inner hair cells. Although our knowledge of inner hair cell physiology is only sketchy, we do have a fairly complete knowledge of the responses of the auditory nerve. This knowledge has accumulated over the last 20 years or so, and has depended on a careful control of stimulus and physiological parameters, together with the surveying of large populations of fibres, sometimes as many as 418 fibres in one animal (Kim *et al.*, 1980). This has been achieved in spite of the inaccesibility of the nerve deep in the bone, and the lack of mechanical stability of the adjacent brain stem, which means that fibres can be easily lost in recording. In fact, it was not until 1954 that the first responses of auditory nerve fibres were published (Tasaki, 1954), and it is now recognized that the records indicate that the cochlea must have been in poor physiological condition. Tasaki's approach was to drill through the temporal bone until the auditory nerve was encountered in the internal auditory meatus. The approach commonly used nowadays is to open the occipital bone at the back of the skull and, by inserting a retractor around the edge of the cerebellum, to retract the cerebellum and brain stem medially away from the wall of the skull until the stub of the nerve running between the internal auditory meatus and the cochlear nucleus becomes visible. Microelectrodes can then be inserted under direct vision. Alternative approaches are to record from cells of the spiral ganglion directly through holes in the cochlear wall, or to record from within the internal auditory meatus by means of microelectrodes inserted stereotaxically through the brain stem. When appropriate measures are taken to stabilize the preparation, fibres can now be recorded for many tens of minutes, compared with the 10 seconds or so managed by Tasaki.

With microelectrodes of tip size 0.3 μm or less, single fibres can be recorded from, and give waveforms corresponding to those in Fig. 4.1. Many fibres show random spontaneous activity. There tends to be a bimodal distribution of spontaneous discharge rates. About a quarter of the fibres discharge at below 20/s, and most of these discharge at 0.5/s or less. The other group has a mean of 60–80 discharges/s, with a maximum of 120/s (Liberman and Kiang, 1968; Evans, 1972).

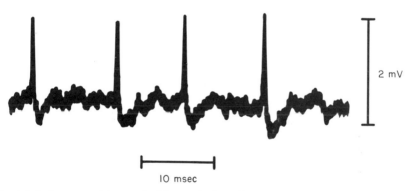

2 mV

10 msec

Fig. 4.1 Action potentials recorded from a single auditory nerve fibre. The waves are initially positive and nearly monophasic. Photography by courtesy of G. Leng.

1. Response to Tones

(a) Frequency selectivity

Fibres are responsive to single tones, and in the absence of other stimuli the tones are always excitatory, never inhibitory. The responses can be demonstrated by means of a Post (or Peri-) Stimulus Time Histogram. In making such a histogram, a stimulus is presented many times, and the occurrence of each action potential is plotted on the histogram by incrementing the count on the column, or bin, corresponding to the time after the beginning of the stimulus. Tone bursts produce a sharp onset response, which drops rapidly over the first 10–20 ms (Fig. 4.2), and then more and more slowly over the next several minutes. The fibres can be characterized by their threshold as a function of frequency of the tone. The intensity of a tone burst is adjusted until an increment in firing is just detectable. This increment is commonly between five and 30 spikes/s, depending on the spontaneous rate of the fibre and the method used to detect the increment. The procedure is repeated for different frequencies of stimulation. Examples of the resulting tuning curves relating threshold to frequency are shown in Fig. 4.3. Each fibre has a low threshold at one frequency, the 'characteristic' or 'best' frequency, and the threshold rises rapidly as the stimulating frequency is changed. Figure 4.3 shows the typical change in shape of tuning curves across frequencies, if the frequency scale is logarithmic. At low frequencies, below 1 kHz, tuning curves are symmetric. At higher frequencies the curves become increasingly asymmetric, with steep high frequency slopes and less steep low frequency slopes. A distinction between two parts of the tuning curve also becomes obvious in high frequency units. There is a very sensitive, frequency selective 'tip' of the tuning curve, and a long, broadly-tuned 'tail', stretching to low frequencies. The tail has a broad dip around 1 kHz. This is probably

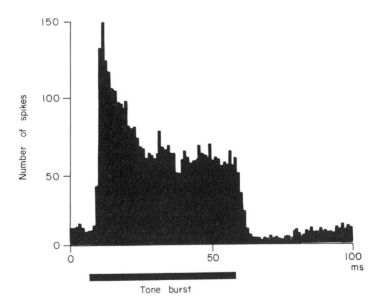

Fig. 4.2 Single fibres of the auditory nerve show an initial burst of activity at the beginning of a tone pip, a gradual decline, and a transient off-suppression of the spontaneous activity at the end of the stimulus. Here, a poststimulus-time histogram was made by presenting tone pips many times, and incrementing the count at the corresponding point on the histogram whenever an action potential occured. Reprinted from *Discharge Patterns of Single Fibers in the Cat's Auditory Nerve* by N. Y.-S. Kiang *et al.*, by permission of The MIT Press, Cambridge, Massachusetts. © The MIT Press, 1965.

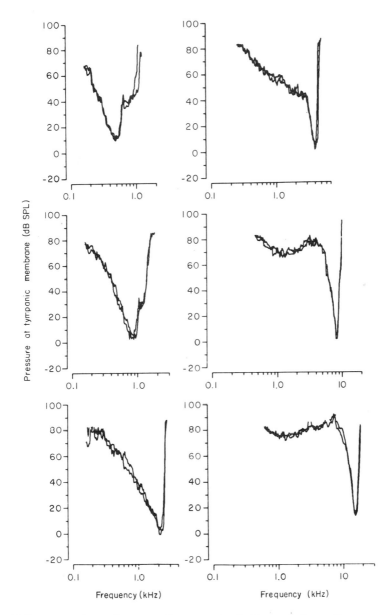

Fig. 4.3 Representative tuning curves (frequency threshold curves) of cat auditory nerve fibres are shown for six different frequency regions. In each panel, two fibres from the same animal, of similar characteristic frequency and threshold are shown, indicating the constancy of tuning under such circumstances. From Liberman and Kiang (1978), Fig. 1.

derived from the boost given to the input by the middle ear characteristics, since it disappears if the stimulus intensity is plotted with respect to constant stapes velocity (Kiang *et al.*, 1967). Single auditory nerve fibres therefore appear to behave as bandpass filters, with an asymmetric filter shape. The frequency selectivity is similar to that of inner hair cells, to which at least the majority of the fibres are connected (Russell and Sellick, 1978), and it is very likely that they derive their frequency selectivity directly from the inner hair cells. The frequency selectivity may well be greater than that of the basilar membrane (compare with Fig. 3.11).

All mammals investigated show tuning curves broadly similar to those of Fig. 4.3, although details such as the degree of frequency selectivity and depth of the tip may vary from species to species.

Our ideas as to the distribution of the fibres' thresholds at the characteristic frequency have had a chequered history. The early report of Katsuki *et al.* (1962) suggested that there was a wide distribution of fibre thresholds. He thought that this could be associated with the different thresholds of inner and outer hair cells, on the then current ideas of cochlear innervation. It was thought that the fibres innervating the outer hair cells had low thresholds, and those innervating the inner hair cells had high thresholds. Later Kiang (1968) showed that when care was taken to calibrate the sound system properly, and when sufficient fibres were recorded from in each animal rather than pooled across animals, the range in any one animal was 20 dB or less. The 'high threshold' units of Katsuki *et al.* (1962) were then probably the high threshold, broadly-tuned tails of the tuning curves of fibres of high characteristic frequency. It has become dogma over the last few years that all fibres have similar, low, thresholds. Now, however, Liberman and Kiang (1978) and Liberman (1978) have shown that there is indeed a 60 to 80 dB spread of fibre thresholds at any one characteristic frequency and in any one animal if precautions are taken to include units with very low spontaneous rates and high thresholds. Nevertheless, the majority, perhaps 70%, of fibres have thresholds within the bottom 10 dB of the range, and 80% within the bottom 20 dB. The remainder, which have particularly low spontaneous rates, are spread over the rest of the range (Fig. 4.4).

The degree of frequency selectivity has been expressed in two ways. One is by the slopes of the tuning curve above and below the characteristic frequency. The slopes are a function of the characteristic frequency of the fibres concerned, with fibres in the 10 kHz region showing the steepest slopes. Here the high frequency slopes measured between 5 and 25 dB above the best threshold range from 100 to 600 dB/octave, and the low frequency slopes from 80–250 dB/octave (Evans, 1975a). Further up the slope of the tuning curves, the low frequency slopes become shallower as the 'tail' is approached, but the high frequency slopes become even steeper, sometimes increasing to as much as 1000 dB/octave (Evans, 1972). These values are considerably greater than those that have been measured for the basilar membrane.

A second way that resolution can be measured is by measuring the bandwidth of the tuning curve at some fixed intensity above the best threshold. By analogy with the practice in the measurement of the bandwidths of electrical filters, it might be thought appropriate to measure the half-power bandwidth, that is, the bandwidth 3 dB above the best threshold. However, because it is difficult to measure threshold sufficiently accurately, bandwidths 10 dB above the best threshold have been used instead. The 10 dB bandwidths plotted as a function of characteristic frequency show a restricted spread (Fig. 4.5A). A related way in which the resolution can be expressed is by analogy with the electrical 'quality' or 'Q' factor of a filter, defined as the centre frequency divided by the bandwidth, the bandwidth here being defined at 10 dB above the best threshold. The quality factor so defined is called 'Q_{10}', and a high quality factor, or high Q_{10}, corresponds to a narrow bandwidth. Figure 4.5B shows that for the cat the minimum relative bandwidth occurs around 10 kHz, where it averages about one eighth of the characteristic frequency. (See however note on p. 70.)

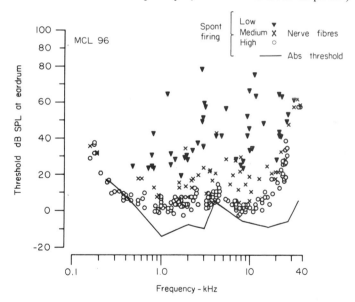

Fig. 4.4 Distribution of best thresholds of auditory nerve fibres in one cat. Fibres with high spontaneous firing rates ($\circ$, ≥ 18/s) have low thresholds, and those with low spontaneous firing rates ($\blacktriangledown$, < 0.5/s) have high thresholds. Fibres with intermediate spontaneous firing rates ($\times$) have thresholds in between.

The behavioural absolute threshold of the cat, expressed in terms of the intensity at the eardrum, lies just below the lowest thresholds of the auditory nerve fibres.

Neural data from Liberman and Kiang (1978), Fig. 2. Behavioural data from Elliott *et al.* (1960).

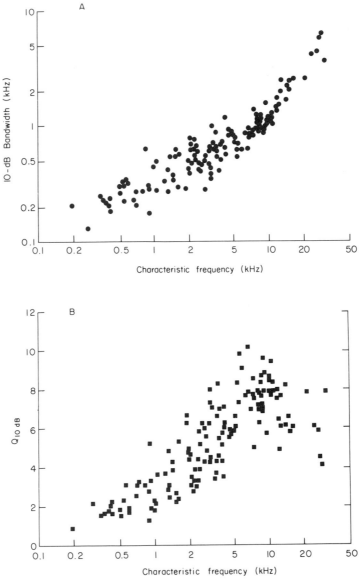

Fig. 4.5 A. The bandwidths of tuning curves of cat auditory nerve fibres are plotted as a function of the fibres' characteristic frequency. Here, the bandwidths were measured 10 dB above the best threshold. Data calculated from Q_{10}s of Evans (1975a).
B. Q_{10}s of auditory nerve fibres are shown as a function of characteristic frequency.
(Q_{10} = characteristic frequency/bandwidth measured 10 dB above best threshold). From Evans (1975a), Fig. 10.

The tuning curves of Fig. 4.3 show the intensity necessary to raise the firing rate above the spontaneous rate by a certain criterion amount, plotted as function of frequency. We can also measure the firing rate as a function of intensity for different frequencies, giving rate-intensity functions (Fig. 4.6). The functions show a sigmoidal shape, saturating at each frequency at an intensity some 20–50 dB above the threshold at that frequency. Thus the dynamic range at any one frequency is limited to 20–50 dB. In some fibres the dynamic range is a little greater for frequencies above the characteristic frequency (Nomoto *et al.*, 1974; Evans, 1975a). The saturation at high frequencies occurs at a lower maximum firing rate than at other frequencies. Inner hair cell potentials show similar behaviour, saturating at relatively low voltages for frequencies above the characteristic frequency.

The suprathreshold response can be plotted in three ways. We can, as in Fig. 4.6, plot the firing rate at a constant frequency for different intensities (rate-intensity functions). We can continue the analogy of the frequency

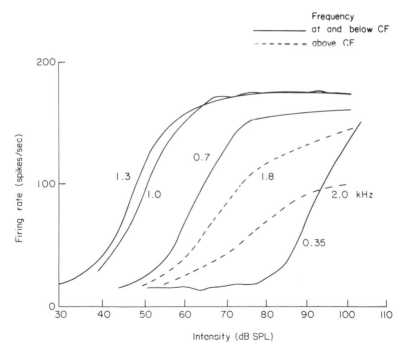

Fig. 4.6 Rate-intensity functions are shown for one auditory nerve fibre for different frequencies of stimulation. At the characteristic frequency (1.3 kHz) the fibre goes from threshold to saturation in about 30 dB. The dynamic range above the characteristic frequency is a little greater. Parameter on curves: frequency of stimulation in kHz. From Sachs and Abbas (1974), Fig. 6.

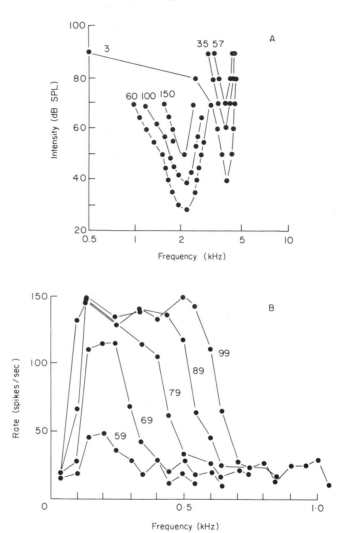

threshold curve to higher firing rates by plotting the combinations of intensities and frequencies necessary to evoke a constant increment in firing rate,
giving iso-response or iso-rate contours (Fig. 4.7A). Or the firing rate can be
plotted as the frequency is varied, the curves being called iso-intensity plots
(Fig. 4.7B–D). Each of the ways is best for showing different properties. The
iso-rate, iso-response, or tuning curves are best at showing the degree of
frequency selectivity, at least for intensities below saturation. The iso-rate
or iso-response curves show that the frequency selectivity generally im-
proves a little as a higher rate criterion is used (Fig. 4.7A), although it later

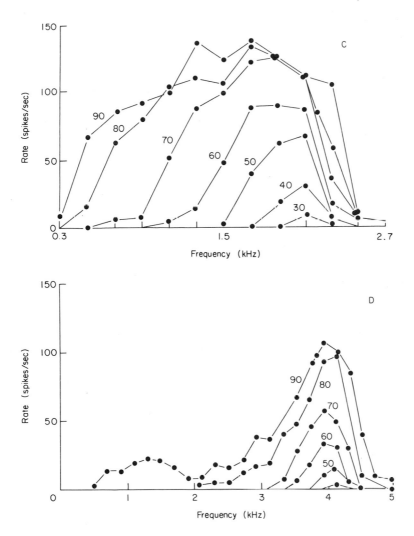

Fig. 4.7 A. Tuning curves constructed at different firing rate criteria (rate shown by parameters on curves) become a little sharper as higher rate criteria are used. From Evans (1975a), Fig. 13. B–D. Iso-intensity functions for auditory nerve fibres show that at the lowest intensity the greatest response is produced by tones near the CF, but that at higher intensities the most effective frequency moves towards 1 kHz. In C the firing saturates at a lower rate at the CF than at lower frequencies. Parameter on curves: intensity in dB SPL. From Rose *et al.* (1971), Figs 1 and 2.

deteriorates as the fibre saturates. The iso-intensity functions show that the frequency evoking the highest firing rate can shift as the intensity is raised, moving upwards for fibres with characteristic frequencies below 1 kHz, and downwards for fibres with characteristic frequencies above (Fig. 4.7B and C).

(b) Temporal relations

At high frequencies, above 5 kHz, the nerve fibres fire with equal probability in every part of the cycle. At lower frequencies, however, it is apparent that the spike discharges are locked to one phase of the stimulating waveform. That is not to say that each fibre fires once every cycle: the fibres fire randomly, perhaps as little as once every hundred cycles on average. But when they do fire, they do so in only one phase of the stimulus. The phase-locking can be most easily demonstrated by means of a period histogram. In making a period histogram, the occurrence of each spike is plotted in time, but the time axis is reset in every cycle at a constant point on the stimulus waveform, perhaps at the positive zero crossings (Fig. 4.8). The period histogram appears to follow a half-wave rectified version of the stimulating waveform. It is reasonable to suppose that this corresponds to deflection of the cochlear partition in the effective direction, if indeed hair cell activation is linked directly to the mechanical events. Deflection in the opposite direction reduces the spontaneous activity of the fibre. It will be shown later that this is the result of actual suppression of the activity by the stimulating waveform, rather than the effect of refractoriness from previous activity. One explanation for the loss of phase-locking at 5 kHz and above is that there is some jitter in the time of initiation of action potentials. While that may be true to some extent, it has recently been suggested by Russell and Sellick (1978), on the basis of their hair cell records, that the phase-locking disappears when the cell's a.c. response becomes small in comparison with the d.c. response, owing to attenuation of the intracellular a.c. component by the capacitance of the cell walls. In this case all the spikes would become initiated by the continuous d.c. depolarization of the cell, rather than the depolarizing half cycles of the a.c. response.

Phase-locking is a sensitive indicator of the activation of a fibre by a low frequency tone. At low stimulus intensities, a tone can produce significant phase-locking even though the mean firing rate is not increased. Tuning curves based on a criterion of a certain degree of phase-locking are similar to those based on an increase in firing rate, although for the above reason they may be more sensitive by 20 dB or so (Evans, 1975a). As the intensity is raised, phase-locking is preserved (Fig. 4.8). Note that, although the total number of spikes evoked does not increase above 70 dB SPL, meaning that the firing rate is saturated, the period histogram still follows the waveform of the stimulus, and does not show any sign of squaring. This may occur because the hair cell's a.c. response is still sinusoidal. Although we do not have any information about the shape of the waveform of mammalian hair cell responses to stimuli near the characteristic frequency, turtle hair cell responses do not show any tendency to square, at least for stimuli near the characteristic frequency (Crawford and Fettiplace, 1980). Alternatively, it is possible that there is a feedback mechanism that maintains the mean firing rate constant in saturation, by influencing the overall tendency to respond. However such a theory would have difficulty explaining how, for any one fibre, the firing often tends to saturate at lower rates for frequencies of stimulation at or above the characteristic frequency (Figs 4.6 and 4.7C).

2. Response to Clicks

A click, which lasts a short time, but which spreads spectral energy over a wide frequency range, can be thought of as the spectral complement of a tone, which lasts a long time but which has only a narrow frequency spread. Figure 4.9 shows the poststimulus–time histograms of the auditory nerve fibres to clicks. The histograms of low frequency fibres show several decaying peaks. It looks as though they would be produced by a decaying oscillation, i.e. as though the cochlear transducer rings in response to a

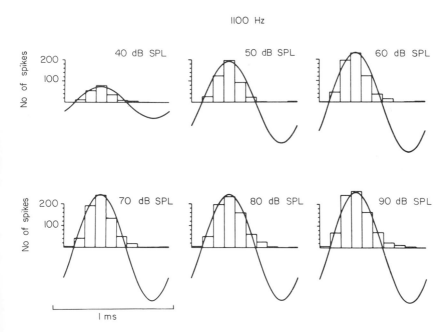

Fig. 4.8 Period histograms of a fibre activated by a low frequency tone indicated that spikes are evoked in only one half of the cycle. The histograms have been fitted with a sinusoid of the best fitting amplitude but fixed phase. Note that although the number of spikes increases little above 70 dB SPL, meaning that the firing is saturated, the histogram still follows the sinusoid without any tendency to square. From Rose *et al.* (1971), Fig. 10.

stimulus. The frequency of the ringing is equal to the characteristic frequency of the cell (Kiang *et al.*, 1965). This ringing at the characteristic frequency is exactly that expected if the tuning of the auditory nerve fibres were produced by an approximately linear filter. We would also expect the rate of decay of the ringing to be inversely proportional to the bandwidth of the tuning curve, so that a sharply tuned fibre would ring for a long time. Although this seems to be roughly true, there are some practical difficulties in making an exact comparison, because the number of spikes in the early peaks tends to limit, just as the response to tones saturates at high intensities. Goblick and Pfeiffer (1969) discuss the difficulty and how it can be obviated.

As with the response to tones, it also appears as though only one phase of the basilar membrane movement is effective. The histogram corresponds to half cycles of the decaying oscillation produced in the transducer. It appears as though an upwards motion of the basilar membrane is responsible for excitation, since at the highest intensities it is a rarefaction click that produces the earliest response. A rarefaction click will move the oval window outwards, and so the basilar membrane upwards. A condensation rather than a rarefaction click reverses the positions of the peaks and troughs of the histogram, as though the basilar membrane were being driven in the opposite direction (Fig. 4.10A). An approximate picture of the excitatory oscillation can be produced by inverting the histogram for a condensation click under that for a rarefaction click, to produce what has been called a com-

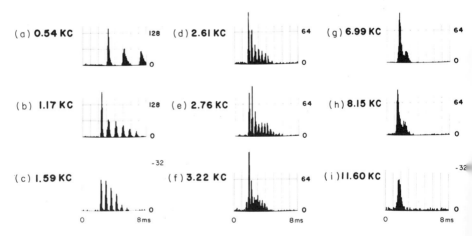

Fig. 4.9 The form of the poststimulus–time histograms to clicks depends on the CF of the fibre. Low frequency fibres show ringing (a–f), high frequency fibres do not (g–i). High frequency fibres also show a later phase of activation (f–h). Reprinted from *Discharge Patterns of Single Fibers of the Cat's Auditory Nerve* by N. Y.-S. Kiang *et al.*, by permission of The MIT Press, Cambridge, Massachusetts. © The MIT Press, 1965.

pound histogram (Fig. 4.10B). The resulting pattern can be compared with the basilar membrane impulse responses of Fig. 3.12. Histograms to clicks can also show that the suppression of activity during the less effective half cycle of the stimulating waveform is not due to refractoriness from previous activity, because the first sign of influence on a fibre can sometimes be a suppression of spontaneous activity produced by the less effective half cycle. At the moment we do not know whether the decaying oscillation is only mechanical on the basilar membrane, or mechanoelectrical, or purely electrical in origin, as though the fibre were being driven by the decaying oscillation of an electrical filter.

As the intensity is raised, earlier, previously subthreshold cycles of activation become effective, and so the histograms for low frequency fibres shift to shorter latencies (Fig. 4.11a). Other complexities are also visible which cannot be fitted into the above scheme. Some fibres, which are of too high a frequency to show phase-locking, can show an earlier phase of activation at high intensities (Fig. 4.11c,d). This must be of different origin, since these units do not show phase-locking to the effective half cycles of the stimulus, and the early phase is more than $1/CF$ (CF = characteristic frequency) before the normal one. Some fibres also show a late phase in the poststimulus–time histogram (Figs 4.11e, 4.9e–h), again far too late to be a result of a cycle of a decaying oscillation at the characteristic frequency of the fibre. The reasons for these changes in the shape of the poststimulus–time histogram are not certain. Auditory nerve fibres of high characteristic frequency have a broad dip in the low frequency tails of their tuning curves. A high intensity click with significant low frequency energy may therefore be able to superimpose a *low* frequency oscillation on the oscillation at the characteristic frequency. This may cause the later or earlier phases of activation in high frequency fibres.

3. Frequency Resolution as a Function of Intensity and Type of Stimulation

The tuning curves of Fig. 4.3 clearly show the degree of frequency resolving power of auditory nerve fibres; that is, they show the extent to which the fibres will respond to one tone rather than another on the basis of frequency. It is reasonable to suppose that this ability is fundamental to the frequency resolution shown by the auditory system as a whole. It is therefore important to consider the ways in which the fibres' frequency resolving power varies for different intensities and different types of stimulation.

(a) Frequency resolution with broadband stimuli

The tuning curves are produced in response to individual tones; yet we know that a considerable frequency selectivity must be shown in the response to

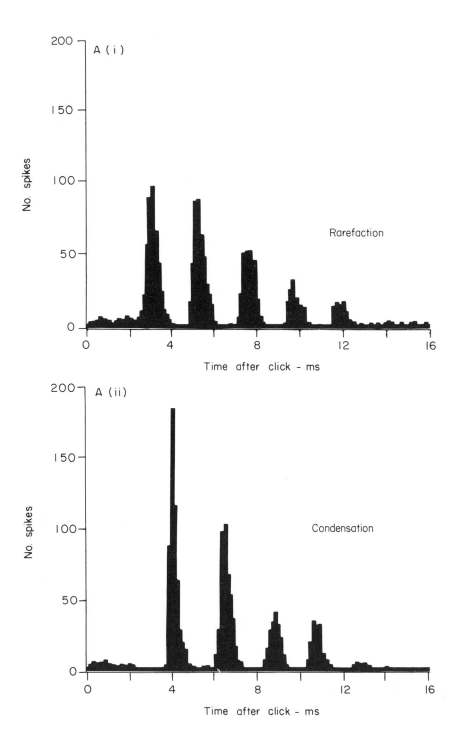

B.

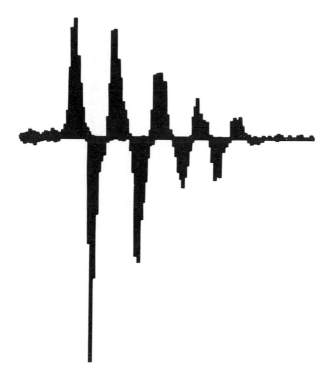

Fig. 4.10 A. Poststimulus-time histograms to (i) rarefaction and (ii) condensation clicks show that the peaks and troughs occur in complementary places for the two stimuli. Fibre CF: 450 Hz. Reprinted from *Discharge Patterns of Single Fibers of the Cat's Auditory Nerve* by N. Y.-S. Kiang *et al.*, by permission of The MIT Press, Cambridge, Massachusetts. © The MIT Press, 1965.
B. A compound histogram is formed by inverting the histogram to condensation clicks under that to rarefaction clicks.

clicks, which have broadband spectra, because of the ringing shown by fibres. In principle, we can calculate the tuning curve of the filter behind the ringing response by taking a Fourier transform of the compound histogram of Fig. 4.10B. If this is done, the frequency selectivity of the tuning curve is found to be approximately comparable to that determined with pure tones (Goblick and Pfeiffer, 1969; Pfeiffer and Kim, 1973). This shows that the frequency selectivity of the auditory nerve is, roughly at least, the same to a broadband stimulus as to a narrowband stimulus, and rules out theories that the sharp tuning is due to lateral inhibition. Lateral inhibition is widespread in sensory systems, and increases the contrast of the peaks and troughs of intensity in a sensory pattern; but a narrow click, which has a broad spectrum, has no spectral peaks and troughs, at least in the frequency range of interest.

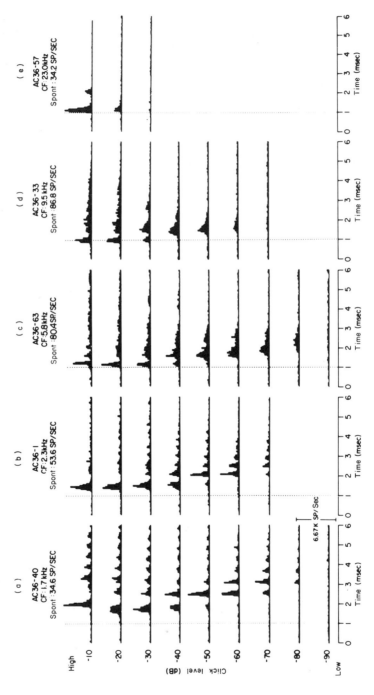

Fig. 4.11 Poststimulus–time histograms to clicks as a function of click level. In *a* earlier cycles of the oscillation become effective. In *c–d* an early wave appears about 0.5 msec before the original peak. In *e* a late phase appears. From Antoli-Candela and Kiang, Fig. 10.

A second way of showing sharp tuning with broadband stimuli involves the correlation of the firing pattern with the input stimulus, which is broadband noise. Broadband noise will of course stimulate the fibre, which will fire with an irregular pattern of discharge. We can imagine the noise as being made of a random collection of waves of different durations, phases and frequencies (Fig. 4.12). If there is a particular wavelet of just the right frequency to stimulate the nerve fibre in question, and if it is of sufficient amplitude, the fibre will be activated and an action potential will be recorded. The action potential will be phase-locked to the stimulating wavelet if the fibre's characteristic frequency is below 4–5 kHz. Of course, because the noise is random, other frequency components will be present, all of which will be in random phase and amplitude relations to the action potential. Therefore if we add together all the samples of the original broadband noise occurring just before the recorded action potentials, all the component wavelets will cancel, *except* those which were in the right frequency and phase relations to fire the fibre. Mathematically, the resulting waveform turns out to be the same as the impulse response (i.e. the response to a click) of the nerve fibre function, only reversed in time. This technique is known as reverse correlation and was first used by de Boer (1969). Once we have obtained the impulse response, we can perform a Fourier transformation on the impulse response to obtain the frequency response, or tuning curve. Figure 4.13 shows the impulse response of two fibres recovered by reverse correlation, and compares the Fourier transform with the tuning curve obtained with pure tones. The transformed impulse responses at all intensities in the 1 kHz fibre, and for the lowest noise intensities in the 2 kHz fibre, showed excellent agreement with the pure-tone tuning curve, at least over the bottom 15–20 dB of the tuning curve, the range of intensities over which the method is reliable. Again, the result shows that the tuning to a broadband stimulus is approximately the same as that to a narrowband stimulus.

(b) Frequency resolution as a function of intensity

We are now in a position to assess how the frequency resolution of auditory nerve fibres changes with intensity. The width of the tuning curve is smallest at low intensities, and this has been taken to mean, erroneously, that the fibres' frequency resolving power is necessarily greatest near threshold, and deteriorates as the intensity is raised and the tuning curve becomes wider. This is not so: if the fibre is not driven into saturation the *relative* importance of stimuli near and away from the characteristic frequency is unchanged. Tuning curves constructed at higher firing rate criteria (iso-rate or iso-response curves) show the same or greater frequency selectivity as the intensity is raised (Fig. 4.7A). It is only when the fibre is driven into saturation that the frequency resolution as shown by the mean firing rate

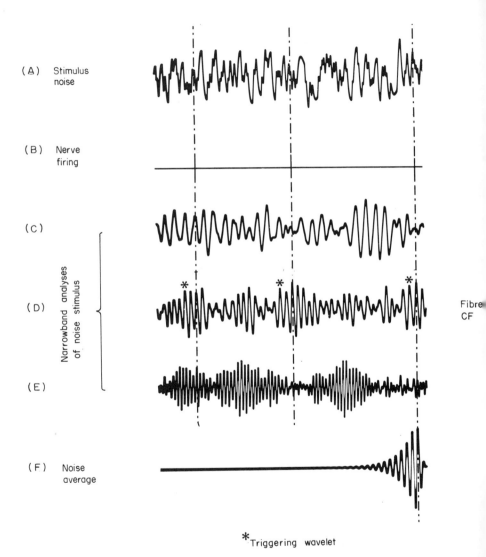

(A) Stimulus noise

(B) Nerve firing

(C)

Narrowband analyses of noise stimulus

(D)

(E)

Fibre CF

(F) Noise average

*Triggering wavelet

Fig. 4.12 The reverse correlation technique is explained graphically. The fibre is stimulated with noise (top trace) and gives action potentials (second trace). In the lower traces the results of passing the noise through narrowband filters of different centre frequencies are shown. One of the filters has the same centre frequency as the fibre. The bottom trace shows the result of adding together all the samples of the original noise waveform that triggered an action potential.

deteriorates. The fibre is now firing as fast as it can, and the firing rate does not change over a wide frequency range. This is shown by the flat tops of the iso-intensity plots of Figs 4.7 B and C.

Does this mean however that the mechanism behind the fibre's filter function has become inoperative? It is possible, using the reverse correlation technique, to calculate the fibre's frequency resolving power in spite of a saturation of the firing rate. Such a calculation is possible because the reverse correlation technique depends only on the *accuracy* of the timing of the action potentials and not on the mean rate. As was shown in the period histograms of Fig. 4.8, the temporal relations of the firings are preserved unchanged at high intensities in spite of saturation of the mean firing rate. The results of the reverse correlation technique in Fig. 4.13 show that although the firing rates were saturated at noise intensities of 60 dB or so, the impulse responses of the fibres' filter functions were substantially unchanged for 40 dB above that. Transformation of the computed impulse responses showed that for the 1 kHz fibre the shape of the tip of the tuning curve was unchanged as the intensity was raised. At low intensities the computed frequency filter function of the 2 kHz fibre of Fig. 4.13B was comparable to that of the tuning curve. At 70 dB, however, when the fibre was 15 dB into saturation, the frequency resolution started to deteriorate, and the best frequency started to move to lower frequencies. Nevertheless, the fibre still showed substantial frequency resolution well into the range of saturation. The different behaviour of these two units appears to be the reflection of a general phenomenon. Møller (1977), using a comparable technique involving the correlation of the firing pattern with the noise stimulus, has shown that fibres with characteristic frequencies near 1 kHz did not change their frequency resolving power or best frequency as the noise level was raised 40 dB into saturation, whereas fibres of higher characteristic frequency deteriorated by up to 60% in their frequency resolving power and shifted to lower frequencies.

These studies are important for auditory physiologists because they show that the mechanism behind the frequency resolution of the auditory nerve is preserved at high intensities. We are therefore in a position to use the data to make theories about, for instance, the relation between basilar membrane motion and transducer resolution over a wide range of intensities. Whether the phenomena shown by these studies is as important for the animal itself is open to question. The animal may well not be able to retrieve the information in the temporal pattern of discharges. As far as we know, it is the mean firing rate that is the main cue for the later stages of the auditory system, and it is precisely this that is constant at high intensities because of saturation, whether or not the filtering process is preserved. Possible ways in which the animal is able to make detailed discrimination at these intensities will be discussed in Chapter 9.

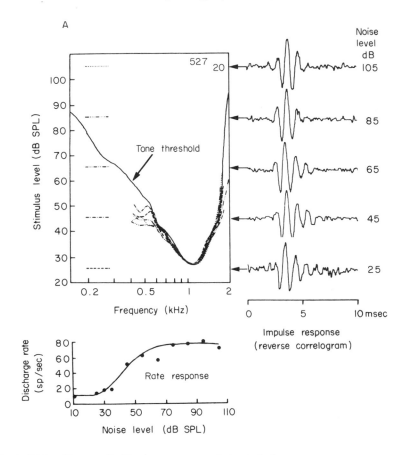

Fig. 4.13 Two fibres studied by the reverse correlation technique.
A. The impulse response recovered by reverse correlation shows little deterioration at the highest intensity, even though the stimulus level is 40 dB above that producing saturation of the firing (rate response: bottom). Fourier transformation of the impulse response shows good agreement with the tuning curve obtained with tones at threshold, over the bottom 15 dB of the tuning curve.

4. Response to Complex Stimuli

(a) Two-tone suppression

It was stated above that single tones produce excitation in auditory nerve fibres, and never sustained inhibition. However the presence of one stimulus can affect the *responsiveness* of nerve fibres to other stimuli, and if the relative frequencies and intensities of two tones are arranged correctly, the second tone can inhibit, or suppress, the response to the first. This can occur, even though the second tone produces no inhibition of spontaneous

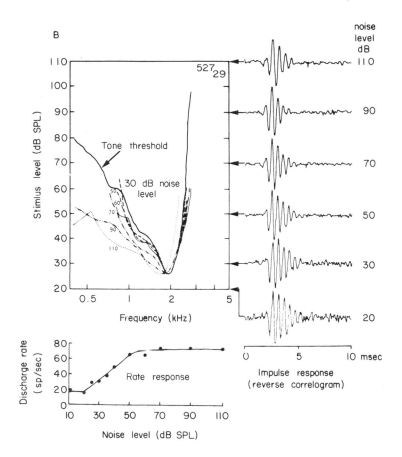

B. The 2 kHz fibre shows some deterioration of tuning as the intensity is raised, together with a downward shift in best frequency. Some tuning is still preserved, even though the intensity is 60 dB above that producing saturation of the firing. From Evans (1977), Figs 4 and 5.

activity when presented alone. Figure 4.14 shows the poststimulus–time histogram produced by a suppressing tone superimposed on a continuous excitatory tone. The pattern of response to the suppressing tone looks like the inverse of the pattern to an excitatory one. The suppressing tone produces an initial maximum of suppression when turned on, and produces a prominent rebound of activity when turned off. The dip in activity at the beginning of the suppressing tone looks like the transient suppression seen at the end of an excitatory stimulus, and the activity at the end looks like the onset burst seen at the beginning of an excitatory stimulus (cf. Fig. 4.2). This suggests that the suppressing tone simply turns the effect of the excitatory tone off. The fact that only stimulus-evoked, and not spontaneous, activity can be suppressed makes the same point. Arthur *et al*. (1971) made detailed measurements of the relative latencies of excitation and suppression. Although the latencies in individual fibres could differ either way by as much as 2.5 ms, on average excitation and suppression only differed in latency by 0.1 ms. These latencies suggest very strongly that suppression is not the result of inhibitory synapses in the cochlea, even if possible synapses had been demonstrated anatomically, because there is no time for synaptic delay (about 1 ms). The latency argument also means that the suppression cannot be a result of the activity of the olivocochlear bundle, the 'feedback' pathway from the brainstem nuclei to the hair cells (see p. 229). Nevertheless, Kiang *et al*. (1965) tested the possibility directly, and showed that suppression survived the sectioning of the olivocochlear bundle. Because it is believed that two-tone suppression is not the result of inhibitory synapses, the more neutral term 'suppression' rather than 'inhibition' is often used. Of

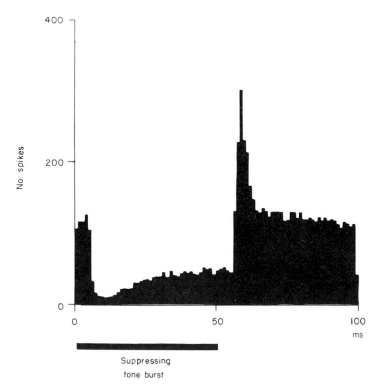

Fig. 4.14 The poststimulus–time histogram of a suppressing tone burst superimposed on a continuous excitatory tone. Reprinted from *Discharge Patterns of Single Fibers of the Cat's Auditory Nerve* by N. Y.-S. Kiang, *et al*., by permission of The MIT Press, Cambridge, Massachusetts. © The MIT Press, 1965.

course, 'inhibition' is still used for the process mediated by inhibitory synapses which is seen in the later stages of the auditory system, in for instance the cochlear nucleus. 'Suppression' is only used for the process occurring in the cochlea. The interpretation of the mechanism is that the presence of one sound will affect the cochlea's responsiveness to another, perhaps by a mechanical interference in the transducer mechanism. It must however be emphasized that two-tone suppression is a weak phenomenon compared with, say, the two-tone inhibition in the cochlear nucleus which is mediated by inhibitory synapses. The frequency and intensity relations of the stimuli have to be precisely adjusted, although under the right circumstances, and with the correct analysis, a reduction of up to 60 dB in the effective driving intensity has been demonstrated (Javel, 1981).

In support of the notion that two-tone suppression is a cochlear phenomenon, two-tone suppression can be demonstrated in inner hair cells. Recordings from hair cells have the advantage that the effects of the exciting and suppressing tones can be assessed separately. In the hair cell shown in Fig. 4.15, the excitatory tuning curve was first assessed from the d.c. response to an excitatory tone. The cell was then stimulated with a continuous tone,

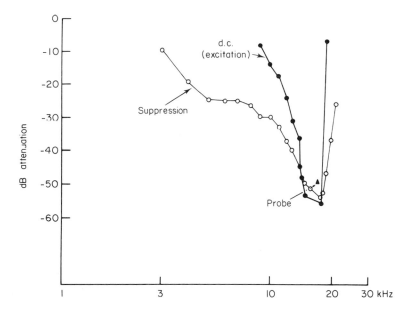

Fig. 4.15 Excitatory and suppressive tuning contours for an inner hair cell. The d.c. contour is the d.c. depolarization to a single tone, and shows the excitatory tuning curve. The triangle shows the frequency and intensity of the probe tone, and the open circles the contour for 20% suppression of the a.c. response to the probe. All stimuli within the excitatory contour excite, and all within the suppressive contour suppress. Stimuli within both contours both suppress and excite. From Sellick and Russell (1979), Fig. 3.

having the intensity and frequency indicated by the triangle in Fig. 4.15. A suppressive tone was then swept across the response area, and the contours for 20% suppression of the a.c. response at the *probe's* frequency, determined (Sellick and Russell, 1979). The results show that the suppressing tone can reduce the response to the exciting tone when presented over a wide range of frequencies. The suppressive area is more broadly tuned than the excitatory response area, and overlaps it at the tip. In other words, a stimulus can suppress even though it does not excite, and will still suppress the response to another stimulus, even though it excites when presented alone. We can suppose that there are two filters in operation. A signal which gets through the first, broadly tuned filter, is capable of both suppressing and perhaps exciting. Only stimuli which get through the second, narrowly tuned filter, are capable of exciting. Searches have also been made for two-tone suppression in the responses of the basilar membrane. Positive results were found by Rhode (1977). This agrees with his results for single tones, since he found nonlinearity such that, say, doubling a tone's amplitude produced less than double the membrane motion. It is not therefore surprising that adding a second tone should reduce the response to the first. Wilson and Johnstone (1975) who found linear basilar membrane responses, did not unfortunately report searching for two-tone suppression, although we would not expect it to be found in view of the linearity of their response.

The overlap of excitatory and suppressive areas that has been demonstrated in inner hair cells can also be shown in auditory nerve fibres, for tones of low frequencies, by taking advantage of the fact that the firing will follow the waveform of the exciting stimulus. If two tones are presented, the firing will follow the waveform of the sum of the two in an appropriate combination of amplitude and phase. By looking at the degree of modulation of the firing pattern at the frequency of one tone in a complex, it is possible to calculate the degree to which the fibre is activated by that frequency component and to measure the extent to which the response to that component is suppressed by the other stimulus. In this way, Javel (1981) showed that the narrow excitatory response area was overlaid by a broader suppressive area.

If, of course, the second tone is in the suppressive area but outside the excitatory area, it will be easy to measure the suppression by measuring the total firing rate to the stimulus complex. The second tone produces only suppression, and does not contribute any excitation. The overall mean firing rate will then be a measure of the activation produced by the excitatory tone and the extent to which it is suppressed. Plots of the combinations of intensity and frequency necessary to reduce the mean firing rate in response to a constant excitatory tone by a certain criterion amount (20% has been commonly taken), show the suppressive areas where they flank the excitatory area (Sachs and Kiang, 1968; Arthur *et al.*, 1971; Fig. 4.16). Of course,

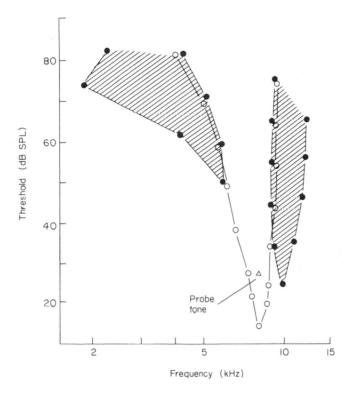

Fig. 4.16 The suppression areas of an auditory nerve fibre (shaded) flank the excitatory tuning curve (open circles). A stimulus in the suppression areas was able to reduce the mean firing rate found with the probe (△) by 20% or more. From Arthur *et al.* (1971), Fig. 2.

when the suppressing tone reaches the boundary of the excitatory area it will begin to activate the fibre on its own account, and so the total number of action potentials will increase. Suppression areas plotted in this way therefore stop at, or near, the boundary of the excitatory area. The plots of Fig. 4.16 nevertheless are able to suggest the shape of the first broad filter in relation to that of the overall tuning curve.

Figure 4.16 indicates that a stimulus is able to reduce the driven response of fibres tuned to neighbouring frequencies. Two-tone suppression is therefore able to increase the contrast in a complex sensory pattern, so that, for instance, the peaks of activation produced by dominating frequencies will tend to stand out in stronger contrast against the background. However, two-tone suppression is not in general a very potent effect, and it is not known whether it is powerful enough to play an important part in psychophysical discrimination. The role of two-tone suppression in auditory discrimination will be discussed in Chapter 9.

(b) Masking

Masking denotes the general phenomenon by which one stimulus obscures or reduces the response to another. Two-tone suppression could therefore provide one mechanism of masking. There is in addition another, and probably more important, mechanism of masking operative as well.

The earliest explanation of masking was that known as the 'line busy' effect. If one stimulus had pre-empted the firing of a fibre, superimposed stimuli would not be able to provoke an increment in firing. In a more modern version of the hypothesis, if the firing was saturated to one stimulus, superimposed stimuli would not be able to increase the rate further (Smith, 1979).

The line busy explanation fell out of favour after Kiang *et al*. (1965) showed that noise could mask a response to a tone pip, even though the tone pip could by itself have produced a greater response than the noise. If the tone pip could produce a greater response than the noise, clearly the firing was not saturated by the noise, and the line busy explanation should not apply. This experiment prompts us to think in terms of two-tone suppression as a mechanism by which noise can mask tones.

The line busy explanation may well however have been more valid than this interpretation of the experiment of Kiang *et al*. indicated. Smith (1979) pointed out that the masker had been left on continuously, so that the evoked firing would have adapted. He showed that if the masker had been intense enough to saturate the firing when it was first presented, the firing would still have been saturated when the rate had dropped through adaptation. It was therefore not surprising that a superimposed tone was unable to produce an increment in firing, even though by itself, and presented to an unadapted fibre, the tone could have produced more firing. Saturation of firing by the masker can explain many cases of masking, once adaptation is taken into account.

The line busy explanation does not of course necessarily require that the firing be saturated. If one signal has a greater effective intensity than the other, the less intense one will add negligible activity of its own. This effect will be greater than might appear at first sight, because the summation of effective intensities will occur on a linear scale rather than the logarithmic scale of decibels. For instance, a signal added 10 dB below another will produce an increase in net stimulus intensity of only 0.4 dB.

Figure 4.17 shows an example of masking by the line busy effect as well as masking by suppression. The figure shows rate-intensity functions for a tone both with and without wideband masking noise. Here the noise was gated, and so adaptation was avoided. The noise alone produced a firing rate of 160/s. Tones less intense than 50 dB SPL did not produce a greater firing rate than this, and so did not increase the response. In this intensity range, the tone was masked by the line busy effect.

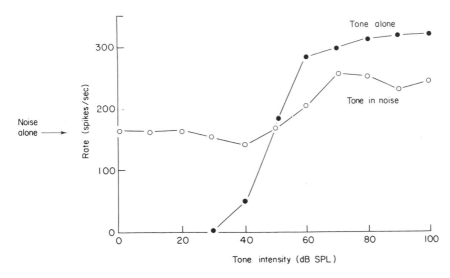

Fig. 4.17 Rate-intensity functions to a tone with and without masking noise. The tone was presented at 2.9 kHz, the CF. Noise band: 2.5 kHz to 4 kHz. Adapted from Rhode *et al.* (1978).

Figure 4.17 also shows the effect of suppression. Noise reduced the maximum firing rate to the tone, even though the tone was able to produce a clear increase in firing (at 60 dB SPL and above). This reduction, which is another case of masking, had the characteristics of two-tone suppression. For instance it is known that two-tone suppression is strongest for suppressors above the characteristic frequency, and in this experiment noise bands above the fibre's characteristic frequency were most effective at reducing the firing. In general, we can expect that where maskers fall on the two-tone suppression areas, suppression will play a part.

We are now in a position to understand some of the complex interactions between the components of multicomponent stimuli. If two stimuli of comparable levels are presented, both well inside the excitatory area, they will each suppress the other strongly, but will both excite the fibre even more strongly. Below saturation, the firing rate in response to both will be greater than that to either one alone, and they will therefore appear to summate in their effects. For low frequency units, the firing will follow a waveform which can be composed of the waveforms of the component stimuli added together with suitable amplitudes and phases (Rose *et al.*, 1971). The relative amplitudes giving the best fit are not necessarily those presented in the acoustic stimulus. The frequency selectivity of the fibre, as well as the mutual suppression of the components, will alter their relative amplitudes. Similarly with the phase: it is known, for instance, that with single tone stimulation the effective phase of the driving waveform varies with the stimulating frequency and its relation to the characteristic frequency of the fibre, and it is possible that the suppressive interactions alter the phase still further.

In a more trivial case, where one stimulus has much less influence over the fibre than the other, the most effective stimulus will dominate both the firing rate and the temporal pattern of the action potentials.

If one stimulus is moved away from the characteristic frequency, both its excitatory and suppressive effects will decline, but the excitatory effects will decline the more rapidly and the balance will be tipped in favour of suppression. A stimulus away from the characteristic frequency will suppress the response to a stimulus near the characteristic frequency, but will add only a little activation of its own. The overall firing rate will therefore be smaller than that to the most excitatory stimulus alone. Now the firing predominantly follows the waveform of the other stimulus (Rose *et al.*, 1971). In the terminology of Rose *et al.*, the suppressing tone now dominates the response.

Some of the different effects of suppression and summation can be seen in the mean firing rates to bands of noise of different widths (Fig. 4.18). As a narrow band of noise of constant spectral density is widened around the characteristic frequency of a fibre, the first effect is for the firing rate to increase, because the greater number of noise components in the excitatory area summate and drive the fibre more intensely (Gilbert and Pickles, 1980). As the bandwidth becomes still broader, the extra noise components added come to fall on the parts of the suppressive area outside the excitatory area, and now not only fail to contribute excitation, but contribute a net suppression. The firing rate therefore comes to a maximum, and then declines. However the effect is not necessarily very large. Over a population of fibres Gilbert and Pickles (1980) found the mean suppression at the widest bandwidths was only 8% of the maximum stimulus-evoked activity.

(c) Combination tones

If the ear is stimulated with two tones at the same time, combination tones may be heard which are not physically present in the stimulus. The presence of combination tones was first demonstrated psychophysically rather than physiologically. They presumably occur as a result of nonlinear distortion somewhere in the auditory system. One combination tone is the *difference tone*, which is at a frequency f_2-f_1, where f_2 and f_1 are the frequencies of the two tones, or primaries, presented. The level of the difference tone at high signal levels is almost completely independent of the frequency separation of the primaries. It was once thought that it originated as an overloading type of distortion in the middle ear (e.g. Helmholtz, 1863). Now the direct measurements of Guinan and Peake (1967) have shown that the middle ear has insufficient nonlinearity, and an intracochlear origin is often assumed.

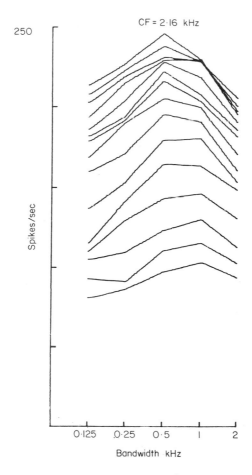

Fig. 4.18 The firing in response to a band of noise shows the effects of both summation and suppression. The noise was of variable bandwidth kept centred on the CF. The contours are at 3 dB intervals of noise spectral density, the lowest being at −25 dB SPL/Hz. From Gilbert and Pickles (1980), Fig. 2.

A second set of combination tones has certain fascinating properties and can be heard even at low sound levels. The best known representative of this group is the tone known as the cubic distortion tone or $2f_1-f_2$, from the frequency at which it is heard. F_2 must be above f_1. Figure 4.19 shows the frequency and level of the cubic distortion tone in relation to the primaries. In this experiment, the level of each distortion tone was measured by introducing a third, cancellation, tone into the stimulus, and altering its level and phase until it just cancelled the sensation of the distortion tone.

The frequency at which $2f_1-f_2$ appears, might be explained by supposing

that the auditory system undergoes a distortion such that the output contains a component that is the cube of the input. If two tones of frequency f_1 and f_2 are inserted, the output distortion component = $(\cos 2\pi f_1 + \cos 2\pi f_2)^3$.
This can be decomposed into a series of cosines containing the frequencies $f_1, 3f_1, f_2, 3f_2, 2f_1, +f_2, 2f_2 + f_1, 2f_1 - f_2$, and $2f_2 - f_1$. Of these, only $2f_1 - f_2$ is at a frequency below the primaries and we can provisionally suppose that the others are masked or filtered out by some hypothetical high reject filter later in the auditory system. Models behind the generation of $2f_1 - f_2$ will be discussed in Chapter 5. At the moment we can note that the name 'cubic distortion tone' arises because the tone can hypothetically be produced by a cubic distortion. However some models behind the process now suppose that the distortion is of the form output = $(\text{input})^r$, where r has a value less than one (e.g. Duifhuis, 1976)*. Such distortion will give rise to the frequencies $3f_1 - 2f_2, 4f_1 - 3f_2$ etc., as well as $2f_1 - f_2$, for the distortion components below

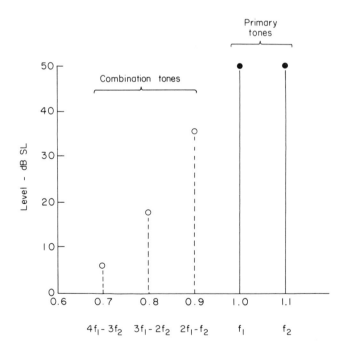

Fig. 4.19 The subjective cubic and related combination tones form a series below the primaries, of frequency spacing equal to the separation of the primaries. The levels indicated were those found by the cancellation method for primaries of 1 and 1.1 kHz, according to Goldstein (1967); 0 dB SL ≈ 0 dB SPL.

*More properly, output = $(\text{input})^r$ for the positive half-wave of the input cycle, and output = $-(-\text{input})^r$ for the negative half wave.

f_1 and f_2 in frequency. Such additional distortion components are detectable psychophysically, although at a lower amplitude than $2f_1-f_2$ (see Fig. 4.19).

Three important psychophysical results about the cubic distortion tone concern the physiologist. One is that the amplitude of the cubic distortion tone, in contrast to that of the high level difference tone, is strongly dependent on the frequency separation of the primaries, declining at a rate of some 100 dB/octave as the frequency ratio of the primaries increases (Goldstein, 1967). This suggests that the site of distortion is *preceded* by some stage of frequency analysis. Secondly, the cubic distortion tone is heard for stimuli near threshold. This suggests that it is not merely an 'overloading' type of distortion, but must be regarded as part of the normal operation of the auditory system. Thirdly, the relative amplitude of the distortion tone with respect to the primaries is almost independent of the amplitude of the primaries if they are both varied in level together. However caution in interpretation is necessary here.

Because the level of the distortion tone was measured by the method of cancellation, it is possible that the cancellation tone will be affected by the same nonlinear process as the primaries, and this means that estimates of the amplitude of the distortion tone relative to that of the primaries will be affected. There are at present two views. One is that the process responsible for the distortion is dominated by the linear component, i.e. output = input $+ k$ (input)^r, where k is small. In this case the cancellation tone itself will be little affected by the nonlinear process, and the amplitudes as determined psychophysically will be a fair reflection of the physiological process (e.g. Goldstein, 1967). We are then left with the considerable problem of devising a model which will produce a distortion tone which bears a constant amplitude relative to the primaries, as the amplitude of the primaries varies. This will not occur on the above formula. For instance, if on the above formula the distortion is cubic, so that $r = 3$, the amplitude of the distortion tone will grow as the cube of the amplitude of the primaries. On the second view, there is no linear component in the relation, i.e. output = (input)^r, where r may be, for instance, less than one (e.g. Smoorenberg, 1972; Duifhuis, 1976). In this case the level of the cancellation tone will itself be strongly influenced by the distortion process. In fact, as was pointed out by Smoorenberg (1972), the above result showing a relative constancy of the distortion tone is just what would be expected on the basis of the above power relation between input and output. The logic is clearly discussed by Green (1976), pp. 246–247.

The search for a correlate of the cubic distortion tone in the responses of fibres of the auditory nerve, has been reported by Goldstein and Kiang (1968) and Kim *et al.* (1980). Goldstein and Kiang presented two tones f_1 and f_2, such that both lay outside the response area of the fibre, neither provoking a response when they were presented singly. If however the calculated frequency $2f_1-f_2$ lay at the characteristic frequency of the fibre, it was possible for the fibre to be excited by both stimuli together. In other words, the fibre could be excited by the combination tone, in the absence of a response to the primaries. The same point was made by studies of the phase-locking to the stimuli for low frequency fibres; it was possible to show significant phase-locking to $2f_1-f_2$ without any phase-locking to f_1 or f_2. Moreover, Kim *et al.* (1980) showed that the fibres' frequency selectivity to $2f_1-f_2$ was the same as that to introduced real tones of the same frequency. This shows that as far as the auditory nerve was concerned, it was as though a real tone at the frequency $2f_1-f_2$ were present in the stimulus. In support of this, it was possible to cancel the response to the combination tone by the addition of a third tone, suitably adjusted in amplitude and phase. Studies of the amplitude behaviour of the combination tone showed a correlate with the psychophysical result: the amplitude of the combination tone calculated from the firing rate was constant relative to the amplitude of the primaries, in one case over a range of over 60 dB (Goldstein and Kiang, 1968). In addition, the response to the combination tone could be found at intensities just above the threshold of the fibre. Neither of these results is consistent with the idea that the response reflects the operation of a high intensity, overloading, type of distortion in the inner ear. In its frequency relations, too, the physiological response paralleled the psychophysical results, since the response to the combination tone dropped rapidly as the frequency separation of the primaries increased. It was only in the phase relations that a clear difference emerged between the phychophysical and physiological results. The psychophysical cancellation tone shifted strongly in phase with changes in stimulus level, but the phase of the physiological distortion tone was almost invariant (Goldstein and Kiang, 1968). The reason for the difference is not clear.

Studies of the cubic distortion tone and related phenomena have great significance for our understanding of cochlear physiology. These studies will be discussed further in Chapter 5.

C. Summary

1. The very great majority, and perhaps all, of the fibres present in the central end of the auditory nerve innervate inner hair cells.

2. Single fibres of the auditory nerve are always excited by auditory stimuli, and never show sustained inhibition to single stimuli.

3. The fibres have lower thresholds to tones of some frequencies than of others. The relation between threshold and stimulus frequency is

known as the 'tuning curve'. Tuning curves show one threshold minimum, at what is known as the 'characteristic frequency'. The threshold rises sharply for frequencies above and below the characteristic frequency. The tuning curve therefore shows a sharp dip in this frequency region.

4.   The great majority (80%) of auditory nerve fibres have minimum thresholds in a 20 dB range near the animal's absolute threshold. The others have thresholds spread over a 60 dB range above that. The low threshold fibres have particularly high rates of spontaneous activity in the absence of sound.

5.   Fibres show a sigmoidal relation between firing rate and stimulus intensity, in many cases going from threshold to maximum rate (saturation) in 20–50 dB at any one frequency.

6.   The frequency resolving power of auditory nerve fibres has been measured by a 'quality' factor, by analogy with a quality factor for filters. The quality factor is the characteristic frequency, divided by the bandwidth of the fibre to tones at an intensity 10 dB above the best threshold. This is called 'Q_{10}'. Therefore fibres with a high Q_{10} have good frequency selectivity. At any one frequency, different fibres have Q_{10}s in a restricted range. In any one animal, the range of Q_{10}s at one frequency is two fold or less. The greatest Q_{10}s in the cat are reached at around 10 kHz, where they have an average value of eight.

7.   During tonal stimulation, auditory nerve fibres fire preferentially during one part of the cycle of the stimulating waveform if the stimulus is below 4–5 kHz. Presumably, the fibres are only excited by deflection of the basilar membrane in one direction.

8.   For fibres with characteristic frequencies below 4–5 kHz, clicks preferentially evoke responses at certain intervals after the stimulus. A histogram of action potentials made with respect to time after the stimulus suggests that the fibres are activated by the half cycles of a decaying oscillation of a resonator. The frequency of the oscillation is equal to the characteristic frequency of the fibre. The resonator corresponds to the tuning properties of the fibre.

9.   One tone can reduce, or suppress, the response to another, even though single tones are always excitatory. This is called two-tone suppression. The suppression probably arises from the nonlinear properties of the

transducer. Two-tone suppression can also be seen in the responses of inner hair cells. Stimuli other than tones cause suppression too.

10. One stimulus can mask the response to another. Masking mainly occurs because the masking stimulus produces a greater firing rate than the masked stimulus. The other main mechanism of masking is the suppression of the response to one stimulus by another.

11. When two-tone stimuli are used, auditory nerve fibres can respond to distortion products as a result of nonlinear interactions in the cochlea. One distortion tone, known as the cubic distortion tone, is at a frequency $2f_1 - f_2$, where f_1 is the lower of the tones presented, and f_2 the higher.

D. Further Reading

The auditory nerve has been reviewed clearly and completely by Evans (1975a).

V. Mechanisms of Transduction and Excitation in the Cochlea

The study of cochlear processing is currently the most exciting area of auditory physiology. New and revolutionary ideas are rapidly replacing the established views. It is hoped that this chapter will be able to convey some of the flavour of an area that is occupying the attention of a large proportion of auditory physiologists today. Cochlear transduction in Chapters 3 and 4 was interpreted in terms of Davis's battery and resistance-modulation theory. Recent intracellular recordings from hair cells have tended to support the broad outlines of the theory. However, we still have no information on the mechanism of the initial stage of resistance-modulation, and many of the other details of the theory are being questioned. The experiments will be reviewed here, as will be experiments on cochlear frequency selectivity, cochlear nonlinearity and distortion products, and the re-emission of mechanical activity from the transducer. The chapter is written at a more advanced level than the rest of the book, and may be omitted without affecting the comprehensibility of the other chapters.

A. Introduction

The fundamental problems of cochlear processing will be considered in this chapter. We have so far interpreted the experimental data in terms of Davis's (1965) battery or resistance modulation hypothesis. Under his hypothesis, the stereocilia are deflected by movement of the basilar membrane (Fig. 3.3). The deflection reduces the resistance of the apical membrane of the hair cells. The positive endocochlear potential (about +80 mV) and the

107

negative intracellular potential (perhaps -40 mV) combine to give a potential of some 120 mV across the apical membrane, which drives current through the varying resistance (Fig. 3.15). This causes both alternating and direct potential changes in the hair cells. The potential changes cause the release of transmitter at the base of the hair cells, so stimulating the nerve terminals. The varying current through the hair cells also produces the extracellularly recordable cochlear microphonic.

The scheme is simple and attractive, and accounts for many of the experimental results in a straightforward way. Nevertheless, all its stages can be, and have been, doubted. For instance, it predicts that the sharpness of frequency tuning of the hair cells will be the same as that of the vertical displacement of the basilar membrane. However there is some evidence that the hair cells are more sharply tuned than the basilar membrane, although that conclusion must still be regarded as controversial. We would also expect the threshold movement of the deforming membrane to be large enough to affect ionic transmission, perhaps of the order of 0.1 nm. Yet depending on the assumptions made about the mode of movement of the basilar membrane, the threshold movement has been calculated to be as low as 2×10^{-4} nm, or 1/500th of the diameter of the hydrogen atom. It is difficult to see how deformations as small as this could affect the flow of ions. Nor does the ultrastructure obviously point to ways in which the permeability of the apex of the hair cells could be altered by deflection of the basilar membrane. A further question concerns the role of the outer hair cells. The vast majority of the afferent nerve fibres are connected to the inner hair cells, whose responses they appear to follow exactly. What then is the function of the outer hair cells? Lastly, there is no direct and conclusive evidence in the *mammalian* cochlea for the key element of the Davis theory, that the intracellular potentials are produced by the battery driving current through a variable resistance at the apex of the hair cells.

These questions and others will be considered in detail and the evidence, if any, evaluated. First, the question of the initial transducer will be discussed. What are the first nonmechanical events to occur in response to the mechanical movements of the basilar membrane? How do these events then lead to neural excitation? Do the characteristics of hair cell and auditory nerve activation follow the passive mechanical movements of the basilar membrane, both in terms of the linearity of the response and the degree of frequency selectivity?

B. Mechanisms of Transduction

1. Cell Membrane Potentials

Before beginning a discussion of the transducer mechanism, it is appropriate to review a few of the basic facts of nerve membrane potentials and their relation to hair cell transduction.

Nerve cell membranes are more permeable to some ions than others — for instance, in the resting state they are many times more permeable to K^+ than to Na^+ ions. A high K^+ concentration is maintained inside the cells by an energy-consuming linked Na^+-K^+ pump. But because the cell membrane is permeable to K^+, K^+ tends to diffuse passively down its concentration gradient, taking positive charge and leaving the inside of the cell negative. This potential is called a diffusion potential. Diffusion stops when the negative potential inside the cell is sufficient to oppose the further movement of ions. This potential is known as the equilibrium potential. However, leakage by some of the other ions will influence the final potential reached. Anything which increases the permeability to any of the other ions will draw the membrane potential towards an analogous equilibrium potential for that ion, and the normal resting potential for cells is therefore rather less negative than the K^+ equilibrium potential.

It is possible to think of various schemes for the modulation of ion flow in hair cells. If for instance the apical surface of the hair cell were faced by an endolymph which, as well as having a low electrical potential, had a low K^+ concentration, similar to that of extracellular fluid, increasing the permeability of the membrane to K^+ alone would generate a negative diffusion potential across the apical membrane of the hair cell. The inside of the cell would then become hyperpolarized, that is, more negative. Increasing membrane permeability to some ions alone does not necessarily therefore produce a *reduction* in the membrane potential; the important point is that the membrane potential moves towards the *equilibrium* potential of the diffusable ion, or to a weighted mean of the equilibrium potentials if more than one ion is involved.

In mammals the K^+ concentration in endolymph is approximately the same as inside the cell, and the Na^+ concentration is very low. No diffusion potential will therefore be produced by ion flow across the apical membrane of the hair cell, and decreasing the resistance will simply pull the intracellular potential towards the endolymphatic potential, producing a depolarization. As a bonus, in mammals the endolymphatic potential is 80 mV or so positive. While this may have evolved secondarily from the mechanism for maintaining a high K^+ concentration in the endolymph, it also serves to increase the driving potential across the apical membrane from 30–40 mV to 110–120 mV.

It is presumably advantageous for the current to be carried by K^+ rather than say Na^+. Because K^+ is in equilibrium across the basal membrane of hair cells, any K^+ entering the cell will diffuse out automatically, and K^+ will not accumulate inside the cell. We must not however forget that the transducer current may also be carried by other ions, for instance Cl^- and Ca^{2+}.

A second relevant property of neuronal membranes is that ionic conductances can be electrically modifiable. If an axonal membrane is depolarized, the K^+ conductivity, for instance, increases with a time lag, and
stays high as long as the membrane is depolarized. Therefore it is quite
possible for the hair cell membrane, presumably including the membrane in
the basal part of the hair cell, to show conductance changes that are *secondary* to the potential changes produced by the 'trigger' action of the transducer mechanisms at the apex of the hair cell. In interpreting experimental
results on resistance changes, we must always be alive to the possibility that
the changes are secondary ones in the basal membrane.

2. The Transduction

The problems of studying the transducer mechanisms of individual hair cells
of the mammalian cochlea are enormous. For instance, the ideal experiment
would be to apply a direct physiological stimulus, a mechanical deflection of
the basilar membrane or of the hairs alone, to a single hair cell in isolation
while recording intracellularly. One would have to be sure that the physiological condition of the hair cell was good, and that the mechanical coupling
was correct at the very low amplitudes of movement that are likely to be
physiologically significant, perhaps 0.1 nm or less. This has so far been
impossible. It is only in the last few years that intracellular records have been
made from hair cells of the mammalian cochlea at all (Russell and Sellick,
1978; Tanaka *et al.*, 1980). In these experiments, auditory stimuli were used.

When the experimental preparation is difficult, it is useful to turn to
biological analogues in the hope of gleaning at least a little information
about the system. Such analogues of the auditory system are provided by
other hair cells of the acousticolateral system, namely the lateral line and
vestibular hair cells. They are morphologically similar to hair cells of the
mammalian cochlea, except for possessing in addition a second type of
cilium called the kinocilium (Fig. 5.1). The kinocilium is composed of
tubulin microtubules, whereas the stereocilia are composed of actin micro-
filaments. Most hair cells of the acousticolateral system nevertheless have
bundles of stereocilia anchored in the cuticular plate at the apex of the cells.
We assume therefore that there will be some similarities in the transduction
process, although the cochlear hair cells may have modifications in view of
their greater sensitivity to movement, their much greater frequency range,
and the high K^+ with which the apical surface is bathed.

(a) Transduction in vestibular hair cells

Vestibular transduction was studied by Lowenstein and Sand (1940) in the
semicircular canals of the ray. They showed that, with the skull stationary,

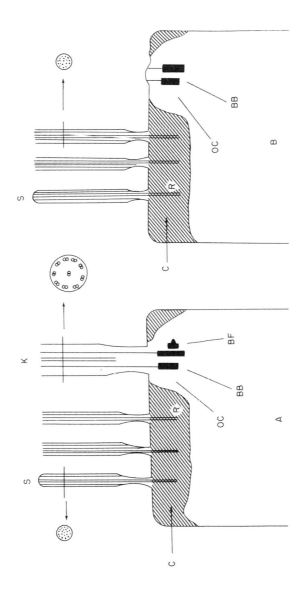

Fig. 5.1 A. Vestibular hair cells possess, in addition to many stereocilia (S), a kinocilium (K) which enters the cell in the opening (OC) in the cuticular plate (C). At the base of the kinocilium there is a basal body (BB) with a basal foot (BF) on the side away from the stereocilia. R: rootlet. B. Cochlear hair cells do not possess a kinocilium when mature, although they may do so in the embryo. In some species the basal body is absent as well, but the opening in the cuticular plate is present in all.

there was a resting discharge in the vestibular nerves fibres. Acceleration of the skull in one direction increased the discharge, and acceleration in the other decreased the discharge. Acceleration produced a fluid flow in the semicircular canals, so that the ampullar cupulae, obstructing the flow like hinged doors, were deflected. It was later shown anatomically that in any one ampullary receptor all the hair cells were oriented the same way, that is, they all had their kinocilia on the edge of the hair cell nearest one particular side of the organ (Lowenstein and Wersäll, 1959). This made it possible to link the deflection of the hairs with the direction for physiological excitation. Deflection of the hairs towards the kinocilium produced excitation, and deflection away from the kinocilium produced inhibition. The same point has been recently made rather more directly by Hudspeth and Corey (1977) in the bullfrog sacculus. Deflection of the hairs by a glass rod in the direction of the kinocilium produced hair cell depolarization, and so was associated with excitation, while deflection in the opposite direction produced hyper-polarization, and so was associated with inhibition (Fig. 5.2).

Hudspeth and Corey (1977) also showed that depolarization of the hair cell was associated with a decrease in the membrane resistance, and hyper-polarization with an increase (Fig. 5.2). This was interpreted as meaning that the permeability of the apical cell membrane was changed by the mechanical stimulus, in accordance with the resistance modulation scheme of Davis. Corey and Hudspeth (1979a) showed by separate perfusion of the apical surface of the hair cells that the depolarization was dependent on ion transfer through the apical surface, making it likely that at least some of the resistance changes were in the apical membrane. The perfusion experiments showed that a range of ions, including K^+, Na^+, and Ca^{2+}, were able to support the current flow. A larger ion, tetramethyl ammonium, was also able to support the flow, although to a lesser extent. This suggests that the channel is nonspecific and that its pore size is at least as large as the hydrated tetramethyl ammonium ion. Its size is therefore similar to that of the channel at the neuromuscular junction, which is also nonspecific.

In Hudspeth and Corey's experiments the solution outside the cell was at zero potential. When the potential inside the cell was held electronically at different levels, deflection of the hairs towards the kinocilium produced an increased inwards current if the intracellular potential were below zero, and an increase outwards current if the potential were above zero. Thus the 'reversal potential' was near zero. This supports the idea that the current was flowing passively between the inside of the cell and the outside. It again supports the idea of a nonspecific increase in permeability, because we would expect the reversal potential to be a weighted mean of the equilibrium potentials of all the ions involved. The preparation was bathed in physio-logical saline, so Na^+ which has a positive equilibrium potential could flow into the cell, and K^+ which has a negative one, out. Similar observations have been made (Fig. 5.3) for hair cells of the turtle cochlea by Crawford and Fettiplace (1979). By polarizing the insides of the hair cells they were able to show that the stimulus-induced voltage change reversed around approximately 0 mV.

It therefore seems that in the bullfrog sacculus and the turtle cochlea deflection of the hairs does indeed cause a nonspecific increase in the permeability of the apical membrane, causing ions to flow down their concentration gradients and so changing the potential inside the cell. It seems that deflection of the hairs in one direction increases the permeability above normal, so depolarizing the cell, and that deflection in the opposite direction decreases the permeability below normal, so hyperpolarizing the cell. Hudspeth and Corey (1977) also showed that the relation between deflection and voltage change was nonlinear, being asymmetric and saturating (Fig. 5.4). The saturation means that in the case illustrated, changes greater than about 8 mV peak-to-peak could not be produced. The asymmetry means that the depolarizing changes were greater than the hyperpolarizing changes. A symmetrical sinusoidal input therefore produced a net depolarization of the hair cells in addition to an alternating voltage change.

We can identify as least three possible stages at which the nonlinearities could have been produced. One, and perhaps the most important, is that the resistance change associated with the transduction process itself was non-linear, following a function like that of Fig. 5.4, as the stereocilia were deflected. Confirmation that this is an important nonlinear stage has been provided by Crawford and Fettiplace (1981b) in hair cells of the turtle

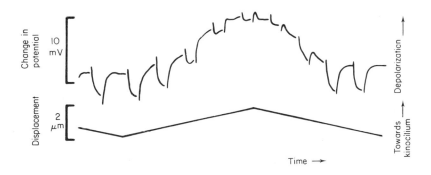

Fig. 5.2 Deflection of the stereocilia towards the kinocilium produced depolarization, and deflection away hyperpolarization, in a hair cell of the bullfrog sacculus. The small pulses on the upper trace show the voltage response to current pulses in the recording electrode. Large voltage changes show that the membrane resistance was high, and small ones that it was low. The membrane resistance was smaller when the cell was depolarized. From Hudspeth and Corey (1977), Fig. 3.

cochlea. They showed similar nonlinear relations between voltage and displacement, and similar changes in resistance, in hair cells that had been poisoned with TEA (tetraethylammonium bromide). TEA abolishes voltage-sensitive changes in K^+ conductance in membranes such as those of nerve axons. Their finding makes it unlikely that a second hypothesis would entirely explain Hudspeth and Corey's observations. That hypothesis is that the changes in membrane resistance were purely *secondary* to changes in transmembrane potential, due to voltage sensitive conductances. Such voltage-sensitive conductances could themselves give rise to nonlinear voltage responses as the stereocilia were deflected. Nevertheless, the hair cells of Hudspeth and Corey's experiment were not so treated. It is possible that in their experiment, the intracellular voltage changes resulting from the

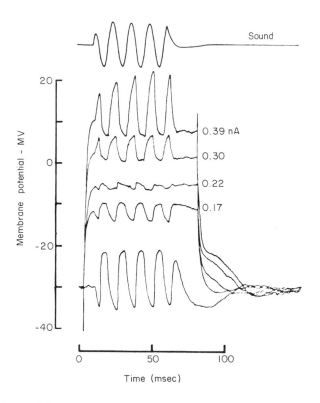

Fig. 5.3 An intracellular record of a hair cell in the turtle cochlea shows reversal of the response to sound by polarizing current. The resting potential of the cell was held at different levels by current passed through the recording electrode. The direction of the alternating voltage changes induced by sound, reversed when the intracellular potential was moved around approximately 0 mV. From Crawford and Fettiplace (1979), Fig. 1.

primary change in resistance at the apex of the hair cells, then caused further changes in membrane resistance, further increasing the nonlinearity of the input–output function. Corey and Hudspeth (1979a) showed that hair cells of the bullfrog sacculus indeed contained just such voltage-sensitive conductances, which they ascribed to a variable K^+ conductance. A third possible nonlinearity follows from the passive properties of a network of resistors, because changing one resistor in a network will not usually produce linear changes in voltage. In Hudspeth and Corey's experiment the circuit parameters were such that this was probably not an important factor, but it may be more important in the cochlea.

The conclusion is that where we do have direct evidence from hair cells in amphibia and reptiles, the essential elements of the resistance modulation scheme of Davis (1958, 1965) seem to be in operation. The aim of the rest of this section is to see whether the evidence supports a similar scheme in mammals. Before doing this, the model to be discussed will be described more explicitly.

(b) Resistance modulation in the mammalian cochlea

The suggested scheme follows the resistance modulation hypothesis of Davis (1958, 1965) exactly, with the exception that the relation between the

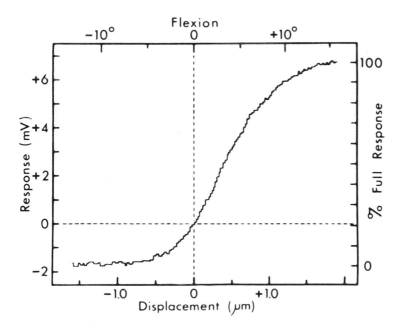

Fig. 5.4 In hair cells of the bullfrog sacculus, the relation between hair deflection and voltage change is asymmetric and saturating. From Hudspeth and Corey (1977), Fig. 3.

resistance of the apical membrane and the deflection of the hairs is non-linear, as it seems to be in the bullfrog sacculus.

The exact nature of the coupling of the movement of the basilar membrane as a whole to the deflection of the stereocilia will be left until later. It is suggested that deflection of the stereocilia towards the remnant of the kinocilium produces a decrease in resistance and so depolarization, and in the opposite direction an increase, and so hyperpolarization. The resistance at any one moment is a function only of the deflection of the stereocilia at that moment.

It is suggested that in inner hair cells the function relating resistance change to deflection is asymmetric, so that the resistance decreases are larger than the resistance increases, with the result that the depolarizations are larger than the hyperpolarizations. This will result in a net depolarization during a sound stimulus, superimposed on an alternating voltage change. The function is probably saturating.

The membrane channels are nonspecific. The currents can be carried by whatever ions are present, and the currents, and so the voltage changes, are proportional to the driving voltage across the apical membrane.

Outer hair cells will be omitted from the model; we have too little information on their properties, and are not sure of their role in transduction.

Finally, the intracellular voltage changes of inner hair cells cause the release of transmitter at the synapse at the base of the hair cells, so activating fibres of the auditory nerve.

How far does the evidence support the model?

(i) *Evidence for resistance modulation in the mammalian cochlea: steady changes in resistance.* It was suggested that in inner hair cells the function relating resistance change and deflection is asymmetric, in the same way that the function in Fig. 5.4 relating voltage and deflection is asymmetric. The result is that sound will produce a drop in mean resistance, as well as an alternating change.

Decreases in the mean resistance of the cochlear partition have been detected during sound stimulation by, for instance, Johnstone *et al.* (1966). They estimated that the resistance across the organ of Corti decreased by about 10% when a 5 kHz tone was presented at 95 dB SPL.

Such a net decrease in resistance would be expected to increase the positivity of the scala tympani and increase the negativity of the scala media, producing what is known as the negative summating potential. It could also produce the depolarization of the inner hair cells in response to sound, measured by Russell and Sellick (1978).

Resistance changes in individual inner hair cells were also found by Russell and Sellick (1978). They measured the voltage response to current introduced through their recording electrodes. In the frequency range studied, around 20 kHz, the alternating changes in resistance were too fast to be detected by the method, but the steady resistance changes could be detected. Their measurements showed that there was a steady decrease in resistance which was proportional to the steady intracellular depolarizing potential (Fig. 3.23).

These changes are exactly those expected in the Davis theory. It can be shown simply (Appendix) that if the intracellular depolarization were due to a decrease in the apical resistance of the hair cell, the intracellular potential would become progressively more positive as the apical membrane resistance, and so the total membrane resistance, fell. The fact that the relation was linear indicates that the resistance of the membrane at the base of the cell was constant.

(ii) *Evidence for resistance modulation in the mammalian cochlea: alternating changes in resistance.* Strelioff *et al.* (1972) measured the resistance of the cochlear partition by measuring the voltages produced in the scala media in response to a 600 Hz current applied between a second electrode in the scala media and an indifferent electrode outside the cochlea. The auditory stimulus was at a much lower frequency, 25 Hz. The voltage produced at 600 Hz was balanced out by a bridge before the sound was applied, and sound unbalanced the bridge. An example of the resulting waveform is shown in Fig. 5.5A. Increases and decreases in resistance could not be distinguished by the technique, but, because we know that there is a net decrease in the resistance of the cochlear partition during a sound stimulus, the resistance change probably followed the waveform of Fig. 5.5B. The waveform followed the sound stimulus, and was asymmetric, as expected from the hypothesis.

In this case the very low frequency of the stimulus provides a limitation to the interpretation of the experiment, because it will have been well below the characteristic frequency of the region measured, within the tail of the tuning curve. It is quite possible that much more complex things are happening at the characteristic frequency, in the tip of the tuning curve.

Hubbard *et al.* (1979) used a rather different and ingenious technique which allowed them to measure resistance changes at higher frequencies. The voltage changes produced by an alternating current (frequency f_1) were used to measure the resistance. If an auditory stimulus (frequency f_2) produces an alternating sinusoidal change in the resistance of the cochlear partition, the voltage changes will have the form $\sin 2\pi f_1 \times \sin 2\pi f_2$. This can be decomposed mathematically into a series containing voltages varying at the sum and difference frequencies ($|f_1 \pm f_2|$). Components of these frequencies were detected by Fourier analysis of the recorded waveforms. The technique had the advantage that the detection was done with frequencies that were not present in the introduced measuring current, so that capacitative leakage did not affect the results. The calculated component of the resistance varying at the frequency of the auditory stimulus followed the microphonic at the stimulus frequency, first increasing approximately linearly, and then saturating with intensity in the same way. This was true up to a stimulus frequency of 3 kHz, the highest that could be used (Geisler *et al.*, 1977). The broad outline of this result agrees with the hypothesis, and suggests, as supposed by the Davis theory, that the micro-

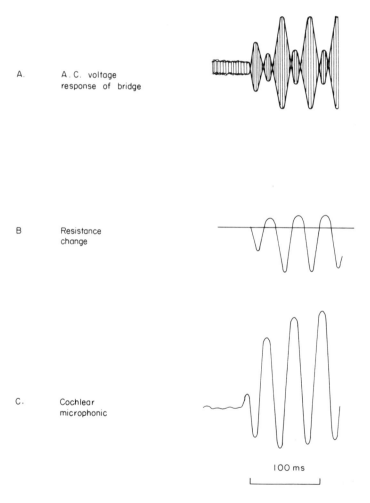

A.   A.C. voltage
response of bridge

B   Resistance
change

C.   Cochlear
microphonic

100 ms

Fig. 5.5 Resistance changes in the cochlea during sound stimulation, as determined from the a.c. voltage produced (trace A) when an a.c. current was applied through an electrode in the scala media. The acoustic stimulus was at 25 Hz. Adapted from Strelioff *et al.* (1972).

phonic is produced by current being driven through a varying resistance at the apex of the hair cells.

However, by a more detailed examination of the data, Hubbard *et al.* (1979) showed that there were departures from the proportionality of cochlear microphonic and resistance expected on the Davis theory. For instance, as the stimulus intensity was raised, the component of the resistance varying at the stimulus frequency increased more slowly than did the component of the microphonic varying at the stimulus frequency. The reason for the discrepancies are not known, and it is difficult to make a model to account for the results. One model the authors suggested involves resistances that vary with the transmembrane voltage differences, perhaps analogous to the voltage-sensitive K^+ conductance discussed above. Until a reasonable biological model of the results can be produced, it is difficult to say whether only a superficial or a radical modification of the Davis theory will be required.

The experiments of Hubbard *et al.* (1979) do however suggest that the nonlinearity of the cochlear microphonic cannot be derived entirely from the passive electrical network properties of the cochlea as suggested by Dallos (1973a). Dallos showed that even if a resistor in a network of resistors representing the cochlea varied linearly, the result would be a nonlinear variation in recorded voltage. Hubbard *et al.* say that the relative phases measured for the harmonics in their experiments do not agree with those expected on Dallos's model. This suggests that the resistor itself must vary nonlinearly, as suggested by the model adopted here.

(iii) *Relation between the d.c. and the a.c. responses of the cochlea.* Under the hypothesis outlined above, the alternating and direct potentials produced in inner hair cells can be related by a single input–output function, similar to that illustrated in Fig. 5.4 for the bullfrog sacculus. By stimulating with a low frequency sine wave, Sellick (1979) showed a portion of a similar input–output function for individual inner hair cells of the mammalian cochlea (Fig. 5.6). We would expect this to produce a distorted output waveform, with direct and alternating voltage components in relative amplitudes predictable from the shape of the function. He showed that this was the case: for low frequency stimuli, the intracellular alternating potential change was several times greater than the intracellular direct potential change, as expected from the function in Fig. 5.6. This was only true at low frequencies. As the stimulus frequency was raised, the d.c. response was unchanged, but alternating current began to leak through the capacitance of the cell walls, attenuating the a.c. voltage, so that by high frequencies the a.c. voltage produced inside the cell was many times smaller than the direct voltage.

In the case of the cochlea, because auditory stimuli have to be used, we cannot be sure that the nonlinearity resides only in the hair cell. For instance, nonlinearity due to eddies in the cochlear fluids may contribute to the shape of the input-output function.

Although a single input–output function seems able to explain the non-linearity of the intracellular inner hair cell responses, the same does not seem true for the gross extracellular responses, namely the cochlear micro-phonic and the summating potentials. Most of the extracellular cochlear microphonic is generated by outer hair cells, and it has been suggested that they show a different form of nonlinearity from inner hair cells (Pierson and Møller, 1980). There may therefore be at least two contributions to the summating potential from the hair cells alone, and, as was indicated in Chapter 3, there may be other contributions to the summating potential, perhaps from neural and metabolic events. While one component of the summating potential can be thought of as a distortion component of the cochlear microphonic (Engerbretson and Eldredge, 1968), the summating

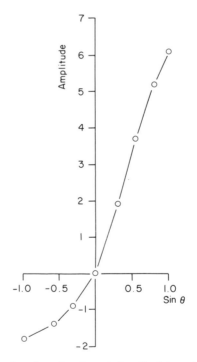

Fig. 5.6 The input–output function of an inner hair cell of the guinea-pig cochlea shows an asymmetric nonlinearity, similar to that of the hair cell of the bullfrog sacculus illustrated in Fig. 5.4. The function shown here was determined by stimulating with sound at 200 Hz, and plotting the instantaneous amplitude of the sound wave (horizontal axis) against the instantaneous amplitude of the response (vertical axis). Stimulus intensity: 100 dB SPL. Maximum response: approximately 20 mV. From Sellick (1979), Fig. 3.

potential as a whole can never be related in a single way to the voltage of the cochlear microphonic.

(iv) *Dependence of the microphonics on the driving voltage.* On the resistance modulation theory, the size of the stimulus related current will be directly proportional to the electromotive force. The driving voltage across the apical surface of the hair cell is about 120 mV, arising from the endocochlear potential of 80 mV and the intracellular potential of some −40 mV. We would therefore expect that varying the endocochlear potential would change the current through the varying resistance, and so change the amplitude of the sound evoked potentials. Tasaki and Fernandez (1952) first showed that positive polarization of the scala media increased the cochlear microphonic, and that negative polarization decreased it. Honrubia *et al.* (1976) showed that the change in the amplitude of the microphonic was linearly proportional to the change in the endocochlear potential. Projection of the linear relation showed that zero microphonic would have occurred when the endocochlear potential had been reduced by about 150 mV, close to (actually rather more than) the hypothesized value of the driving potential. In a second experiment, in order to reduce the endocochlear potential to this value, the animal was first made anoxic. Anoxia reduced the endocochlear potential to −20 mV, and then a polarizing voltage was superimposed. They showed that the cochlear microphonic reversed sign if the endolymph were driven below −50 mV with respect to the perilymph.

Although this experiment very strongly suggests that an auditory stimulus changes the resistance of the cochlear partition, and that microphonics can result from the flow of current driven through the variable resistance by the voltage across the apex of the hair cells, its interpretation is unfortunately limited by the use of anoxia. It is now believed that even the mechanical movement of the cochlear partition is affected by anoxia, and it is known that the intracellular hair cell responses are particularly vulnerable. Therefore it is unlikely that Honrubia *et al.* were investigating the process involved in the sensitive, low-level, and physiologically vulnerable part of the transduction process.

(v) *The functional polarization of cochlear hair cells.* In the suggested scheme, cochlear hair cells are functionally polarized in the same way as the other acousticolateral hair cells; that is, deflection of the stereocilia towards the kinocilium or its remnants produces a decrease in the apical resistance of the hair cell, and so a depolarization. The available evidence in the mammal supports this view.

The gross cochlear microphonic is dominated by outer hair cells (p. 53). The middle trace of Fig. 5.7 shows the gross microphonic response, recorded just below the reticular lamina, to trapezoidal displacements of the basilar membrane, indicated on the bottom trace. It is evident that upward movement of the basilar membrane is associated with positivity below the reticular lamina, and so with depolarization of outer hair cells. Because hair cells in the mammalian cochlea are oriented with the remnants of their kinocilia away from the modiolus, upwards movement of the basilar membrane bends the stereocilia towards the remnants of the kinocilium. This direction is associated with intracellular depolarization, and so the functional polarization of outer hair cells is the same as that of other hair cells of the acousticolateral system.

Figure 5.7 also shows the intracellular response of an inner hair cell. Here there is a large response to the *velocity* of the displacement of the basilar membrane. Nevertheless, an intracellular depolarization appears while the basilar membrane is moving towards the scala vestibuli, showing that inner hair cells also have the same functional polarization as other hair cells.

The results of Fig. 5.7 indicate that the gross cochlear microphonic, and hence the responses of outer hair cells, depend on the *displacement* of the cochlear partition, whereas the responses of inner hair cells depend on the velocity. Such a velocity sensitivity might be expected from the anatomy. Whereas the stereocilia of outer hair cells touch the tectorial membrane, the stereocilia of inner hair cells do not make contact, or if they do, then only very lightly (Engström and Engström, 1978). We would therefore expect the stereocilia of the outer hair cells to be deflected by the displacement of the cochlear partition, and the stereocilia of the inner hair cells, being moved by

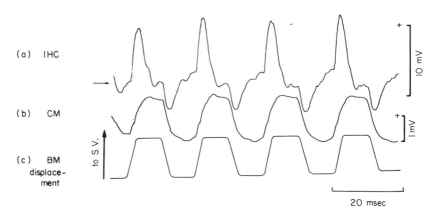

Fig. 5.7 The cochlear microphonic (CM: trace b), dominated by outer hair cells, follows the *displacement* of the basilar membrane (trace c), whereas inner hair cells (trace a) follow the *velocity*. In both cases, movement towards the scala vestibuli caused positivity below the reticular lamina, indicating a similar morphological polarization for inner and outer hair cells.

The cochlear microphonic was here recorded extracellularly in the organ of Corti. The displacement of the basilar membrane was calculated from the rate of change of sound pressure. Adapted from Sellick and Russell (1980), Fig. 1.

viscous drag, to be deflected by the velocity. This difference in the response mode of inner and outer hair cells however only seems to hold at low frequencies of stimulation; above about 250 Hz inner as well as outer hair cells seem to respond to displacement (Sellick and Russell, 1980).

(c) The site of transduction

The weight of evidence seems to be in favour of some stage of resistance modulation in the apical membrane of the hair cell, although this may not be adequate to explain all the evidence. Where in the apical surface does the resistance modulation and transduction occur? Such information as we have, suggests that the transduction is associated with the stereocilia themselves. Vestibular hair cells have a kinocilium in addition to their stereocilia. Hudspeth and Jacobs (1979), working with hair cells from the bullfrog sacculus, were able to free the kinocilium from the bundle of stereocilia by means of a glass rod in a micromanipulator. They showed that deflection of the kinocilium did not produce receptor potentials, whereas deflection of the stereocilia alone did. If transduction is associated with the stereocilia rather than the kinocilium in vestibular hair cells, it is very likely that the same conclusions can be applied to cochlear hair cells, which do not possess a kinocilium, but only remnants of the structures supporting it (Fig. 5.1).

In some cases it was possible to deflect some but not all of the stereocilia. Here, smaller receptor potentials were produced than during deflection of the whole bundle. This suggests that each stereocilium makes some contribution to the receptor potential.

Identifying the transduction with the stereocilia makes it difficult to account for the functional polarization of hair cells. Each stereocilium does not seem to be *morphologically* polarized, and this suggests that the *functional* polarization of the hair cell as a whole arises from the relations of the stereocilia to each other or to the structure of the hair cell. At the moment it is not possible to go further than this, and say where in the stereocilia and hair cell the transduction and resistance modulation occur.

(d) The amplitude of the movement at threshold

Some of the greatest objections to the simple resistance modulation hypothesis have arisen from the estimated magnitude of the movement of the basilar membrane at threshold. It was originally calculated from the measurements of von Békésy (1960) that the displacement of the basilar membrane at threshold was 2×10^{-4} nm, or 1/500th of the diameter of the hydrogen atom. The distortion of the critical structure would probably be even less. If the movements are very much less than those found necessary elsewhere for controlling ion flow, it is difficult to see how the resistance model could be sustained.

Part of the answer may lie in the noise of the system. Brownian movements, if sufficiently great, will sometimes push the transducer over the critical displacement, and we would expect this displacement to be reached more readily if there is a superimposed signal present. The result will be, that in the presence of noise, there need never be an ultimate threshold, if the noise induced displacements are comparable to the critical displacement. Indeed, electronic digitizing systems sometimes add a 'dither' signal to produce such an effect. The sensitivity will then depend on the signal retrieval system employed, presumably an averaging over time and over a number of stereocilia or hair cells. But even with noise in the signal, there are limits as to how far the threshold can be lowered. Because the amount of averaging necessary increases as the square of the noise level, the retrieval system rapidly becomes uneconomic. This sets a limit to the possible signal-to-noise ratio, and hence to the ratio of the mean displacement at threshold to the critical displacement of the transducter.

A second part of the answer may arise from the assumptions behind the calculation of the threshold displacement. Von Békésy's estimate of 2×10^{-4} nm, referred to above, was obtained by extrapolation from measurements at sound pressure levels of 130 dB SPL. The assumption behind this calculation is that the movement of the basilar membrane is linear. As will be described in Chapter 5, Section E, there is increasing evidence that this assumption will have to be modified.

Let us attempt to calculate the displacement of the basilar membrane at threshold from more recent measurements. Firstly, the data of the two groups who found linear movements in the guinea-pig at physiological sound pressure levels will be used (Wilson and Johnstone, 1975; Johnstone *et al.*, 1970). The behavioural threshold of the guinea-pig at 20 kHz, corrected for the influence of the outer ear, is approximately 10 dB SPL at the eardrum (Heffner *et al.*, 1971). Linear extrapolation of the basilar membrane response at 20 kHz to this level gives 5×10^{-3} nm peak-to-peak, larger than calculated from the results of von Békésy, but still rather small.

On the other hand, Rhode (1978) in the squirrel monkey at 7 kHz found nonlinearity near the peak of the basilar membrane response at sound pressure levels of 70 dB SPL and above. The squirrel monkey's absolute threshold at this frequency is about 20 dB SPL at the tympanic membrane, if corrected by 10 dB for the influence of the outer ear on the assumption that it is like that of the cat (Fujita and Elliott, 1965). If it is assumed that the basilar membrane moves linearly below the range investigated by Rhode, this corresponds to 6×10^{-2} nm peak to peak. If the nonlinearity continues below 70 dB at the same rate as above (Rhode, 1978), then the figure will be 20–50 times greater than this, or 1–3 nm peak to peak.

A further assumption behind the calculation is that the measured movement adequately mirrors the critical movement as transmitted to the hair cells. It has been suggested by Zwislocki and Kletsky (1980) that the tectorial membrane acts as an additional tuned mechanical resonator, vibrating on top of the organ of Corti and increasing the response at the characteristic frequency. If there is such a mechanical resonator, the shearing displacement at the hair cells will be greater than that expected from the displacement of the basilar membrane. The shear at threshold may therefore be greater than that expected from the 1–3 nm displacement quoted above.

Neglecting such a mechanical resonator for the moment, on Davis's scheme the displacement of the basilar membrane will be directly translated into a displacement of the stereocilia, by a factor that depends on the geometry of the organ of Corti. The angle of deflection of the stereocilia will be greater than the angle of deflection of the basilar membrane, by a ratio equal to the height of the organ of Corti divided by the length of the stereocilia. A threshold displacement of the basilar membrane by 1 nm will deflect the stereocilia by about 10^{-2} degrees. Such an angle of rotation will produce a stretch of a hypothetically possible critical amount of 0.1 nm in a structure 0.6 μm thick. This figure is comparable to the thickness of many structures at the apex of the hair cell, for instance of the stereocilia. This very rough calculation therefore shows that the calculated displacement of the basilar membrane at threshold, may well be physiologically reasonable.

(e) Theories of transduction

Davis did not specify the exact way in which the mechanical deformation would increase the permeability of the transducing membrane. One possibility is that the packing of the components of the membrane is reduced, opening spaces between them. Another possibility is that preformed channels in the membrane are opened.

In common with the channels in postsynaptic membranes, we might expect such channels to be chemically controlled, perhaps by the conformation of, say, proteins in the membrane. This would explain the finite, though small, delay in channel opening observed in the bullfrog sacculus by Corey and Hudspeth (1979b). The possibility then exists that the mechanosensitivity exists in the controlling molecules themselves. It is moreover quite possible in view of the known complexities of the factors controlling membrane conductance, that important components of the sensitivity and amplification of auditory transduction occur at this point. For instance, Hendry *et al.* (1978) have shown with artificial lipid bilayers, that changes in the thickness of the membrane by a few percent, can increase the conductance by more than a hundredfold. Tasaki (1960) suggested that a polarized membrane in a K^+-rich medium was unstable, and could show large resistance changes when the conditions were changed. There may be factors such as these, at present unknown, which are essential for the high sensitivity of the transducer process. That some process of this sort may be occurring is suggested by the high vulnerability of inner hair cell and neural potentials to certain drugs and anoxia.

In contrast to the theories put forward so far, there have been theories that the cochlear microphonic is a direct physical expression of the displacement of the basilar membrane, and is not dependent on tapping the biological energy of the endolymph. De Vries (1948) suggested that in the vestibular system the microphonics were the result of piezoelectric effects. Christiansen *et al.* (1961) suggested that the stereocilia contained molecules of potassium hyaluronate which produced electric potentials to mechanical stress. Dohlman (1960) similarly suggested that the stereocilia were covered by a film of highly charged mucopolysaccharide, which produced electric potentials when deformed and which then triggered the synapse directly. All these theories can be countered by an experiment of von Békésy (1960). Von Békésy displaced the basilar membrane with a needle, and showed that the generated potential lasted as long as the membrane was deformed. Sustaining a deflection did not require a further input of work, yet the resulting current was maintained. Clearly, if the experiment were continued for a long time, the energy produced could exceed that put in by an indefinite amount. The cochlear microphonic therefore needs an extra source of energy.

What theories does the most recent evidence suggest? The author believes that the advantages of the resistance modulation theory outweigh its disadvantages. The main electrical phenomena of the cochlea are simply explained. Because we do not know the nature of the deformation causing the resitance change, or the exact nature of the mechanical movements of the basilar membrane at resonance, it is not possible to test whether the magnitudes of the displacement at threshold are sufficient. However, recent measurements of basilar membrane motion suggest that the induced shear within the apical structures of the hair cell may well be of a size that would be able to affect ion flow. It is quite possible that as yet unknown membrane processes increase the sensitivity and gain of the response to deformation. Identifying the transducing structure is difficult. It is possible that the membrane along the length of the stereocilia, or only near the roots, is involved.

C. Active Movements in the Cochlea: the Evoked Cochlear Mechanical Response

Kemp (1978) sealed both a loudspeaker and a microphone into the ear canal of human subjects. An acoustic click presented through the speaker of course produced a brief wave of pressure in the ear canal. However, a second much smaller sound wave, delayed by 5–15 ms, could also be recorded. The results of a recent replication of his experiment by Wilson (1980b) are shown in Fig. 5.8. The 'echo', which arose from the cochlea, was strongest relative to the input for low intensity clicks. The suggestion was made that the mechanical impulse travelling up the basilar membrane at some point met a jump in the impedance of the basilar membrane. This caused a certain proportion of the energy to be reflected, setting up a pressure wave which travelled back to the base of the cochlea. The fact that the delayed response could be affected by ototoxic agents and was absent in sensorineurally deaf subjects indicated a cochlear origin for the effect. With suitable signal retrieval techniques it could be measured well below the sensory threshold. Moreover, it preserved many details of the stimulus waveform, and inverted its waveform when the stimulus was inverted. These suggest that it was generated by a stage before the synapse, and suggest that it was not the result of the middle ear muscle reflex (Wilson, 1980a; Anderson, 1980). Analogous echoes can be seen with other types of stimuli.

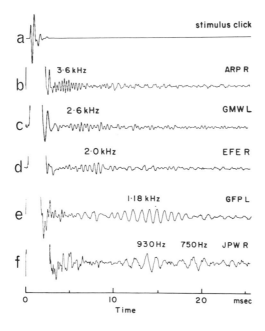

Fig. 5.8 When the ear is stimulated with a click, the cochlea returns an acoustic echo to the external auditory meatus. The form of the echo is different for each subject.

The original stimulus in the meatus is shown in trace a. In traces b–f, shown with a much magnified vertical scale, the stimulus has clipped but the waveform of the echo is visible. Each trace is the average of many responses. From Wilson (1980b), Fig. 2.

If for instance the ear is stimulated with a continuous tone, the cochlea reflects a tone back into the ear canal. With two-tone stimulation (frequencies f_1 and f_2) a distortion product at the frequency f_2-f_1 can also be detected in the ear canal. Mountain (1980) showed that the amplitude of the reflected distortion tone could be affected by stimulation of the crossed olivocochlear bundle, and this suggests that the hair cells themselves are involved in the reflection. Further experiments suggest that the reflections occur from a rather late stage in the transduction process. For instance, it is possible to mask the echo to a click by a continuous tone. The frequency and intensity relations of the tone necessary to mask any particular frequency component of the echo show that the generators behind the echo must be very sharply tuned.

In themselves, these observations are not necessarily very radical, although it is surprising that mechanical reflections can be obtained from as late a stage of the auditory system as the hair cells. However, one observation with much more fundamental implications is shown in Fig. 5.9. It was found that in certain subjects with a tendency to subjective tinnitus of cochlear origin, a short tone burst was able to trigger a long chain of sound pressure fluctuations in the ear canal. The subjects at this point were able to hear an augmentation of their tinnitus. This is very strong evidence that not only are intracochlear events able to affect the sound pressure in the ear canal, but that an amplifying and *mechanically active* physiological process must be involved. The necessity for an amplifying stage was also shown by Kemp (1978), who calculated that even when a click did not evoke tinnitus, more energy could be produced by the cochlea than was originally introduced. The obvious, but revolutionary, hypothesis that must be put forward is that when the hair cells are stimulated, the cochlear partition is actively moved in return.

The mechanism for the reflex movement of the cochlear partition is not known. It is possible, for instance, as was suggested by Wilson (1980c), that during activation the hair cells or supporting cells undergo volume changes, perhaps as a result of solvent following ions passing in and out of the hair cells. A second hypothesis is that hair cells are actively motile, as a result of an interaction of actin and myosin in the stereocilia. Stereocilia are composed of actin filaments, and also contain myosin (Tilney *et al.*, 1980; Macartney *et al.*, 1980). It is quite possible that such an interaction in the stereocilia, as in muscle cells, is able to generate movement. It is likely, for instance, that Ca^{2+}, which is known to be necessary for sensory transduction, enters hair cells when they are activated. Calcium ions could then stimulate the interaction, resulting in movement of the stereocilia. A similar activation of the interaction by sound could also cause a stiffening of the stereocilia, and this may possibly explain some of the nonlinearities of the mechanical response of the cochlea, and explain why the nonlinearity disap-

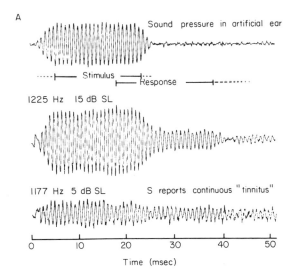

A

Sound pressure in artificial ear

······┣━━━ Stimulus ━━━┫···
                      ┣━━ Response ━━━┫━━━━ ┫········

1225 Hz   15 dB SL

1177 Hz   5 dB SL   S reports continuous "tinnitus"

0   10   20   30   40   50

Time (msec)

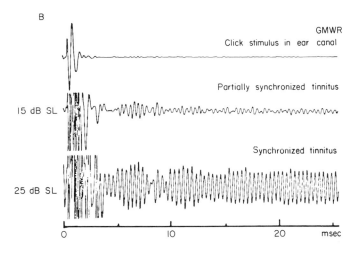

B

GMWR
Click stimulus in ear canal

Partially synchronized tinnitus

15 dB SL

Synchronized tinnitus

25 dB SL

0   10   20   msec

Fig. 5.9 Acoustic waveforms, recorded in the external auditory meatus, of tinnitus of cochlear origin.
A. A tone pip at 1225 Hz and 15 dB SL evoked an echo that outlasted the stimulus. But at 1177 Hz and 5 dB SL the tone pip induced a prolonged ringing, and the subject heard continuous tinnitus.
B. Continuous tinnitus was detectable in the external auditory meatus of this subject, although because it was not phase-locked to the stimulus it did not appear in the averaged trace. Clicks of increasing intensity phase-locked the tinnitus to some extent at 15 dB SL and completely at 25 dB SL. From Wilson (1980b), Fig. 5.

pears during anoxia or after death.

Both hypotheses for the origin of the evoked cochlear mechanical response are highly speculative at the moment. Both would predict severe high frequency limits for the active response, in one case because of the time taken for the diffusion of water molecules, and in the other because of the time constants of the molecular interaction. At the moment, we do not know if either model is reasonable.

D. Hair Cells and Neural Excitation

Having considered the ways in which hair cells may be activated by sound, and the ways in which they may respond, we now turn to the way in which their activity is transmitted to the fibres of the auditory nerve.

1. Inner Hair Cells

There are synaptic terminals at the base of both inner and outer hair cells. The terminals of one type, known as Type 2, are large and granulated and are particularly prominent on outer hair cells (Fig. 3.5). They are the endings of the efferent pathway to the cochlea called the olivocochlear bundle, the 'feedback' pathway by which the brain stem is able to affect the activity of the hair cells. These terminals are not our main object of interest in this section. The other type, known as Type 1 terminals, are more prominent on inner hair cells, although they are also present on outer hair cells. They are the endings of the primary afferent fibres of the auditory nerve. As was described above, at least 90–95% and perhaps all of the fibres of the central end of the auditory nerve synapse directly on the inner hair cells. The influence seems to be straightforward, because inner hair cells and auditory nerve fibres have similar response properties.

The presynaptic membrane under the afferent terminals of inner and outer hair cells has a presynaptic structure consisting of a synaptic bar, which may be rod-like or spherical, or which may consist of an invagination of the membrane into the cell (Ades and Engström, 1974). Similar presynaptic bars are seen in all the hair cells of the acousticolateral system, as well as some of the synaptic contacts of the retina. They are surrounded by vesicles, which may be attached by a matrix of fine filaments (for a review, see Finlayson and Osborne, 1975). The function of these special structures is not known, although it is likely that they are analogous to the presynaptic structures seen generally in synapses. Presynaptic structures of this form seem to be associated with what have been called 'high gain' synapses, which need only a few mV of depolarization to be activated (Llinas, 1979).

Postsynaptic potentials have not been recorded locally in the organ of

Corti. Such potentials have however been recorded in the postsynaptic structures of other hair cell systems. Furukawa and Ishi (1972) for instance recorded graded postsynaptic potentials intracellularly in the giant afferent terminals of the goldfish sacculus. They showed that there was a continual barrage of spontaneous miniature excitatory postsynaptic potentials, as would be expected from the quantal release of neurotransmitter contained in vesicles. Crawford and Fettiplace (1980) in the cochlea of the turtle, recorded similar miniature brief depolarizations together with spiking activity as they advanced their electrode through the area of the nerve terminals. Russell and Sellick (1978) did not record such action potentials in the organ of Corti, and this has suggested that action potentials in the cochlea are generated not in the organ of Corti itself, but more centrally. The obvious site is just beyond the habenula perforata, where the axons gain their myelin sheath (Fig. 3.1). At this point they become severely constricted, and we would expect the current density to rise. This is in accordance with the concept of an 'initial segment' found in many nerve cells, a point some way along the axon at which action potentials are initiated. It would also allow the nerve fibres to be affected by other structures in the region, such as the terminals of the sympathetic innervation (Spoendlin and Lichtensteiger, 1966; Pickles, 1979b).

The transmitter at the afferent synapse has not been identified.

2. Outer Hair Cells

Outer hair cells are by far the most numerous of the hair cells, outnumbering the inner hair cells by over three to one. The outer hair cells also generate nearly all the recordable microphonic. Yet it appears that the auditory nerve responses entirely follow the properties of the inner hair cells. The outer hair cells must be doing something. The most widely held hypothesis is that they somehow increase the sensitivity of auditory nerve fibres. Figures 5.10 and 10.1B show two different patterns of auditory nerve fibre responses recorded from regions of outer hair cell loss and apparent inner hair cell normality, following the administration of ototoxic agents. It is possible that the short sharp dip on the upper slope of the tuning curve in Fig. 10.1B is the remnant of the sharply tuned, low-level, tip. Whether or not these fibres can be said to retain much frequency selectivity, it is obvious that there has been a great shift in the threshold sensitivity. This suggests that the outer hair cells somehow contribute low-level sensitivity to the auditory nerve fibres, by means of a boost around the characteristic frequency.

The outer hair cells may have low thresholds because their stereocilia actually touch the tectorial membrane.

Inner hair cells show thresholds and frequency selectivity comparable to those of auditory nerve fibres, and it is likely therefore that the contribution of the outer hair cells has already been made by that stage. Nevertheless, it is rather difficult to think of a mechanism by which the outer hair cells confer sensitivity and probably frequency selectivity on inner hair cells.

One possibility is that the interaction is electrical. The outer hair cells do not show obvious d.c. responses (Tanaka *et al.*, 1980). At high frequencies we would expect the alternating receptor currents, as in inner hair cells, to be short-circuited through the capacitance of the cell walls. The outer hair cells will therefore show neither large a.c., nor large d.c. potentials intracellularly, and so will act merely as current shunts. They would therefore have their effect on the inner hair cells by altering the local electrical environment of the inner hair cells. Nevertheless, when the details are taken into account, it becomes difficult to devise a convincing way in which

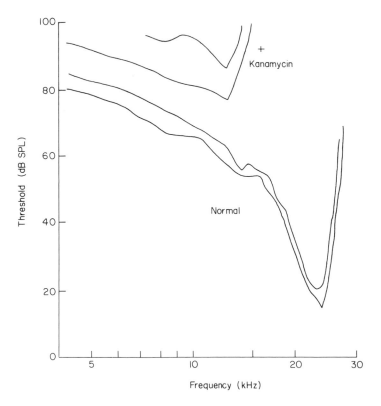

Fig. 5.10 When outer hair cells are destroyed by kanamycin, auditory nerve fibres can lose their sensitivity and frequency selectivity, and can shift to lower best frequencies. In this experiment, single neurones of the spiral ganglion (auditory nerve cell bodies) were recorded in the guinea-pig at a site 2.2 mm from the base of the cochlea. Adapted from Robertson and Johnstone (1979).

this could substantially lower the thresholds of inner hair cells around the characteristic frequency, but not at other frequencies.

A second hypothesis is that the interaction is mechanical. Zwislocki and Kletsky (1980) have suggested that the tectorial membrane acts as an additional mechanical resonator, sitting on top of the organ of Corti. The tectorial membrane on this hypothesis undergoes expansion and compression vibrations in the radial direction. It is coupled to the organ of Corti by means of the stereocilia. Such a resonator could increase the deflection of the stereocilia near the tip of the tuning curve, and increase the frequency selectivity of the stimulus to the hair cells (Allen, 1980). However the outer hair cells, by means of their stereocilia, are relegated to providing a merely mechanical restoring spring for the resonator, and it is difficult to explain why therefore they show so many of the morphological characteristics of transducing structures. The role of the cochlear microphonic is also unexplained. Moreover, we would expect the outer hair cells, and so the cochlear microphonic, to be as sharply tuned as the inner hair cells, which is not the case. The theory does, however, explain how destruction of the outer hair cells could affect the sensitivity and selectivity of inner hair cells, because we would expect the resonator to be disrupted. It also explains how the crossed olivocochlear bundle could affect the response of inner hair cells. If the mechanical properties of the stereocilia are modifiable by activation of the efferent synapses, perhaps as a result of changing actin–myosin interactions in the stereocilia, then this also would be expected to change the mechanical properties of the resonator.

A hypothesis that has been suggested in the past is that the interaction is neural, between the nerve fibres innervating the outer hair cells and those innervating the inner hair cells, perhaps in the habenula perforata where they come into close proximity. The function of the afferent nerve fibres innervating outer hair cells certainly needs explanation, but it now appears that the interaction has already occurred at the inner hair cells, and the hypothesis can no longer be held.

Whatever the basis for the interaction, it has been suggested that both inner and outer hair cells are able to excite auditory nerve fibres, but that at low frequencies they do so in phase opposition (Sokolich *et al.*, 1976). That is, if during one phase of the sound wave the inner hair cells excited a fibre, the outer hair cells would inhibit it, although generally to a different extent, and vice versa. For most auditory nerve fibres, this probably only occurs for frequencies well below the characteristic frequency. The mode of interaction near the characteristic frequency, where the outer hair cells substantially boost the sensitivity of the inner hair cells, is not known.

E. The Linearity of Cochlear Function

1. Introduction

An area of current debate concerns the linearity of the cochlear responses, as reflected both in the mechanics of the basilar membrane and in the electrical responses of the hair cells and auditory nerve.

As was described in Chapter 3, the evidence on the linearity of the movement of the basilar membrane is conflicting. Rhode (1978) using the Mössbauer technique and Lepage and B. M. Johnstone (1980) using the capacitive probe have both shown a nonlinearity of the saturating type, such that the movement became relatively smaller at high intensities. On the other hand Wilson and J. R. Johnstone (1975) using the capacitive probe in the guinea-pig and Evans and Wilson (1975) using the same probe in the cat found complete linearity. Lepage and Johnstone indicated that a good physiological condition of the cochlea was essential for the detection of the nonlinearity, and this may explain why the nonlinearity has not always been found. Nonlinearity is also supported by much of the indirect evidence. Therefore, while the evidence is by no means conclusive, many investigators would favour a nonlinearity of the movement.

According to Rhode (1978), the nonlinearity is severe and extensive. His data in Fig. 5.11 indicate that the amplitude of the movement could increase with a slope of 0.3 or less when plotted on log–log scales, over a range of 50 dB. On linear scales, therefore, the rate of growth of movement became less and less as the stimulus intensity was increased. Such a nonlinearity is known as a compressive nonlinearity. It may serve to increase the dynamic range of hearing, and may account for its astonishing range of 120 dB or more.

The origin of the nonlinearity is unknown. Some of it may be purely mechanical, with perhaps the short stereocilia on the hair cells giving progressively more and more support to the long ones as the stereocilia are deflected. The nonlinearity seems to depend on the physiological condition of the cochlea, and it is possible that the stiffness of structures such as the stereocilia is actively modifiable, perhaps by actin-myosin interactions in the stereocilia. Furthermore, at low amplitudes of vibration, it is possible that the evoked cochlear mechanical response can amplify the movement. At very high levels, models have shown that the cochlear fluids themselves move nonlinearly (Tonndorf, 1973).

Further nonlinearities can be expected to occur in the transmission between the movement of the basilar membrane and the electrical responses of the hair cells. One source may be the geometry of the linkage between the basilar membrane and the stereocilia (Johnstone and Johnstone, 1966). It is also likely, as was suggested above, that the relation between hair deflection and resistance change is nonlinear, in the way that it seems to be for vestibular hair cells (p. 113).

Many models attempt to reproduce the nonlinearity of the cochlea by only one nonlinear stage, although as the above list shows, there are likely to be more.

Testing the nonlinearities directly, by measuring the movement of the basilar membrane or the intracellular potentials of hair cells, is technically difficult. A lot of the evidence for nonlinearities in the cochlea has been provided by studying the nonlinear interactions between two-tone stimuli, as revealed in the responses of single fibres of the auditory nerve. There are two such phenomena that have been studied extensively, namely two-tone suppression and the production of combination tones.

2. Two-tone Suppression

Two-tone suppression was described in Chapter 4 (p. 92) and an example for an inner hair cell was shown in Fig. 4.15, and for an auditory nerve fibre in Fig. 4.16. It was suggested that these results could be interpreted in terms of a nonlinearity, such as might exist in the movement of the basilar membrane

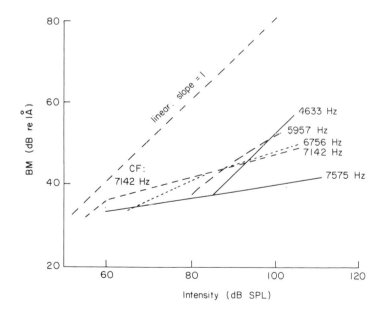

Fig. 5.11 Intensity functions for the basilar membrane of the squirrel monkey, determined by the Mössbauer technique for different frequencies of stimulation. Many of the curves have a slope less than one, indicating that the output did not grow in proportion to the input, and representing a saturating type of nonlinearity. From Rhode (1978), Fig. 10.

or in the transduction process, sandwiched between two linear filters. This is known as the 'Band Pass Nonlinear' network (BPNL) model, one form of which was due to Pfeiffer (1970). The input–output function of the nonlinear stage is saturating (Fig. 5.12). The first filter might be comparatively broadly tuned, and determined by the mechanical travelling wave on the basilar membrane. The second filter might be more sharply tuned, and is at the moment purely hypothetical. It should be explained that this scheme is a matter of current debate, and is merely being used as a convenient model.

Consider how such a model would explain two-tone suppression. Suppose a steady tone is introduced into the whole system at a frequency such that it is transmitted by both the first and the second filters. Imagine then super-imposing a second tone, at a frequency which will be transmitted by the first filter, but not the second. Because the nonlinearity is of the saturating type, the output of the nonlinear stage to both stimuli together, will be less than the sum of the responses to the two stimuli individually. Each stimulus has the effect of reducing the response to the other. At the second filter, our second tone will be filtered out, leaving only the first tone at a reduced amplitude. In other words, a tone which gets through the first filter, but not the second, will contribute suppression but not excitation. This explains the suppression areas of Figs. 4.15 and 4.16. The outer edges of the two-tone suppression areas indicate the outer edge of the first filter, and the excitatory tuning curve approximates to the product of the first and second filters. Figure 4.16 also shows that the supression areas are asymmetric. We can provisionally suppose that this occurs because the two filters are tuned to different frequencies, the second filter being tuned to a rather lower frequency than the first.

The evidence from two-tone suppression indicates that the cochlea operates nonlinearly at some stage before the synapse. The nonlinearity continues to the lowest intensities, because two-tone suppression can be demonstrated right down to threshold.

3. Combination Tones

A second line of evidence for nonlinear interactions in the cochlea arises from the response of auditory nerve fibres to combination tones. If a system is entirely linear, its output waveform will contain only the same frequency components as the input. If a system is nonlinear, single tones will also produce harmonics. A pair of input tones will in addition produce combination tones, that is, tones whose frequencies depend on the frequencies of *both* of the input tones. The pattern of such harmonics and combination tones immediately tells us a great deal about the form of the nonlinearity. If the input–output function through the nonlinearity is symmetric around the line at input = 0 (otherwise called even-order), we shall have even har-

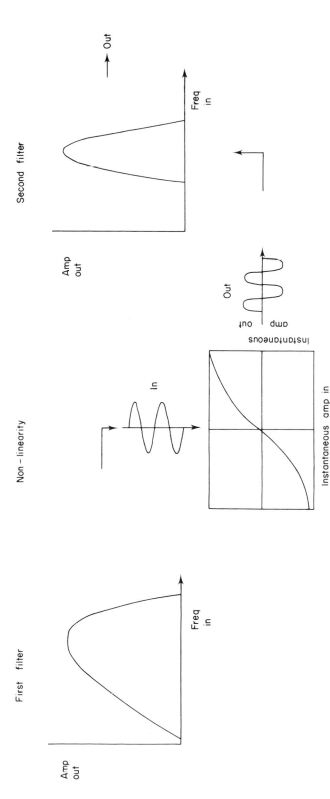

Fig. 5.12 In the 'BPNL' (Bandpass nonlinear) network model, a nonlinearity is sandwiched between two bandpass filters. The particular nonlinearity illustrated here is antisymmetric and saturating, and so clips the peaks of the sine wave evenly.

monics ($2f_1$, $4f_1$, etc.) and sum and difference tones of the form $f_2 \pm f_1$, $2f_2 \pm 2f_1$, etc. (Fig. 5.13). If the input–output function through the non-linearity is antisymmetric, or odd-order, we shall, in addition to the original frequencies, have odd harmonics and combination tones of the form $2f_1 \pm f_2$, $3f_1 \pm 2f_2$, etc. Combination tones of the form $f_2 - f_1$ (the difference tone) and $2f_1-f_2$ (known as the cubic distortion tone) can be demonstrated both psychophysically and electrophysiologically (Goldstein, 1967; Hall, 1972; Goldstein and Kiang, 1968; Kim *et al.*, 1980). This suggests that the input–output function through the nonlinear stage is a sum of both symmetric and antisymmetric components.

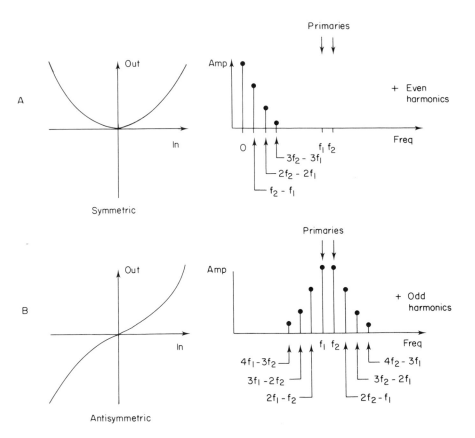

Fig. 5.13 Combination tones produced by different nonlinearities.
A. A nonlinearity with an input–output function symmetrical about the line: input=0 (even order function) produces an output with terms of the form $n(f_1 \pm f_2)$, and even harmonics of the primaries.
B. An antisymmetric input-output function (odd-order function) produces the primaries, combination tones of the form $nf_1 \pm mf_2$, and odd harmonics. All input–output functions can be made by combinations of even order and odd order functions.

It has to be explained why, for the antisymmetric or odd-order contribution, the dominant cubic distortion or combination tone is $2f_1 - f_2$, and not $2f_2 - f_1$, where $f_2 > f_1$. Figure 5.13 suggests that they should be present with equal strength. As a provisional hypothesis, we may again invoke the second filter. If as was suggested in the last section, the second filter is tuned to a rather lower frequency than the first one, then it will pass the combination tones that are lower in frequency, but reject those that are higher. The same second filter also explains why no harmonics are seen after the nonlinear stage, because they also are filtered out.

Responses to such combination tones may be detected in the firing of single fibres of the auditory nerve. Goldstein and Kiang (1968) showed that fibres tuned to the frequency of the combination tone $2f_1 - f_2$ would respond to the combination tone when the primaries f_1 and f_2 were presented. They were able to show this by detecting changes in the mean firing rate to the compound stimulus. A second method that has been used extensively for detecting the response to the combination tones depends on the finding that, for low frequency stimuli, the period histogram of the firing pattern follows a half-wave rectified version of the stimulating waveform. If a waveform corresponding to a half-wave retified version of the combination tone can be shown in the period histogram, then it follows that the fibre must have been responding to the combination tone. Again, auditory nerve fibres have been shown to respond to combination tones when the primaries are presented (Kim *et al.*, 1980).

One result of Goldstein and Kiang (1968) has rather interesting implication. They showed that when the combination tone $2f_1 - f_2$ was at the characteristic frequency of a fibre, it could excite the fibre even though f_1 and f_2 separately produced no response in that fibre. A moment's reflection will show the surprising nature of this result. The combination tone must have been generated where f_1 and f_2 overlapped, and so the primaries must have been present in the cochlea at the site where the combination tone was produced. But the fibres were able to respond to a combination tone at their characteristic frequency without any response to the primaries. The primaries must have been separated from the combination tone by some form of filter, tuned to the characteristic frequency of the region, and occurring *after* the basilar membrane.

There are two current hypotheses explaining this result. One is that there is an explicit second filter, tuned to the characteristic frequency of the region, and situated after the nonlinearity. The other is that the combination tone is generated as a physical movement of the basilar membrane at the site where the primaries overlap; and just as an external tone sets up a travelling wave on the basilar membrane, the resulting oscillation produces a travelling wave of its own, peaking at the place in the cochlea corresponding to its frequency. There, the combination tone is transduced just as though it were a tone that had been introduced from outside. The evidence favours the second alternative.

There is strong evidence that the combination tone is propagated *from* the site of transduction of the primaries. Smoorenberg (1972) found that a subject with a sharp high frequency hearing loss was unable to detect the combination tone psychophysically, when the primaries were in the area of hearing loss, but the combination tone was not. A similar point has been made in electrophysiological experiments by Dallos and Harris (1978). This suggests that the normal operation of the cochlea at the point of transduction of the primaries is necessary for the generation of the combination tone, and suggests that this point is different from the site of transduction of the combination tone.

Kim *et al.* (1980) demonstrated the propagation of the combination tone by recording the responses of auditory nerve fibres to a two-tone stimulus. They sampled the responses of a large number of fibres in each animal, so producing a 'neurogram', or picture of activity in the whole nerve fibre array. They measured phase-locking to the two fixed primaries and to the combination tone. Figure 5.14 shows the neurograms for the primaries, and for the $2f_1 - f_2$ combination tone. Note that the two primaries produced separate peaks of activity at their characteristic place in the cochlea, and that the combination tone produced a peak at *its* characteristic place in the cochlea.

The phase data in the neurogram produced very strong evidence that the distortion component was transmitted along the basilar membrane by a travelling wave, just as though it were an externally introduced tone. For externally introduced tones, the phase of activation of auditory nerve fibres increases steadily along the cochlea, because of the time taken by the travelling wave (line f_s in Fig. 5.15). Apical to the site of generation, the phase of the response to the combination tone varied in exactly the same way, after an arbitrary phase shift necessary because we have no reference phase (line $2f_1 - f_2$ in Fig. 5.15). We are forced to conclude that the distortion tone is propagated along the cochlea just as though it were an externally introduced tone, to produce a resonance in the cochlea at the characteristic point associated with its frequency.

What is the mechanism behind the nonlinear stage generating the combination tone? The generation of the combination tone seems to occur after one stage of the frequency filtering, because the amplitude of the combination tone depends strongly on the frequency separation of the primaries. We can therefore suppose that the overlap occurs only if both primaries get through the same first filter, perhaps to be identified with the mechanical resonance of the cochlear partition. Mechanical energy will then have to be fed back to the basilar membrane. This is not an entirely novel idea, and we have already met such a reverse flow of energy from the transducer in the evoked cochlear mechanical response. In that case, the energy was detected in the ear canal.

We are not certain of the mechanism of the re-emission of the distortion tone, whether it depends on a purely passive reflection of mechanical energy from a mechanically nonlinear stage, or depends on an active mechanical process, such as a motility of the stereocilia. Whatever the process, it would have to act very quickly, because there is no indication that combination tones become weaker at high frequencies. It does however seem that the

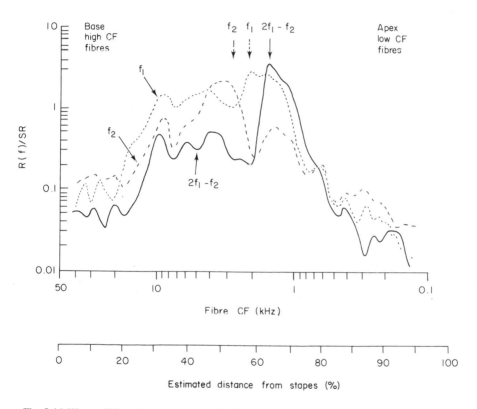

Fig. 5.14 Kim and his colleagues presented a picture of the activity evoked in the auditory nerve fibre array by a two-tone complex stimulus. For each of a large number of nerve fibres, they calculated the number of spikes phase-locked to the stimulus tone or combination tone of interest, divided by the number of spontaneous spikes. The results were then sideways averaged over fibres of a small range of characteristic frequencies, to produce the running averages illustrated here.

The activity phase-locked to the primaries (f_1 and f_2) was most prominent in fibres of those characteristic frequencies (arrows). Activity phase-locked to $2f_1 - f_2$ was most prominent in fibres tuned to $2f_1 - f_2$. (There was also phase-locking to $f_2 - f_1$, which was deleted for the purposes of the illustration.) The frequencies of f_1, f_2, and $2f_1 - f_2$ are indicated by the arrows. Note that fibres of high characteristic frequency are plotted to the left of the figure, so that points on the left refer to the base of the cochlea. From Kim *et al.* (1980), Fig. 4.

reflection depends on the hair cells, because Mountain (1980) showed that the magnitude of an acoustic combination tone reflected into the ear canal was altered when the olivocochlear bundle was stimulated.

Because we do not yet know the exact stage from which energy is reflected, we are not able to say which of the possible nonlinearities is the one responsible for the combination tone. For instance, the nonlinearity generating the combination tone could be purely mechanical. The observation that it is affected by the olivocochlear bundle would then be explained by supposing that activation of the olivocochlear bundle changed the linearity of the passive mechanical properties of the stereocilia. On the other hand, if the electrical responses of the hair cells could somehow generate mechanical movements, the nonlinearity of the transducer itself could be involved.

The hypothesis that energy is fed back to the basilar membrane neatly

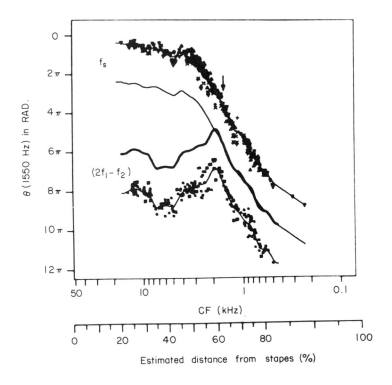

Fig. 5.15 The phase of the neurogram of the $2f_1 - f_2$ combination tone increases with distance apically to the site of generation, in just the same way as does the phase of an introduced tone (f_s). The points for the individual neurones are shown as well as the means; in the centre the mean curves have been shifted so as to coincide at the frequency indicated by the arrow. From Kim *et al.* (1979), Fig. 6.

explains why, of the two possible cubic distortion tones, it is the one that is lower in frequency ($2f_1 - f_2$, where $f_2 > f_1$) that is prominent. It is known that travelling waves in the cochlea move more readily in the apical than in the basal direction. Because the $2f_1 - f_2$ distortion tone is lower in frequency than the primaries, its travelling wave will readily move apically to the point in the cochlea at which it can produce a large resonance. The other distortion tone, $2f_2 - f_1$, is of higher frequency than the primaries, and to reach its resonant point would have to produce a wave travelling towards the base of the cochlea. Note that this explanation, unlike the provisional one suggested earlier, does not require a separate second filter.

The theory requires that a mechanical travelling wave corresponding to the distortion tone be present on the basilar membrane. It has not so far been detected by direct measurements. This may be because they do not have the required sensitivity. The position is controversial, and the reader is referred to a discussion on pp. 39–41 of Evans and Wilson (1977). However a microphonic response to $2f_1 - f_2$, with a small peak in the place in the cochlea tuned to that frequency, has been seen in the cochlear microphonic (Dallos *et al.*, 1980).

4. Conclusion

Auditory nerve fibre and hair cell responses both show that the cochlea behaves nonlinearly over the whole of its dynamic range, right down to threshold, even though the nonlinearity has not always been visible in the mechanical measurements. The nonlinearity may serve to increase the dynamic range of the auditory system.

F. Frequency Selectivity and the Second Filter

An idea that has been used several times so far, is that the initial stage of frequency filtering due to the travelling wave is followed by a second stage of filtering before the stage of neural excitation. The idea was originally suggested because auditory nerve fibres semed more sharply tuned than the travelling wave on the basilar membrane. At the moment the sharpness of tuning of the basilar membrane mechanics is uncertain, and it may well be that as techniques improve the tuning may be shown to be as sharp as that of auditory nerve fibres. The existence of the second filter is controversial, and some do not believe that it is necessary. Others who do, suggest that it may be purely mechanical, arising perhaps from the 'microresonance' of an extra resonator sitting on the organ of Corti, or following from the directional sensitivity of the stereocilia to deflection. Yet others believe that the second filter is a physiologically active process, perhaps dependent on a resonant electrical tuning of the hair cells themselves.

Because the existence of the second filter is controversial, the direct evidence for its existence will be described first. Then an example will be given from the turtle, where a distinct second filter is known to exist. Finally, indirect evidence for the second filter in the mammalian cochlea will be examined.

1. Direct Evidence for the Second Filter: Comparisons of Mechanical and Neural Frequency Selectivity

The basilar membrane tuning curves of Fig. 3.11 show consistently less frequency selectivity than the auditory nerve tuning curves of Fig. 4.3. This discrepancy has been viewed in two ways. One group, including Evans and co-workers (e.g. Evans, 1975b; Evans and Wilson, 1975) have suggested that the difference arises from the existence of a second filter between the travelling wave and the neural synapse. The other group, including particularly Pfeiffer, Kim and co-workers, have suggested that the difference arises from the nonlinearity of the basilar membrane's responses (e.g. Kim *et al.*, 1973; Goblick and Pfeiffer, 1969). Note that Rhode's basilar membrane results in Fig. 3.11D show that the tip becomes sharper at low levels. This arises because the effect of the nonlinearity is greatest at the tip. It prompts the thought, that were it possible to measure the mechanics at still lower intensities, in fact in the region where the neurones were generally measured, the tip would become even more prominent and the degrees of mechanical and neural selectivity would become equal.

Geisler *et al.* (1974) measured the response of single auditory nerve fibres in the squirrel monkey, in the same frequency and intensity range as the basilar membrane motion had been measured. The comparison is shown in Fig. 5.16. If there is a difference, it is confined to the tip. It must be remarked that this basilar membrane response is one of the sharpest that has been recorded, and that the neural threshold is rather high and the tip segment rather short, at least compared with the cat. Depending on their point of view, some workers are fond of pointing out the similarities between these two sets of data, and others the differences.

All the direct evidence on basilar membrane motion is at present in question. The techniques used for measuring the movement may not be accurate, or may involve disturbing the sharpness of the resonance. Given that, many workers have turned to indirect evidence to demonstrate the existence of the second filter. Before doing the same however, an example will be given from the turtle, where a second filter is known to exist, and resides in the membrane properties of the hair cells. (See also note on p. 70.)

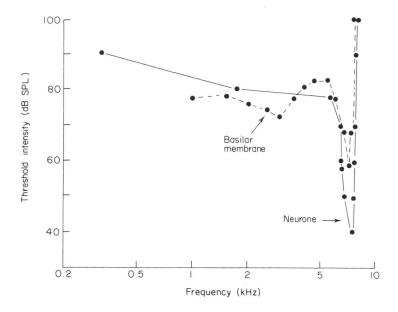

Fig. 5.16 In the squirrel monkey, there is some degree of agreement between the tuning of the mechanical response of the basilar membrane, and the tuning of single auditory nerve fibres. But is the difference at the tip significant? From Rhode (1978), Fig. 15.

2. A Second Filter in the Cochlea of the Turtle

The turtle possesses a basilar papilla, directly analogous to the mammalian organ of Corti, situated on a short basilar membrane. There are many hair cells across the width of the basilar papilla, with no differentiation corresponding to inner and outer hair cells. Crawford and Fettiplace (1980) recorded intracellularly from hair cells in the turtle *Pseudemys scripta elegans*. The response to a tone was an approximately sinusoidal voltage change with no sustained depolarization. The tuning curve showed great frequency selectivity, with 10 dB bandwidths averaging 125 Hz over the frequency range of the basilar papilla, which stretches from some 20 Hz to 800 Hz. The highest Q_{10} was 7.5, higher than that of mammals in the same frequency range. Evidence for an electrical second filter within the hair cell is shown in Fig. 5.17. Current pulses were injected into the hair cell through the recording electrode. The hair cell showed an electrical ringing at, or near, the characteristic frequency of the cell. It therefore appeared as though the hair cell contained a tuned electrical resonant circuit, which allowed it to oscillate in response to stimuli of the characteristic frequency.

Such an electrical resonance has been described before for both nerve cell and receptor cell membranes. Hodgkin and Huxley (1952) showed similar ringing in squid giant axon fibres. Bennett (1967) showed that fish electro-receptors could show dramatic and prolonged ringing under suitable conditions. Hopkins (1976) showed that this was associated with a sharp frequency selectivity for electrical detection. The explanation can be given in terms of electrically generated conductance changes in the cell membrane. Hodgkin and Huxley (1952) showed that when a nerve cell membrane was depolarized, the K^+ conductance increased with a time lag. The increase in K^+ conductance pulled the membrane voltage down towards the K^+ equilibrium potential, which is in the opposite, i.e. hyperpolarizing, direction. The cell would hyperpolarize, again with a time lag, this time given by the electrical time constant arising from the resistance and capacitance of the cell walls. Because the cell hyperpolarized, the K^+ conductance would then fall, causing the membrane potential to rise again, and so on. If the gains and time lags were right, the system would show a damped oscillation. This membrane resonance substantially accounts for the frequency response of the turtle hair cells (Crawford and Fettiplace, 1981a).

In the model, therefore, there is an initial trigger of an alternating voltage in the hair cell, which is amplified in a frequency selective way by the resonant properties of the cell membrane. The initial voltage change will, we presume, be produced by a mechanically-induced alternating resistance

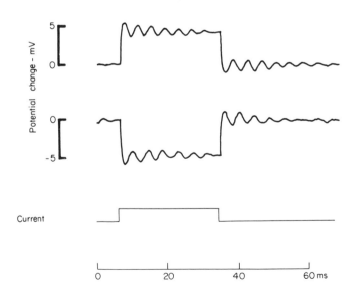

Fig. 5.17 Hair cells of the turtle cochlea show an electrical ringing at their CF, in response to step changes in membrane potential. Such ringing substantially accounts for the tuning of the hair cells. From Fettiplace and Crawford (1980), Fig. 2.

change in the apical cell membrane. We would expect this to be caused by deflection of the hairs, as found for the bullfrog sacculus (Hudspeth and Corey, 1977).

Elegant as this scheme is, there is reason to believe that it does not apply to the mammalian cochlea, at least over the greater part of its frequency range. In the turtle cochlea, the alternating voltage changes in the hair cell are a key stage in driving the membrane oscillator. Mammalian hair cells show sharply tuned direct as well as alternating voltage responses. Such direct voltage changes in the above model can only arise from a rectification of the alternating voltages, and so cannot exceed them. However, at high frequencies hair cells of the mammalian cochlea show direct voltage responses that are much larger than the alternating ones. Therefore the alternating changes cannot drive the direct ones, and the sharp tuning of the latter must arise from a different source.

3. Indirect Evidence for the Second Filter

(a) The vulnerability of the second filter

It has been suggested that the second filter is an active physiological mechanism, occurring after the purely passive first filter. In this case we might expect that agents which affected the normal metabolism of the cochlea might abolish the second filter, and that the neural and mechanical tuning curves would then match. Such a view was supported by the effects of kanamycin (Fig. 5.10) and by the effects of hypoxia and agents such as cyanide and loop diuretics. The tuning curves became rather like those of the basilar membrane shown in Fig. 3.11. This correspondence has been taken as evidence for a second filter (Evans, 1975b).

More recent work, however, has shown that the position is less clear than it once appeared to be. Firstly, the mechanical responses of the basilar membrane are sensitive to the physiological condition of the cochlea (Lepage and Johnstone, 1980). Manipulations intended to damage the hypothetical second filter may have affected the first. Secondly, kanamycin damage in the chinchilla can leave a sharply tuned tip or notch on the high frequency edge of the tuning curve (Fig. 10.1B). This has suggested the alternative hypothesis that the notch, or in other words the sharp tuning, arises from the first filter, and that the effect of the vulnerable element is to boost the sensitivity around the tip (Dallos and Harris, 1978). Although this boost can be thought of as a filtering process in that it is frequency dependent, it is rather a departure from the original notion of a second filter needed for sharp tuning. Third, kanamycin in the guinea-pig alters the tuning curves so markedly, that match with even the broad tuning curves of Wilson and Johnstone (1975) becomes impossible. This can be seen particularly clearly with the place-frequency maps of the cochlea, which relate the distance along the basilar membrane to the characteristic frequency of the region. In the normal animal there is close agreement between the mechanical and neural place-frequency maps. After kanamycin damage, when fibres can lower their characteristic frequency by as much as an octave, this match becomes lost (Robertson and Johnstone, 1979). But if a second filter normally exists, the neural place-frequency map should match the mechanical one especially well when the second filter has been abolished. Figure 5.10 shows additional evidence that the neural tuning curve after kanamycin is unlikely to be the same as the mechanical one. The characteristic frequency of the normal tuning curve is well beyond the high frequency cutoff of the abnormal one. If the abnormal tuning curve was equal to the mechanical one, then this frequency mismatch would in the normal animal lead to a large and maladaptive loss in sensitivity.

It should be added that not all treatments shift the characteristic frequency to this extent; for instance cyanide and anoxia in the cat abolish the sharply tuned tip of the tuning curve with very little effect on the best frequency (Evans, 1975b).

The conclusion is that, although the cochlea has to be in a good physiological condition to show normal frequency selectivity and sensitivity, this cannot be taken as evidence that there is a broadly tuned mechanical first filter and a sharply tuned, physiologically vulnerable, second one.

(b) Evidence from nonlinearities

In explaining some of the nonlinearities of the cochlea, models using two filters were introduced several times. It is worth therefore examining those arguments, to see how strongly they suggest a second filter.

One of the most successful of the two filter models, the BPNL model, suggests that there is a frequency-independent nonlinearity sandwiched between two linear filters. On this model, a second filter is required to explain how some tones can suppress but not excite—they get through the broadly tuned first filter to the nonlinearity and so contribute suppression, but are then filtered out by the second filter and so do not contribute excitation. Nevertheless, two filters are not necessarily required to explain the observed frequency relations of two-tone suppression. A *single* filter, if it itself behaves nonlinearly, can generate the suppression areas shown in Figs. 4.15 and 4.16 (Crawford and Fettiplace, 1981b).

Another nonlinear phenomenon for which a second filter had to be introduced was that of the generation of combination tones. A first filter was necessary to explain why the intensity of the combination tone produced was dependent on the frequency separation of the primaries. This suggested that the stage generating the combination tone occurred after a first stage of frequency filtering. A second filter was required to explain how neurones could respond to the combination tone without a response to the primaries. However, in order to explain further aspects of the data, it was necessary to suppose that the combination tone itself produced a mechanical travelling wave on the basilar membrane. Such a travelling wave would then act as a filter, and do the job of filtering out the combination tone from the primaries. In this case, the 'second' filter is the 'first' one appearing for the second time. A separate second filter is therefore not required (pp. 139-143).

In conclusion, although two filters have been incorporated in models of nonlinear phenomena, on examination the second filter turns out not to be required.

4. Models for the Second Filter

In the past, several models for the second filter have been proposed. Because new models are being proposed all the time, and because it is not even certain that a second filter is necessary, they will be listed only briefly.

(a) An electrical resonance in hair cells

In the turtle cochlea, there is good evidence that the second filter depends on electrical resonances in the hair cell membrane (Crawford and Fettiplace, 1981a). The oscillator can be derived from the known characteristics of nerve membranes. In its original form, the model does not apply to the mammalian cochlea because inner hair cells of the mammalian cochlea show sharply tuned d.c. potentials that are larger than their a.c. potentials (see discussion on p. 147).

(b) Directional sensitivity of hair cells

Duifhuis (1976) suggested that the second filter existed because hair cells were most sensitive to a shear in the radial direction. The mechanical travelling wave shown by von Békésy produced not only a vertical displacement of the basilar membrane, but a radial one. The radial displacements were more sharply tuned and peaked more basally in the cochlea. The model generates the tuning of hair cells and the nonlinear phenomena of the cochlea in a very natural way. However it requires that neurones be tuned to a frequency some 20% lower than the vertical displacements of the mechanical travelling wave at the same point, and this does not seem to be the case (Robertson and Johnstone, 1979).

(c) Spatial differentiation on the basilar membrane

Some workers have suggested that factors such as the slope and curvature of the basilar membrane rather than its displacement are related to hair cell excitation. Such parameters, which depend on the *gradient* of displacement along the basilar membrane, and its higher spatial derivatives, are more sharply tuned than the displacement, and could constitute a second filter. Hall (1980), for instance, proposed such a second filter to explain two-tone suppression. No physical explanation was given of why excitation should be related to the slope of displacement or the curvature of the basilar membrane; however, it is a reminder that we do not have any *direct* evidence for the hinging scheme of Davis, illustrated in Fig. 3.3, in which basilar membrane displacement in the vertical direction alone is the critical factor.

(d) Microresonance on the basilar membrane

Zwislocki and Kletsky (1980) suggested that the tectorial membrane could undergo elastic vibrations in the radial direction, forming a resonator sitting on top of the organ of Corti and increasing the shear at the hair cells in a frequency-dependent way. In this model, the mass in the resonator is provided by the mass of the tectorial membrane, and the spring by the stiffness of the stereocilia. Allen (1980) showed that such a model could account not only for sharp tuning, but also for some of the odd notches seen in the tuning curves of auditory nerve fibres (e.g. in Fig. 4.3, in the fibre of characteristic frequency 500 Hz, at 700 Hz). It also explains how outer hair cells could affect the response of the inner hair cells, because their stereocilia are necessary for the resonator. But it does not say why outer hair cells have many of the morphological characteristics of transducing structures, nor does it give a function for the cochlear microphonic.

G. Summary

1. Davis's battery or resistance modulation hypothesis forms a framework for theories of transduction in the cochlea. Under this hypothesis, the travelling wave on the basilar membrane causes deflection of the stereocilia, reducing the resistance of the apical membrane of the hair cells. The endolymphatic potential and the negative intracellular potential combine to form a battery driving current through the varying resistance, producing the cochlear microphonic and exciting the nerve endings at the base of the hair cell.

2. The evidence points to the stereocilia, either at their base or along their length, as containing the membrane at which resistance modulation occurs. However that does not explain why deflection of the stereocilia in one direction causes excitation, and deflection in the other, suppression.

3. It is likely that deformation opens channels in the membrane which are not specific to any particular ions. It is also possible that the particular nature of the channels contributes to the very high sensitivity of the transduction process.

4. It is likely that the relation between deflection of the stereocilia and resistance change is nonlinear, so that a sound stimulus will produce a net decrease in resistance as well as an alternating one, and a direct potential change as well as an alternating one. This is supported by measurements of resistance across the whole cochlear partition, as well as by measurements of resistance changes in single inner hair cells. However, measurements of the resistance of the cochlear partition also show some changes that cannot be fitted into Davis's scheme, and it is possible that voltage-sensitive ion channels are present as well.

5. The amplitude of movement of the basilar membrane at threshold is probably much greater than had been suggested by the early measurements of von Békésy. This may be because the basilar membrane moves nonlinearly, the amplitude of vibration increasing to a smaller and smaller extent as the stimulus intensity is increased.

6. The origin and extent of the nonlinearity of the basilar membrane's vibration is a matter of current debate. The basilar membrane may move nonlinearly over the whole of its range, right from threshold to the highest intensities. The nonlinear movement depends on the cochlea being in good physiological condition. The nonlinearity serves to increase the dynamic range of hearing.

    The evidence for the nonlinearity comes from direct mechanical measurements of the movement of the basilar membrane, particularly by Rhode. Others however have not shown the nonlinearity. Strong evidence for nonlinearity comes from the responses of inner hair cells and auditory nerve fibres. When two tone stimuli are used, they show evidence of nonlinear interactions, resulting in two-tone suppression and responses to combination tones.

7. When the hair cells are activated, mechanical energy is returned to the basilar membrane. The return of energy may be a purely passive reflection, but there is some evidence that a stage of amplification is involved. The mechanism behind the return of the energy is not known, except that it depends on the function of the hair cells. The return of mechanical energy to the basilar membrane sets up a traveling wave on the basilar membrane, which travels apically in the normal way. Such a travelling wave carries, for instance, the distortion tone $2f_1 - f_2$, which is

generated by nonlinearities where f_1 and f_2 overlap, to its more apical site of transduction.

The return of mechanical energy by the transducer also sets up a pressure wave travelling towards the base of the cochlea. Some of the energy is transmitted through the middle ear and can be measured as sound in the external auditory meatus. A proportion of the energy is reflected back from the base of the cochlea. It is thought that multiple reflections, together with a mechanically amplifying stage, can sometimes lead to sustained oscillations in the cochlea which can be heard as tinnitus and which can be recorded objectively as sound pressure fluctuations in the external ear canal.

8. Both inner and outer hair cells are necessary for the normal responses of auditory nerve fibres. The responses of auditory nerve fibres closely follow the responses of inner hair cells, to which the great majority are connected. Outer hair cells are necessary for the low threshold and perhaps sharp tuning of inner hair cells and so of auditory nerve fibres. This can be shown by the application of ototoxic agents to the cochlea, some of which differentially affect outer hair cells. Such agents abolish the low-threshold sharply-tuned tip of the tuning curves of auditory nerve fibres. The mechanism for the interaction between inner and outer hair cells is not known: it could possibly be electrical, by means of local currents in the organ of Corti, or mechanical, the stereocilia of the outer hair cells possibly affecting the mode of vibration of structures on the basilar membrane.

9. It has been suggested that at low frequencies inner and outer hair cells interact in phase opposition; if in one phase of vibration of the basilar membrane the inner hair cell was activating the nerve fibre, the outer hair cell would be contributing inhibition, and vice versa. There are further complications, because at low frequencies inner hair cells respond to velocity, and outer hair cells to displacement. This probably stems from the different modes of coupling of the stereocilia to the tectorial membrane in the two cases. The stereocilia of outer hair cells actually touch the tectorial membrane, whereas those of inner hair cells do not, and so will be moved by viscous drag.

10. Auditory nerve fibres show sharper tuning than does the basilar membrane. This difference may be real, or may reflect inadequacies of the present techniques for measuring basilar membrane movement. Because all mechanical measurements of the basilar membrane vibration are at present in doubt, the necessity for a second filter is problematical. Many models of other phenomena in the cochlea, such as

two-tone suppression and the response to combination tones, incorporate a second filter. But on closer examination the second filter can be dispensed with in the models, and so the phenomena cannot be used as evidence for a second filter. Some recent measurements have shown the basilar membrane and auditory nerve fibres to have comparable tuning. See note on p. 70.

11. The mechanism of the second filter, if it exists, is not known. It has been suggested that the second filter arises from the interrelation of the mechanical movements of the basilar membrane with the directional sensitivity of hair cells, or from a 'microresonance' of the tectorial membrane on top of the organ of Corti. In the turtle cochlea, a definite second filter is known to exist. It depends on an electrical oscillation of the hair cell membrane, arising from voltage-sensitive ionic conductances in the membrane. But there is reason to believe that the same mechanism does not apply in the mammalian cochlea.

H. Further Reading

Dallos (1973a), Chapter 5 and especially pp. 366–390 has a useful discussion of transducer processes. Particularly penetrating discussions, although not having the benefit of the more recent observations, will be found in Flock (1971) and Fex (1974). Some of the newest ideas of cochlear functioning are discussed in articles in the *J. Acoustical Soc. Am.* 1980, **67**, 1679 — 1735. Articles by Zwislocki, Lim, Rhode, Kim *et al.*, Hall and Geisler *et al.*, are recommended. Dallos (1981) also has a good review of recent work.

VI. The Brain Stem Nuclei

The responses of the brain stem auditory nuclei will be described in terms of the neural temporal firing patterns, neural frequency resolution, excitatory–inhibitory interactions, response to complex stimuli and, where appropriate, binaural interactions. Auditory brain stem reflexes and what little information we have on the involvement of brain stem auditory nuclei in learning will be described.

A. Considerations in Studying the Central Nervous System

Many experiments have shown that single auditory nerve fibres have qualitatively uniform properties, although the fibres may vary quantitatively in factors such as bandwidth, spontaneous firing rate, and threshold. It is therefore comparatively easy (but still difficult!) to describe the properties of the whole population from a small number of experiments. In the cochlear nucleus however there are many different cell types and regions. Therefore, giving a complete description is already very difficult, and it is much easier to undertake experiments and analyse the results, if we have some theories as to the function of the system.

Three themes can be discerned in the analysis of sensory systems. One concerns 'feature detection'. In such an analysis, we suppose that certain features of the sensory environment are selectively extracted. In the visual system, the scheme of Hubel and Wiesel (1962) has had great appeal. Here, cortical cells were described as responding selectively to lines and edges in various orientations. In the auditory system, it has unfortunately been difficult to describe any critical features beyond the rather elementary ones, either from psychological experiments aimed at finding important features

154

to look for, or from electrophysiological experiments in which neuronal responses to complex stimuli were analysed. For instance, at a simple level, lateral inhibition seems to emphasize the contrast in the neuronal representation of a spectral pattern. This could be said to be one example of feature detection. At a slightly more advanced level, cells in the dorsal cochlear nucleus have been found, which give particularly strong responses to stimuli, which are either amplitude or frequency modulated. But even here, there seems to be continuum in the complexity of neuronal responses, and it is very difficult to decide the extent to which such features are preferentially extracted. It is therefore difficult to decide whether we are entitled to think of such modulated stimuli as forming specific 'features' of particular significance for the nervous system. These problems are compounded further, when the analysis of complex sounds such as those of speech is considered in a high level structure such as the auditory cortex.

A second theme is the localization of functions to the activity of individual cells. In the context of feature detection, it involves finding cells that respond to specific features, so that the detection of a feature can be defined by the activity of single cells studied in isolation. At the other end of a continuum, detection might only be defined by the pattern of activity over many cells. In a common analogy, the first case might be compared to a photograph, in which each point on the photograph represents one point in space, whereas the opposite end of the continuum might be compared to a hologram, in which each point on the hologram represents many points in space, and in which individual points in space can be reconstructed only by the integration of information from many points on the hologram. Undoubtedly, many of the more complex features will only be represented in the second form, and at any level of the auditory system we might expect to find many coexisting stages in between the two extremes. In the context of feature detection, features that are not represented by the activity of individual cells can only be represented by the pattern of activity over many cells. A simple example is seen in the auditory nerve. The fibres of the auditory nerve, by their sharp tuning, appear to be specialized for the detection of specific frequencies. Sharp tuning in such a quasi-linear system is necessarily correlated with poor temporal resolution. Yet sound localization experiments show the auditory system is able to detect temporal disparities of the order of 10 μs, and it is generally hypothesized that such accuracy is achieved by the integration of activity over many fibres.

A third theme is that of hierarchical processing, in which successively more complex analyses are performed at ascending levels of the nervous system. If the only points of interest in an acoustic environment are, say, vowel formants, then it is obviously economical to extract the formants at an early stage in the system, reject all other information, and perform further processing on the information given by the formants.

Schemes for sensory analysis based on the logical extremes of each of the three themes, that is, on the extraction of specific features, on the representation of the features in the activity of single cells, and on hierarchical analysis, naturally spring to mind. But it is likely that the auditory system operates far from these logical extremes on all three points. Such a mode of operation has contributed greatly to the difficulty of the electrophysiological analysis of the central auditory nervous system.

B. The Cochlear Nuclei

1. Anatomy

In view of the diversity of the properties of cochlear nucleus neurones, anatomical studies are vital in aiding the physiologist in his analysis of the functions of the nuclei.

Each fibre of the auditory nerve branches on entering the nucleus, sending one branch rostrally and the other caudally. The rostral branch innervates the division known as the anteroventral cochlear nucleus, whereas the caudal branch innervates both the posteroventral division of the nucleus and the dorsal cochlear nucleus (Fig. 6.1A). We might expect the orderly arrangement of the incoming fibres to be reflected in an orderly arrangement of characteristic frequencies of the neurones they innervate, leading to a 'tonotopic' frequency map. Such maps are indeed found (Rose *et al.*, 1960). But instead of two maps, one for each branch of the auditory nerve, there are in fact three, one corresponding to each of the above-named divisions of the nucleus. One map is supplied by the rostral branch of the

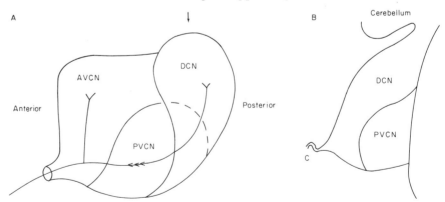

Fig. 6.1 A. A sagittal section of the cat cochlear nucleus shows the three divisions of the nucleus, innervated by a branching auditory nerve fibre. AVCN: anteroventral cochlear nucleus; PVCN: posteroventral cochlear nucleus; DCN: dorsal cochlear nucleus.
B. Transverse section of the cochlear nucleus, at the point marked by the arrow in A; C: choroid plexus.

auditory nerve, and the other two by the caudal branch. Figure 6.1C shows two of the tonotopic maps, encountered as an electrode was moved from the dorsal to the anteroventral cochlear nuclei.

These three divisions of the cochlear nucleus show broadly different response properties, and it is very likely that they have correspondingly different functions. In general, neurones of the anteroventral cochlear nucleus have properties rather similar to those of auditory nerve fibres, and may well function much as a simple relay for afferent information. Cells of the dorsal cochlear nucleus on the other hand have very much more complex response properties, and may therefore contribute to complex signal analy-

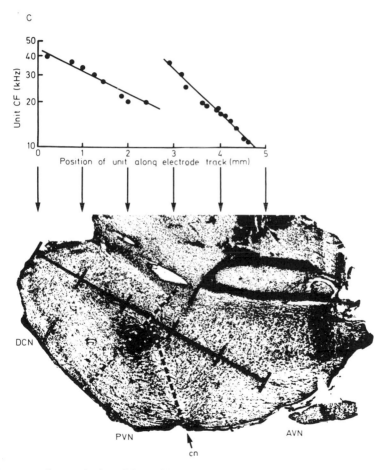

C. The tonotopic organization of the cochlear nucleus. Two separate high–low sequences were seen as a recording electrode was moved from the dorsal to the anteroventral cochlear nucleus. Sagittal section. From Evans (1974a), Fig. 28.

sis. Their output axons bypass the next nucleus in the auditory pathway, the superior olivary complex, and end in the nuclei of the lateral lemniscus and the inferior colliculus. The properties of many neurones of the posteroventral nucleus are intermediate to those of the other two. Interestingly, the dorsal cochlear nucleus is comparatively small in primates.

The detailed study of the cells of the cochlear nucleus has led to the hope that different functional characteristics can be associated with the different cell types. The mapping of cell types is due to Osen (1969) and Brawer *et al.* (1974), both in the cat. The schemes are generally similar; the terminology used here is that of Osen.

Certain areas can be defined as most obviously being occupied by certain cells. In the anterior pole of the anteroventral cochlear nucleus there is an

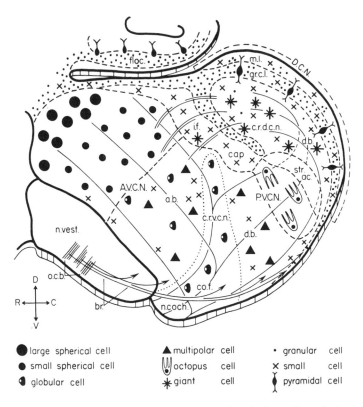

Fig. 6.2 A cytoarchitectural map of the cochlear nucleus is shown in sagittal section. The predominant cell types in each region are represented. AVCN: anteroventral nucleus; cap: peripheral cap of small cells; crdcn; central region of DCN; crvcn: central region of ventral nucleus; DCN: dorsal nucleus; floc: floculus (cerebellum); gcl: granular cell layer; if: intrinsic fibres; ml: molecular layer; PVCN: posteroventral nucleus; strac: dorsal and intermediate acoustic striae. From Osen and Roth (1969), Fig. 1.

area of large spherical cells (Fig. 6.2), although there are other cells among them. Auditory nerve fibres contact the large spherical cells by means of particularly large synaptic endings known as end-bulbs of Held, as well as by smaller endings. Caudal to this area there is an area of smaller spherical cells, and then one of globular cells (Fig. 6.2). Octopus cells, known as such from the pattern of their dendrites, although Morest *et al.* (1973) remark that they look more like ostrich cells (Fig. 6.3), occupy a region of the posteroventral cochlear nucleus called the octopus cell area. The area consists almost entirely of octopus cells. The other areas of the postero-ventral cochlear nucleus contain a variety of cells. The dorsal cochlear nucleus caps the posteroventral nucleus both dorsally and caudally. It contains a striking layer of cells with double processes, one orientated towards the surface of the nucleus and one towards the centre. The cells have been called fusiform cells or pyramidal cells in different terminologies. There are also 'giant' cells deep in the dorsal nucleus. Many other smaller cells are distributed throughout the whole cochlear nucleus, some of which are likely to be interneurones.

2. Physiology

(a) Classification on the basis of responses in time

In an electrophysiological experiment, Pfeiffer (1966a) classified cells of the cochlear nucleus by the apparently arbitrary, but in fact useful, criterion of the time pattern of the response to short tone bursts, delivered just above threshold at the neurone's characteristic frequency.

(i) *Primary-like cells*. These have poststimulus time histograms (PSTHs) to tones similar to those of auditory nerve fibres, with an initial peak at the onset, declining gradually to lower levels (Fig. 6.4A). Such units are found throughout the ventral cochlear nucleus. In particular, those in the antero-ventral cochlear nucieus resemble auditory nerve fibres in other ways, for instance in the shape of the tuning curve, the degree of phase-locking to low frequency stimuli, monotonic rate-intensity functions, lack of inhibitory sidebands, and relative independence of response classification on intensity. There is evidence that some of the spherical cells of the anteroventral nucleus form at least some of the primary-like neurones. For instance, primary-like responses are obtained from the spherical cell area. Stronger indirect evidence comes from the waveform of the extracellular action potential. Many such recordings show a positive deflection just before the usual monophasic or diphasic waveform recorded from a cell body, and Pfeiffer (1966b) suggested that this corresponded to the depolarization of the large end-bulbs of Held, the presynaptic endings on the auditory nerve fibres on the cells. The primary-like responses, together with the short

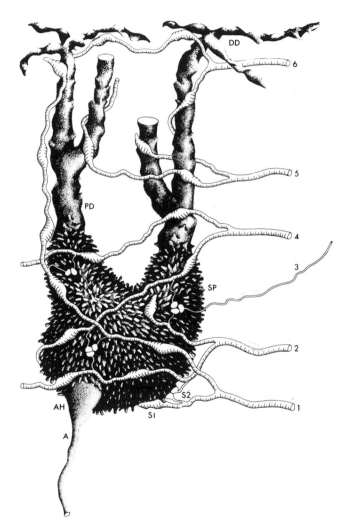

Fig. 6.3 An octopus cell. The thick auditory nerve fibres ((1,2,4,5,6) give rise to large endings (S1) on the cell, and branch to give thin fibres, which, together with thin afferent auditory nerve axons (3) give rise to small secondary endings (S2). The cell is covered with stubby appendages (SP). AH: axon hillock; a: axon. From Morest *et al.* (1973), Fig. 2.

synaptic delay on these cells, as well as the time pattern of the spontaneous activity, suggests the existence of what have been called 'secure' synaptic connections, in which each afferent action potential produces an action potential in the output. This suggests that the cells act to relay the activity of auditory nerve fibres to the higher centres in a straightforward manner.

(ii) *Onset responses*. Cells showing onset responses produce a sharp peak in the PSTH at the beginning of a tone burst, and then either no activity, or a low level of sustained activity (Fig. 6.4B). Such cells are found throughout the cochlear nucleus. However, one region has proved of particular interest. The octopus cell area produces only onset responses, and the area consists almost entirely of octopus cells. It is therefore very likely that octopus cells generate onset responses (Godfrey *et al.*, 1975a). We might suppose that there is an excitatory input, and then a delayed inhibitory input. Kane (1973) found that in fact single auditory nerve fibres gave rise to two types of synapse on octopus cells. There are large, primary, endings covering much of the cell surface. But the afferent axons branch, sending finer processes with smaller boutons to the same cells (Fig. 6.3). It was suggested that a single axon could produce both the initial, rapid, excitatory effect, and the delayed inhibitory effect, by the two types of terminal. It is unfortunate for this story that intracellular recording has not so far found a period of hyperpolarization during the inhibition after the initial onset response (Britt and Starr, 1976a).

Presumably the inhibition following the onset response will inhibit a response to the next stimulus if the stimuli are presented rapidly enough. Such units will follow every click in a rapid train of clicks up to a certain click rate, beyond which the response drops precipitously (Godfrey *et al.*, 1975a). Such cells behave similarly to those investigated more extensively by Møller (1969). They may code the periodicity of complex stimuli, although there are some theoretical objections to the idea that they may be responsible for periodicity pitch (Chapter 9). The cells have wide tuning curves, and this may be a correlate of the great degree of synaptic convergence in their inputs.

(iii) *Chopper Responses*. Chopper units tend to fire repetitively during a sustained tone burst at a rate that is unrelated to the period of the stimulus waveform. The PSTH therefore shows a series of peaks, which, because the timing of the spikes becomes rather ragged during the latter part of the tone burst, declines towards the end (Fig. 6.4C). The increasing raggedness is better seen in the raster diagram showing the timing of the spikes during each tone burst (Fig. 6.4D). Presumably such cells receive a large number of synaptic inputs, which summate to produce a smooth depolarizing membrane potential, with firing and resetting whenever it reaches threshold. Identification of chopper responses with any particular cell type is not

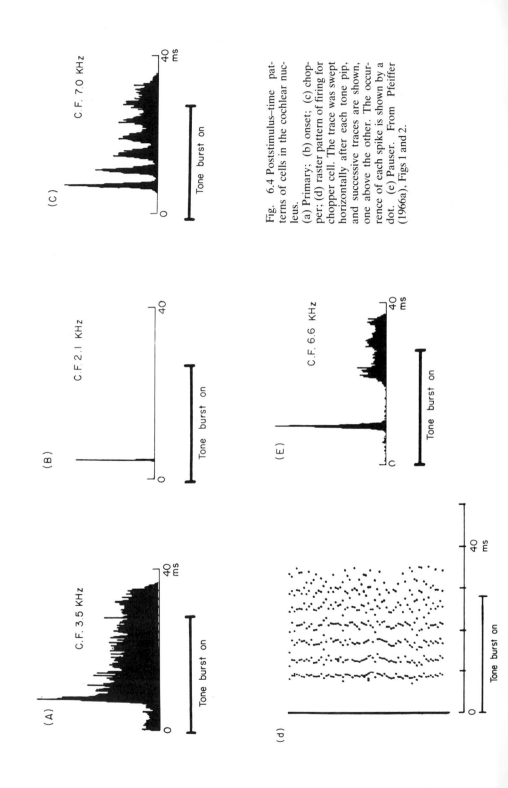

Fig. 6.4 Poststimulus–time patterns of cells in the cochlear nucleus.
(a) Primary; (b) onset; (c) chopper; (d) raster pattern of firing for chopper cell. The trace was swept horizontally after each tone pip, and successive traces are shown, one above the other. The occurrence of each spike is shown by a dot. (e) Pauser. From Pfeiffer (1966a), Figs 1 and 2.

possible, since the responses are found throughout the cochlear nucleus. However, they are strongly represented in some regions of the posteroventral nucleus and the deep layers of the dorsal nucleus (Godfrey *et al.*, 1975a,b).

(iv) *Pauser and Buildup responses.* Pauser cells show an initial onset response, a silent period, and then a gradual resumption of activity (Fig. 6.4E). Buildup units were identified by Rose *et al.* (1959) as those that did not show the initial onset component, but whose activity increased slowly with time. Cells with these two patterns of response are found particularly in the fusiform layer of the dorsal cochlear nucleus (Godfrey *et al.*, 1975b). The response properties change markedly with changes in stimulus parameters, and it is likely that the temporal pattern is an indication of the complex excitatory and inhibitory inputs playing on the cells. It is therefore possible that such cells may be extracting certain complex features from the auditory stimulus.

(b) Patterns of excitation and inhibition

No neural inhibitory responses are seen in single fibres of the auditory nerve. All suppressive phenomena arise from the nonlinearity of the excitatory transduction process, or follow a period of excitation. However, cells of the cochlear nucleus show strong inhibition arising from inhibitory synapses. In contrast to the auditory nerve, spontaneous as well as stimulus-evoked activity can be reduced. In general, least inhibition is found in the anteroventral division of the cochlear nucleus, where the cells seem to be closest to auditory nerve fibres in their response characteristics, and increasing degrees of inhibition are found as the posteroventral, and then dorsal cochlear nuclei are approached.

Evans and Nelson (1973a) carried out an extensive investigation of the excitatory–inhibitory properties of cells of the cochlear nucleus of the cat. At one extreme, cells were found with properties very similar to those of auditory nerve fibres, with similar response areas and no inhibitory responses beyond those arising from suppression in the auditory nerve (Fig. 6.5A). Although Evans and Nelson did not make the correlation, it is reasonable to suppose that these corresponded to the primary-like cells of Pfeiffer (1966a). An intermediate type of cell showed an excitatory tuning curve surrounded by inhibitory sidebands (Fig. 6.5B). At high intensities, the inhibitory sidebands could overlap the excitatory response area, and served to narrow down the region of excitation. Thus lateral inhibition could at high intensities increase the frequency resolving power of the cochlear nucleus, at least for tones. This only applies to the response well above threshold. It seems that the *tips* of the tuning curves are no narrower in the dorsal cochlear nucleus than in the auditory nerve (Goldberg and Brownell, 1973).

These increasing degrees of inhibition seen at high intensities are often associated with nonmonotonic rate-intensity functions (Fig. 6.6).

Still stronger inhibitory phenomena were found as the sampling electrode moved towards the dorsal cochlear nucleus. In the dorsal nucleus of chloralose-anaesthetized or decerebrate animals, neurones were found whose response areas were entirely or almost entirely inhibitory, perhaps possessing a narrow island of excitation (Fig. 6.4 C and D). Such particularly

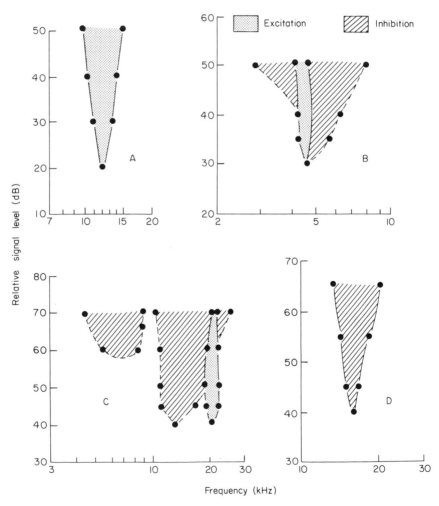

Fig. 6.5 Tuning curves of excitation and inhibition in the cat cochlear nucleus are shown in order of increasing amounts of inhibition (A–D). Purely excitatory responses as in A are predominant in the AVCN. Greater amounts of inhibition are found in the DCN (B–D). From Evans and Nelson (1973a), Figs 2, 5, 7 and 9.

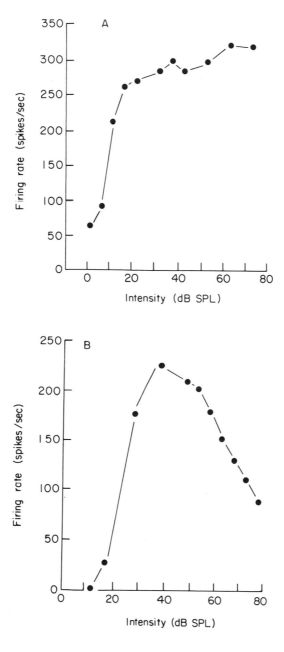

Fig. 6.6 Monotonic (A) and nonmotonic (B) rate-intensity functions in the cochlear nucleus. A is typical of neurones showing only weak inhibitory sidebands, and B of those with strong ones. Adapted from Greenwood and Goldberg (1970).

strong inhibition was blocked by barbiturate anaesthesia and therefore was not seen in earlier experiments. Pfeiffer's classification, performed in experiments under barbiturate anaesthesia, did not include any wholly inhibitory classes, but it is likely that his onset, buildup and pauser types resulted from delayed inhibitory inputs.

Evans and Nelson (1973b) suggested, in contrast to the ideas then current, that the functionally dominant input of the cells of the dorsal cochlear nucleus, that is, the inhibitory input, did not arise from the fibres of the auditory nerve directly innervating the dorsal nucleus, but was relayed from the ventral nucleus by an intranuclear association pathway. The dorsal cochlear nucleus would then be essentially a second order rather than a first order relay nucleus. However, such a conclusion is still rather controversial. Voigt and Young (1980) presented evidence that the predominantly inhibitory neurones of the dorsal cochlear nucleus received their inhibitory input from interneurones in the dorsal nucleus itself.

The analysis of excitation and inhibition suggests that a functional division between two components of the auditory pathway has already occurred at the cochlear nucleus. One pathway, arising from the ventral cochlear nucleus, preserves in many ways the response characteristics of primary auditory nerve fibres. That pathway feeds directly by secure, short-latency, synapses to the superior olivary complex, where, among other things, spatial information is extracted. The other, arising from the dorsal nucleus, introduces extensive complexity early in the auditory pathway, and by bypassing the superior olivary complex feeds directly to higher centres, such as the nuclei of the lateral lemniscus and the inferior colliculus. There the results of the complex frequency analyses are combined with the results of the spatial analyses performed at the superior olive.

(c) The analysis of complex stimuli

We might expect the complex response areas of the dorsal cochlear nucleus to be appropriate for the analysis of complex stimuli. It is unfortunate that most of the experiments with complex stimuli have been performed under barbiturate anaesthesia, which reduced the amount of inhibition.

Stimuli which spread onto the inhibitory sidebands of neurones possessing them will, of course, reduce the firing rate. If therefore a band of noise is centred on the characteristic frequency of such a neurone, and increased in width, the firing rate will at first increase, as more noise falls into the excitatory response area, and then decrease, as some of the noise falls in the inhibitory sidebands. Such effects, which are analogous to those occurring in the auditory nerve as a result of suppression, were described by Greenwood and Goldberg (1970) in the cochlear nucleus. They are of course much stronger in the nucleus than the nerve, as might be expected from the greater strength of inhibition.

When a tone is presented in wideband noise, we might expect that the inhibitory sidebands would suppress the weaker parts of the stimulus pattern, so emphasizing the stronger parts. We would therefore expect them to enhance the response, relative to the background, of a tone in wideband masking noise. Although there have been comparatively few studies of this important phenomenon, Greenwood and Goldberg (1970) showed with certain narrowband background stimuli that lateral inhibition could indeed lead to the expected increase in emphasis of the stronger parts of the stimulus pattern. We would also expect that under such circumstances the firing would depend on the contrast in the stimulus pattern rather than on the overall intensity; such a point was confirmed in a cell of the dorsal cochlear nucleus by Evans and Palmer (1975). A similar point was made by Evans (1977): the response to a spectrally complex pattern of constant contrast was constant over a very wide range of overall stimulus intensity.

More detailed investigation shows that, although this picture may be representative for those cells with an excitatory centre and inhibitory sidebands, it may not be so for cells with more complicated response areas, similar for instance to those shown in Fig. 6.5C. Young and Brownell (1976) in unanaesthetized cats showed that broadband noise was able to drive such cells more strongly than any tone. In some cases, both tones and noise were excitatory near threshold, but at higher intensities tones became inhibitory and noise was excitatory. Such a finding is rather paradoxical, since we would expect that the interplay of excitation and inhibition in a complex response area would *reduce* the response to broadband stimuli in comparison with that to tones. Voigt and Young (1980) showed that these units were themselves inhibited by those cells with the simpler organization of an excitatory centre and an inhibitory surround. Broadband stimuli therefore inhibited an otherwise inhibitory input, and led to excitation. Such cells may, therefore, be specialized for the detection of broadband stimuli. However, it is clear that we do not have the evidence to assess the role of cells with complex response areas in the detection of complex features.

In view of the interplay of excitation and inhibition in the responses of single cells, and the likelihood of different latencies for the different inputs, it is not surprising that interesting responses can be obtained with stimuli which vary in time, such as for instance tones swept in either frequency or intensity across the response area. Dynamic factors were shown to be important in determining the responses of such cells, because the responses to time-varying stimuli could not be predicted from the responses to static tones. In this, they were in contrast to cells with simpler response areas, or primary nerve fibres (Britt and Starr, 1976b). Moreover, neurones with either complex and asymmetrical response areas, or many with buildup or pauser time patterns, showed marked asymmetries as a tone was swept in frequency across the response area (Nelson and Evans, 1971; Britt and

Starr, 1976b). In some extreme cases, neurones were found which responded to a frequency sweep in one direction and not to one in the other. Britt and Starr (1976b) by intracellular recording showed that two different types of inhibition were involved, one arising from stimulation of the inhibitory surround, and the other arising from the off-inhibition following a period of excitation.

Møller (1978) has shown that in certain cells of the cochlear nucleus frequency-modulated tones could produce stronger responses than steady tones. Sometimes the cells were responsive to very small changes in the stimulus parameters. Similar, though less dramatic, selectivities were shown for amplitude-modulated tones. Many of these cells responded to the stimulating waveform in a relatively unchanged way over a wide range of stimulus intensities. It has been hypothesized that a regulating mechanism, perhaps negative feedback from inhibitory interneurones, tends to keep the mean firing rate constant while allowing rapid changes to be transmitted (Møller, 1976).

What is uncertain is the extent to which we are able to think in terms of feature detection in the cochlear nucleus. There seems to be a continuum of response characteristics along every category of response that has been analysed. It is not therefore certain that we are justified in asserting that the degree to which any one feature is extracted, results from anything other than a random arrangement of excitation and inhibition on the constituent neurones. However, as a provisional hypothesis, we can assume that the cell types that have been demonstrated form the functional basis for a sensory analysis, that lies in between the logical extremes of the completely holistic and the completely nonholistic.

In the alert animal, the situation is even more complicated. Centrifugal connections from the higher centres innervate the nucleus, and the activity of the nucleus is likely to reflect later sensory processing, and the central state of the animal.

C. The Superior Olivary Complex

1. Innervation and Anatomy

There are three main outflows from the cochlear nucleus, as shown in Fig. 6.7. The fibres in the dorsal acoustic stria arise in the dorsal cochlear nucleus, and those in the intermediate acoustic stria in the posteroventral cochlear nucleus. However, the greatest outflow runs in the ventral acoustic stria or trapezoid body, and arises in both the anteroventral and posteroventral nuclei. The pathways of the dorsal acoustic stria bypass the superior olivary complex and end in the next highest nuclei, the nuclei of the lateral lemniscus and the inferior colliculus, predominantly on the opposite side (Fig. 6.8). The outflows in the ventral and intermediate striae end in the superior olivary complex of both sides, as well as to a lesser extent in the nuclei of the lateral lemniscus. Within the superior olivary complex itself, several subnuclei can be distinguished (Fig. 6.9), all receiving different distributions of fibres from the different regions of the cochlear nuclei. The main nuclei associated with the ascending auditory system are the lateral and medial nuclei of the superior olive (LSO and MSO), and the medial nucleus of the trapezoid body (MTB). The nuclei are surrounded by other nuclei, known as the pre-olivary and peri-olivary nuclei, which are mainly associated with the centrifugal auditory system, although they receive an ascending input as well. They will be discussed in Chapter 8. As far as the ascending system goes, the MTB is a relay carrying information from the opposite cochlear nucleus to the ipsilateral LSO. The MSO is a disc-shaped structure, and receives direct fibres from the cochlear nuclei of both sides. It is involved in detecting the direction of a sound source by means of the temporal disparities of the stimuli at the two ears. The LSO is the largest of

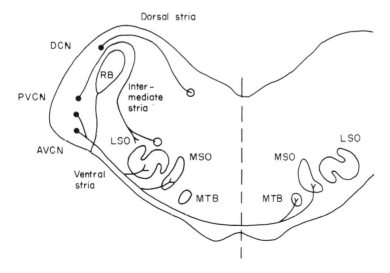

Fig. 6.7 The three main outflows of the cochlear nucleus are shown on a transverse section of the cat brain stem. The dorsal and intermediate acoustic striae pass dorsally around the restiform body (RB), or inferior cerebellar peduncle. The largest outflow is in the ventral acoustic stria or trapezoid body. AVCN: anteroventral cochlear nucleus; DCN: dorsal cochlear nucleus; MSO: medial nucleus of the superior olive; LSO: lateral nucleus of the superior olive; MTB: medial nucleus of the trapezoid body; PVCN: posteroventral cochlear nucleus. The small circles indicate fibres passing to higher levels. The fibres are represented diagramatically, and do not necessarily branch or join as indicated.

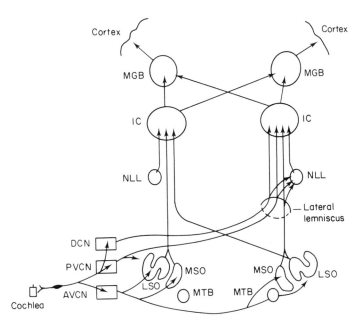

Fig. 6.8 The main ascending auditory pathways of the brain stem. Many minor pathways are not shown. IC: inferior colliculus; MGB: medial geniculate body; NLL: nucleus of the lateral lemniscus. For other abbreviations see Fig. 6.7. The branching and joining of arrows does not mean that the fibres branch or join.

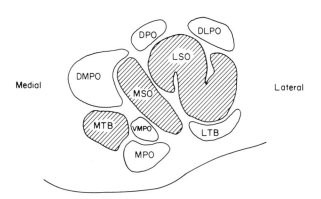

Fig. 6.9 The nuclei of the superior olivary complex are shown in a transverse section in the cat. The main nuclei associated with the ascending system are shaded. DLPO: dorsolateral perioli-vary nucleus; DMPO: dorsomedial periolivary nucleus; DPO: dorsal periolivary nucleus; LSO: lateral superior olivary nucleus; LTB: lateral nucleus of the trapezoid body; MPO: medial preolivary nucleus; MSO: medial superior olivary nucleus; MTB: medial nucleus of the trapezoid body; VMPO: ventromedial periolivary nucleus. From Harrison and Howe (1974b), Fig. 8.

the component nuclei, and has a characteristic structure of a folded sheet, which in the cat is S-shaped in transverse sections, but which in other species appears more like a boxing glove. It receives direct connections from the ipsilateral cochlear nucleus, and indirect ones from the contralateral nucleus via the MTB. In so far as this nucleus plays a role in sound localization, it detects disparities in interaural intensity.

2. Physiology and Function

(a) Introduction

Analysis of the dorsal cochlear nucleus has demonstrated that it may be difficult to assess the functional significance of a nucleus from the response characteristics of its neurones. However, the superior olive shows an advance in sensory processing, that of receiving information from the two ears, which surely must be of functional significance. It is reasonable to suppose that the nucleus plays a part in sound localization.

(b) The lateral superior olive (S-segment)

The principal cells of the LSO have dendritic trees joining the two surfaces of the folded sheet of the nucleus, with afferents from the ipsilateral cochlear nucleus and the ipsilateral MTB contacting the two branches (Fig. 6.10A). The cell characteristic frequencies are arranged tonotopically (Fig. 6.10B), although for a long time this was difficult to detect because of the complex folding of the structure (Tsuchitani and Boudreau, 1966). In the anaesthetized preparation, the responses to ipsilateral stimuli are entirely excitatory with tuning curves similar to those of primary fibres, best thresholds in the range 10–20 dB SPL, and chopper time patterns (Tsuchitani, 1977). Brownell *et al.* (1979) have more recently shown that when unanaesthetized cats are used, inhibitory sidebands can be seen to ipsilateral stimuli, and the chopper pattern disappears. Figure 6.11 shows an example of the response to a stimulus at the excitatory centre, and in the inhibitory sidebands. The organization of the excitatory response was more complex than that of the inhibitory one, since it was followed by a rebound. Unlike the responses to ipsilateral stimuli, the responses to contralateral stimuli were predominantly inhibitory in both anaesthetized and unanaesthetized animals. Therefore the majority of binaural neurones in anaesthetized animals were excited by ipsilateral stimuli and inhibitied by contralateral ones, forming the so-called 'EI' neurones. The threshold and tuning of the ispsilateral excitatory and contralateral inhibitory effects were often comparable, although the inhibitory response areas tended to be a little wider. We might, therefore, imagine that the LSO responds to difference in intensity at the two ears, defined on a spectral basis. The LSO might use these differences as a cue in

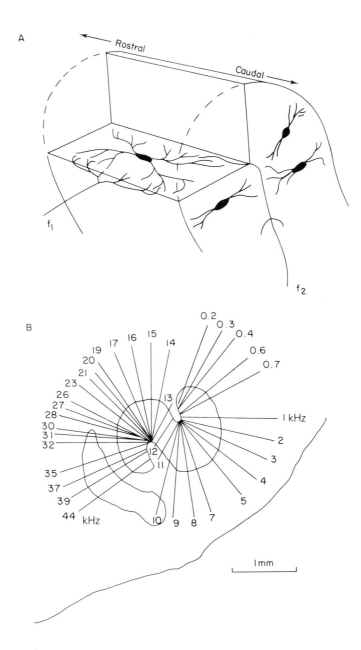

A

Rostral

Caudal

f₁

f₂

B

0.2
0.3
0.4
0.6
0.7
15
16 17 14
19
20
21
23
26
27 13
28
30
31 1 kHz
32
2
12 3
11
35
37 4
39
44 kHz 5
10 9 8 7

1 mm

Fig. 6.10 A. The neural organization of the LSO. f₁, f₂: afferent fibres. Adapted from Scheibel and Scheibel (1974).

B. The tonotopic organization of the LSO. A high proportion of the nucleus is devoted to high frequencies. The numbers denote the characteristic frequencies of the sectors. From Tsuchitani and Boudreau (1966), Fig. 6.

sound localization. The intensity differences will be largest at high frequencies, where the degree of diffraction around the head will be small. In accordance with this, most of the LSO is devoted to high frequencies (Fig. 6.10B).

(c) The medial superior olive (accessory olive)

The MSO receives a direct innervation from the anteroventral cochlear nucleus of both sides. The axons innervate opposite sides of the sheet of cells constituting the MSO. It will be remembered that most cells of the anteroventral cochlear nucleus have short-latency, secure, synaptic connections by means of the large end-bulbs of Held, and so the cells of the MSO are able to receive temporally matched and temporally accurate signals from the two ears.

Single unit studies of the MSO face severe difficulties, because the sheet of cells is thin, and because gross potentials from neighbouring cell groups tend to swamp the single unit action potentials. Such studies as have been successful in identifying cells in the nucleus, found that most were excited by stimuli at both ears, with relatively simple tuning curves and simple temporal patterns of discharge (Guinan *et al.*, 1972; Goldberg and Brown, 1968, 1969). In the dog, which has a particularly large MSO, Goldberg and Brown found that almost all the cells were binaural. Three-quarters of the cells were excited by both ears (EE cells), and the remainder were excited by one and inhibited by the other (EI cells). Many of the low frequency units with CFs less than 1 kHz were responsive to the relative phases of the stimulating sinusoids at the two ears. Figure 6.12A shows the discharge rate of an MSO neurone as a function of interaural time delay. The firing rate showed a cyclic dependence. The period of the cycle was equal to the period of the sound stimulus. The neurone was therefore responsive to the interaural time

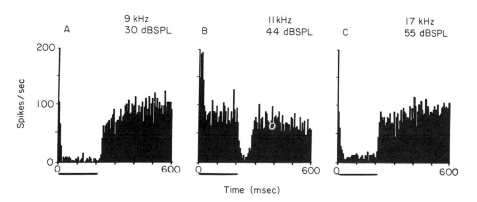

Fig. 6.11 Poststimulus-time histograms of a cell in the LSO. From Brownell *et al.* (1979), Fig. 1.

difference. This interpretation was supported by experiments in which the stimulus frequency was varied. The time disparity for the optimal response was independent of stimulus frequency, showing that the cells were responsive to time disparity, rather than phase disparity (Fig. 6.12B). We might suppose that this arose from a difference in the speed of transmission of signals from the two ears. Such a position was supported by the timing of the discharges in response to stimuli at the two ears separately (Fig. 6.13). The two delays calculated for ipsilateral and contralateral stimuli separately could be used to predict the optimal interaural phase disparity. In this way, when the relative phases of the two stimuli were adjusted so that their excitatory effects coincided, there was a large binaural response (Goldberg and Brown, 1969; Moushegian *et al.*, 1975). This was true for neurones where both stimuli had a net excitatory effect (EE neurones), as it was for many EI neurones. Such experiments lead to the notion of a *characteristic delay*, different for each cell, and resulting from differences in the speed of transmission of signals from the two ears. Overall, there does not appear to be any preference for the ipsilateral ear leading or lagging (Fig. 9.14).

It appears that the stimuli in the two ears cause cyclic phases of inhibition as well as excitation for both EE and EI neurones, because the response to binaural stimuli in the most effective phase relation could be larger than, and in the least effective smaller than, the response to either monaural stimuli alone (Fig. 6.12A). In the excitatory phase relation, the interaction between stimuli was one of facilitation, because binaural stimuli could drive the neurones far harder than could even more intense monaural stimuli (Fig. 6.14).

A sound wave arising from an object in space will reach one ear before the other. If this temporal difference matches the characteristic delay of neurones in the MSO, large responses will be generated. The different neurones possessing different characteristic delays will then be responsive to sounds originating in different directions, and so could be said to map the direction of the sound source.

One of the problems with this simple and obvious formulation is that the characteristic delays of MSO neurones are generally far greater than required to match the interaural time disparity arising from a real sound source. Many neurones therefore do not map direction in the way that might be initially thought. The implications of this will be discussed further in Chapter 9.

If such neurones indeed have a role in sound localization, we can summarize by describing two binaural mechanisms. In the LSO most cells are EI cells and so respond to intensity *differences* between the two ears. The majority of the cells are high frequency cells, and so have characteristic frequencies in the range where a sound source to one side will produce significant differences in interaural intensity. Such high frequency cells will

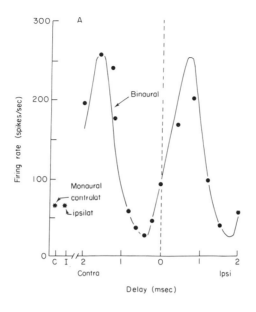

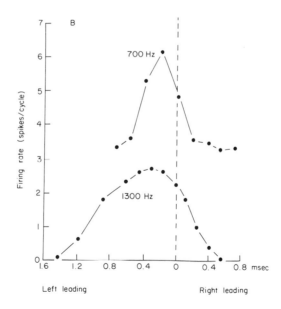

Fig. 6.12 A. The cyclic function relating firing rate to interaural delay for a cell in the MSO.
CF = 444 Hz, period of stimulus = 2.25 ms. From Goldberg and Brown (1969).
B. Firing rate as a function of interaural delay for sinusoids of two different frequencies. The
delay giving the greatest response is independent of stimulus frequency. Kangaroo rat MSO.
From Crow et al. (1978), Fig. 2.

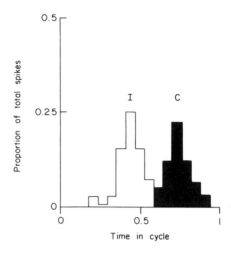

Fig. 6.13 The histograms of latencies of firing to ipsilateral (I) and contralateral (C) stimuli, made with respect to constant phase of the stimulus waveform, indicate different delays in transmission from the two ears. From Goldberg and Brown (1969), Fig. 7.

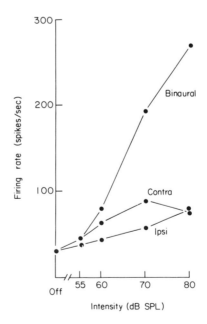

Fig. 6.14 Rate-intensity functions are shown for monaural and binaural stimuli in the dog superior olive. The binaural stimulus was in the optimal phase relation, and could produce a greater firing rate than could either monaural stimulus. From Goldberg and Brown (1969), Fig. 11.

best respond to sounds which are above the frequency range for phase-locking. By contrast, in the MSO the majority of cells are EE cells, and so will not be responsive to interaural intensity differences. They are able to respond to direction on the basis of interaural temporal cues, and in general are most responsive to low frequencies, in the range in which phase information is preserved. Anatomical evidence suggests a similar picture. Animals with large heads and poor high frequency hearing, who might be expected to favour temporal cues, have large MSO nuclei and small LSO nuclei, whereas animals with small heads and good high frequency hearing, tend to have the reverse (Masterton and Diamond, 1967).

(d) The medial nucleus of the trapezoid body

The medial nucleus of the trapezoid body is the relay conveying information from the cochlear nucleus of the opposite side to the ipsilateral superior olive. The afferent axons are the largest fibres of the trapezoid body, and end as large end-bulbs of Held. The principal cells therefore receive secure, short-latency, synaptic inputs, as indeed do the cells of the anteroventral cochlear nucleus from which the axons arise, and so are able to influence the LSO with only a short delay. As we might expect, cells of the MTB have simple discharge characteristics, similar to those seen in the anteroventral cochlear nucleus (Goldberg *et al.*, 1964). In addition to the pathways described above, the nucleus receives projections from the fibres projecting to the LSO, and sends axons not only to the ipsilateral LSO but to the surrounding subnuclei as well. Other types of cell and other types of response have also been described. For instance, the olivocochlear bundle, the centrifugal pathway to the cochlea, with its complex response characteristics, also arises partly from the MTB (Warr, 1975). The olivocochlear bundle will be discussed further in Chapter 8.

D. The Ascending Pathways of the Brain Stem

The principal ascending pathways were shown diagramatically in Fig. 6.8.

The main receiving station for the ascending pathways from the superior olivary complex is the inferior colliculus. The LSO projects bilaterally to the inferior colliculus, whereas the MSO projects only ipsilaterally (Adams, 1979; Elverland, 1978). The fibres run in the tract known as the lateral lemniscus. Some send collaterals to the nuclei of the lateral lemniscus. The ventral nucleus of the lateral lemniscus receives a unilateral input and projects unilaterally to the inferior colliculus, whereas the dorsal nucleus of the lateral lemniscus receives a binaural input and projects bilaterally to the inferior colliculus (Aitkin *et al.*, 1970). The inferior colliculus also receives direct afferents from the contralateral dorsal cochlear nucleus, from the contralateral posteroventral nucleus, and to a lesser extent from the contralateral anteroventral nucleus (Adams, 1979). Most paths that cross, do so at or near the level of the trapezoid body, although the fibres from the dorsal cochlear nucleus cross further rostrally. There is also a smaller uncrossed projection from these nuclei. Interestingly, the direct projection of the cells with simpler response properties, such as the large spherical cells, the globular cells and the octopus cells, to the inferior colliculus seems particularly small. The inferior colliculus is therefore a site of convergence of projections with complex frequency responses but a monaural input from the dorsal cochlear nucleus, and projections with rather simpler frequency responses but a binaural input, from the superior olive. Because the inferior colliculus is tonotopically organized, fibres from different sources but of the same characteristic frequency manage to meet at the appropriate site.

E. The Inferior Colliculus

1. General Anatomy

The inferior colliculi form the rear pair of a set of four lobes on the dorsal surface of the brain stem. The anterior pair, the superior colliculi, are an important visual reflex centre. The inferior colliculi are an auditory relay and reflex centre. There are three main divisions to the inferior colliculus (Fig. 6.15A). The central nucleus, an oblate spheroid occupying most of the body of the nucleus on each side, is the main auditory relay. Some authors (e.g. Rockel and Jones, 1973a) refer to a dorsal cap as a separate nucleus, the pericentral nucleus, although Geniec and Morest (1971) believe it in man to be part of the central nucleus. The external nucleus, in contrast to the rest of the inferior colliculus, is primarily a somasthetic and auditory intergrative area rather than an auditory relay (Robards, 1979; Aitkin *et al.*, 1978).

2. The Central Nucleus

(a) The spatial organization of the nucleus and its afferents

The central nucleus has a pronounced laminar structure. The sheets are arranged like the skin of an onion, and are formed by layering of the afferent axons and the dendrites of the intrinsic neurones (Rockel and Jones, 1973a). The sheets in the very dorsal part of the nucleus form complete spheroids, but those situated more ventrally are incomplete and become flatter and flatter (Fig. 6.15B). Semple and Aitkin (1979) associated these sheets with

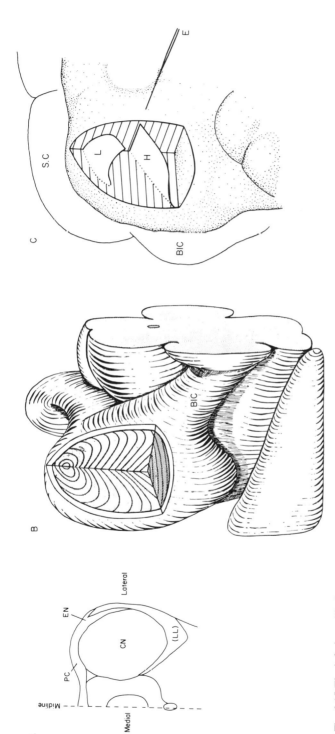

Fig. 6.15 The inferior colliculus.

A. Transverse section of the inferior colliculus. From Rockel and Jones (1973a), Fig. 21.

B. Rostrolateral view of the inferior colliculus, showing laminae. From Rockel and Jones (1973a), Fig. 22.

C. Low frequency (L) and high frequency (H) iso-frequency sheets in the central nucleus of the inferior colliculus, seen in caudolateral view. From Semple and Aitkin (1979), Fig. 5.

BIC: brachium of inferior colliculus; CN: central nucleus of inferior colliculus; E: electrode; EN: external nucleus of inferior colliculus; LL: lateral lemniscus; PC: pericentral nucleus of inferior colliculus; SC: superior colliculus.

iso-frequency sheets of cells, although perhaps because of difficulties in sampling closely enough they did not reproduce the sharply curved sheets in the dorsal part of the nucleus (Fig. 6.16C). Low frequencies were found in the dorsal sheets, and high frequencies in the ventral ones.

Interesting overlaps and segregations have been described in the innervation of the central nucleus. Mention has already been made of the wide range of nuclei that project to the inferior colliculus. Roth *et al.* (1978) showed that any particular injection of horseradish peroxidase (HRP) into a confined area of the central nucleus led to reaction product, transported in a retrograde direction, in only some, but never at once all, of the nuclei labelled by large injections. They suggested that the afferents from the contributing nuclei arrive in the inferior colliculus in a patchy, rather than an even manner. Adams (1979) showed a similar patchiness in the origin of projections from the anteroventral cochlear nucleus. Retrograde transport of HRP showed alternate labelled and unlabelled columns of cells in the cochlear nucleus. Therefore, while there must be a great deal of convergence onto the inferior colliculi, there seems to be a microstructure in the sites of both the origin and termination which could well be of functional significance.

A similar patchiness was found electrophysiologically by Roth *et al.* (1978). It often appeared that groups of adjacent cells had similar response properties, so that a microelectrode might meet groups of several intensity sensitive EI cells together, then several time sensitive EE cells, and so on, even if all were of the same characteristic frequency. A similar point was made over a larger scale by Semple and Aitkin (1979) who showed that neurones with different types of binaural interaction were segregated into different parts of the iso-frequency sheet. EE neurones were most common medially, whereas EI neurones were most common rostrally. Monaurally driven units were encountered more caudally, ventrally and laterally. Binaural time sensitive neurones were almost completely segregated from the ones sensitive to intensity differences, and were encountered rostrally, dorsally and laterally. It seems that there is a considerable segregation of function within each iso-frequency sheet, both generally across the nucleus and on a much smaller scale.

(b) Electrophysiology

In response to single tones, tuning curves and temporal response patterns can be described. Tuning curves show a wide range of bandwidths, some being very broad and some very narrow. The early report of Erulkar (1959) of some neurones which were very sharply tuned (Q_{10} values about 10) for the frequency range (1–2 kHz), may have been due to the inadequate standards of calibration of time. However, a more recent and presumably adequately calibrated study by Aitkin *et al.* (1975) showed extraordinarily high Q_{10} values of 25–40 for a frequency range around 10 kHz. Such tuning is unrivalled elsewhere in the auditory system. The whole question of a progression to sharper and sharper tuning at higher levels of the auditory system is controversial. Katsuki *et al.* (1958, 1959) suggested that tuning curves became sharper and sharper from the auditory nerve to the medial geniculate body, after which they became broader. Kiang (1965), and Aitkin and Webster (1972) contradicted this progression at the levels of the cochlear nucleus and the medial geniculate body, respectively. It should be pointed out that when we analyse frequency resolution it is important to distinguish the frequency resolving power shown by the tip, described by the Q_{10} measure, from that shown well above threshold. Q_{10}s indicate, except for the above report of Aitkin *et al.* (1975), similar or deteriorating tuning at the higher levels of the nervous system. Any such increase in resolution could be produced only by as yet unknown mechanisms, that increased the fundamental resolving power of the auditory system. In contrast, well above threshold, some high level neurones show narrow bandwidths of excitation to tones, much narrower than for instance those shown by primary auditory nerve fibres (e.g. Fig. 6.5B). Here it seems that a simple mechanism of lateral inhibition could help preserve at high intensities the resolution seen at low intensities, by narrowing down the response area. Katsuki *et al.* (1958, 1959) may have sampled such neurones selectively in their report; other reports indicate that the proportion of broadly tuned neurones *increases* at higher levels of the nervous system.

Complex excitatory–inhibitory interactions have been found in the inferior colliculus, although they have been described in less detail than in, say, the cochlear nucleus (e.g. Ryan and Miller, 1978). Half of the neurones showed the nonmonotonic rate-intensity functions suggestive of complex excitatory–inhibitory interactions. Temporal patterns of response showed many onset and pauser types (Rose *et al.*, 1963), with transitions between the types as the stimulus intensity was varied (Ryan and Miller, 1978). For instance, Ryan and Miller describe a common transition from primary-like to pauser, and then to onset, with changes in intensity. Unanaesthetized animals may show sustained excitatory and inhibitory responses rather than onset or pauser ones (Bock *et al.*, 1972), although this has more recently been disputed (Ryan and Miller, 1978). Some neurones were found to be sensitive to amplitude or frequency modulation and were specifically responsive to a certain speed or direction of modulation (Nelson *et al.*, 1966). As in the dorsal cochlear nucleus, the response to time-varying stimuli could not necessarily be predicted from the response to tones. But we do not have enough information to decide whether the processing of complex monaural stimuli in the inferior colliculus shows significant advances over that in the dorsal cochlear nucleus.

As in the various nuclei of the superior olive, many neurones were sensitive to interaural phase or intensity differences (Rose *et al.*, 1966; Kuwada *et al.*, 1980; Nelson and Erulkar, 1963). However, in contrast to the MSO, most of the neurones were predominantly sensitive to sounds on the contralateral side. In so far as the sensitivity to interaural time disparity depends on input from the MSO, this is puzzling, since the MSO codes both sides evenly and yet projects almost exclusively ipsilaterally. This may reflect differences in species, or sampling, or may be real, due to as yet unknown mechanisms.

As in the MSO, time sensitive neurones seemed to have a characteristic delay, which was independent of the frequency of stimulation (Rose *et al.*, 1966). Again as in the MSO, the characteristic delays of the majority of neurones appeared to be too great to match the interaural time disparity expected for a real sound source in space, at least in the kangaroo rat (Stillman, 1971). However, by moving a speaker around a cat's head, Bock and Webster (1974) found that many of the neurones indeed represented the direction of a real sound source. Intensity cues as well as time cues may therefore have been playing a role. An apparently detailed map of auditory space has been found in the barn owl, in its homologue of the inferior colliculus, the lateral dorsal mesencephalic nucleus (Knudsen and Konishi, 1979). Neurones in the lateral rim of the nucleus coded the direction of a real sound source. Points high in space were represented high in the nucleus, and points low were represented low. Points forward were represented anteriorly, and points to the side were represented posteriorly. Each nucleus represented space on the contralateral side although in front, the field crossed 15° over to the ipsilateral side. Knudsen and Konishi did not analyse whether time or intensity cues were the critical ones. However, they noted that most of the neurones were high frequency ones, for which intensity cues would have been able to play a part.

The inferior colliculus therefore seems to combine the complex frequency analysis of the dorsal cochlear nucleus with the sound localizing ability of the superior olive. Very little is known of the details of the interactions between the inputs from the two sources. There is evidence from Roth *et al.* (1978) that while some inputs were represented directly in the responses of the inferior colliculus, some were not represented directly and therefore must have served only to modulate the others. Thus, many cells had the properties of ipsilateral MSO neurones, being sensitive to interaural time disparities, or of contralateral LSO neurones, being ipsilaterally inhibited EI cells. However, there were *no* cells with the properties of the ipsilateral LSO, that is, ipsilaterally excited EI cells. But the ipsilateral LSO is known to project to the inferior colliculus. Roth *et al.* suggested that whereas some cells receive a direct input from the MSO or the contralateral LSO, the function of the projection from the ipsilateral LSO was to *modulate* the responses of the other cells.

Clearly, we are far from having a complete picture of the response properties of cells in the inferior colliculus in anaesthetized, let alone in unanaesthetized, animals. Nor do the neuronal responses alone give us much idea about a special function for the inferior colliculus. Such a special function may arise from the convergence that we have already noted in the input to the inferior colliculus. Localizing sound by interaural time disparities requires the preservation of accurate time relations. These are lost in the dorsal cochlear nucleus by the circuitry needed for complex amplitude and frequency analysis. It is therefore appropriate that the direction of the sound should be extracted separately. The inferior colliculus, by combining information from both sources, might therefore be able to code simultaneously the complexity of sounds and their direction in space.

The inferior colliculus has an important role in many auditory reflexes. They will be discussed below in Section G of this chapter (p. 188).

3. The External Nucleus

The external nucleus is an extension of the intercollicular area, the region in between the inferior and superior colliculi (Robards *et al.*, 1976). As mentioned above, it is primarily a somaesthetic and integrative area rather than an auditory relay. Tuning curves to auditory stimuli are very broad, so much so that the definition of a best frequency is often arbitrary (Fig. 6.16). Aitkin *et al.* (1978) found that 54% of neurones recorded were bimodal, most of these being excited by auditory, and inhibited by somatosensory, stimuli. Very little is known about the functions of the nucleus.

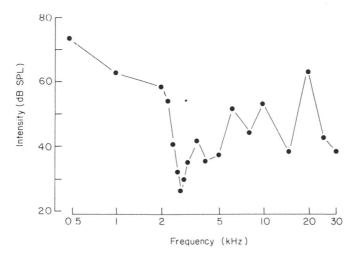

Fig. 6.16 The broad tuning curve of a neurone in the external nucleus of the inferior colliculus. From Aitkin *et al.* (1978), Fig. 5.

F. The Medial Geniculate Body

1. Anatomy

The medial geniculate body is the specific thalamic auditory relay of the auditory system, receiving afferents from the inferior colliculus, and projecting to the cerebral cortex. The medial geniculate body has been divided in different ways by different anatomists. According to the scheme of Morest (1964), there is a ventral (or lateral) medium celled, principal division (Fig. 6.17), a dorsal division, and a medial, large-celled division. Of these, only the ventral division has any claims to being a specific auditory relay. Its afferents run mainly ipsilaterally from the central nucleus of the inferior colliculus, although there are some crossed ones. The fibres run in the brachium of the inferior colliculus, a bulge on the lateral surface of the brain stem between the inferior colliculus and the geniculate bodies (Fig. 6.15B). The medial and dorsal divisions receive a multiplicity of inputs, the former receiving auditory afferents from the inferior colliculus and the lateral tegmental system running just medial to the brachium of the inferior colliculus, as well as somatosensory afferents, and the latter receiving afferents from the region medial to the brachium, the superior colliculus, and the somatosensory system (e.g. Harrison and Howe, 1974a).

The ventral division projects principally to the AI area of the auditory cortex, and in addition to the AII and Ep areas. In contrast, the medial

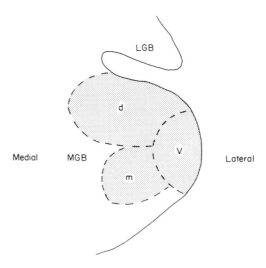

Fig. 6.17 Divisions of the Medial Geniculate Body (MGB). d; dorsal division of MGB; LGB: lateral geniculate body; m: medial division of MGB; v: ventral division of MGB. From Harrison and Howe (1974a), Fig. 8.

division projects to the auditory cortex, in a less specific way, and the dorsal division projects to the 'association' auditory cortex.

The ventral division itself shows a laminar structure, the laminae being flat sheet-like layers consisting of both the afferent fibres and the dendrites of the constituent neurones (Morest, 1965). Over much of the nucleus the sheets are curved and oriented vertically. Tonotopic organization in this division of the nucleus produces high frequencies located medially and low frequencies laterally, and it is very likely therefore that the sheets of cells detected anatomically are iso-frequency planes (Aitkin and Webster, 1972; Merzenich *et al.*, 1977).

The ventral division contains only two cell types, the principal cells, which project to the auditory cortex, and Golgi type 2 cells, which are short axon interneurones (Morest, 1975). The principal cells have characteristically tufted dendritic trees (Fig. 6.18A) (Majorossy and Kiss, 1976). This comparatively simple cellular complement is, however, associated with a great deal of complexity in the local synaptic and dendritic organization, which has now been worked out in detail (Morest, 1975; Majorossy and Kiss, 1976). The interneurones make dendro-dendritic synapses with the principal neurones in terminal clusters called 'synaptic nests', containing three-way synaptic contacts between the different cell types. These could lead to gating by descending fibres from the cerebral cortex, as well as to complex transformations of the afferent activity (Fig. 6.18B).

2. Physiology

Neurones in the ventral division, the specific auditory relay, show responses to sound. Tuning curves range from the very broad to the relatively sharp, although only a very small proportion seem more sharply tuned than primary auditory nerve fibres, and then by only a small amount (Aitkin and Webster, 1972). Aitkin and Webster did not report any cells with extraordinarily sharp tuning, as in the inferior colliculus. In their temporal firing patterns, many cells were onset or pauser types in the anaesthetized preparation, although sustained excitation or inhibition were more common in the unanaesthetized preparation (Aitkin and Prain, 1974). Inhibitory sidebands existed in the medial geniculate body, as in other brain stem nuclei (Whitfield and Purser, 1972) and as the stimulus frequency was changed, complex excitatory–inhibitory interactions became visible. In general, the neurones with complex temporal properties had nonmonotonic rate-intensity functions and complex frequency response areas, as would be expected from neurones with a multiplicity of excitatory and inhibitory inputs (Aitkin and Prain, 1974).

As in the inferior colliculus, a high proportion of neurones were binaurally sensitive (Aitkin and Webster, 1972). Some, mainly high frequency units,

A

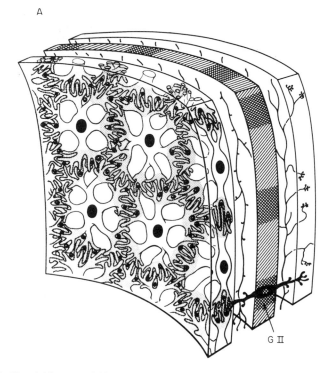

G II

Fig. 6.18 A. Dendritic trees within the laminae of the medial geniculate body. G II: Golgi type II interneurone. From Majorossy and Kiss (1976), Fig. 7.

were predominantly sensitive to interaural intensity differences. Others, mainly low frequency units, were predominantly sensitive to interaural time differences. The tuning curves for stimuli at the two ears separately were approximately similar, although not exactly so (Fig. 6.19). Units sensitive to differences in interaural intensity may show very sharp sensitivity to the intensity differences, sometimes being driven over 80% of their firing range by a change of only 2 dB in interaural disparity.

Such studies, again, give very little idea of the sensory transformations occurring in the medial geniculate body. Thus attempts have been made to find neurones specifically responsive to the features of complex sounds. Whitfield and Purser (1972) reported that some units responded only to complex sounds and not to tones. Smolders *et al.* (1979) compared the responses of both medial geniculate and cochlear nucleus neurones to tones and the complex sounds produced by cat's vocalizations. They reported that, at least for the neurones studied in the posteroventral cochlear nucleus, the response to complex sounds could be reasonably well predicted from the response to tones. This was however not the case in the medial geniculate

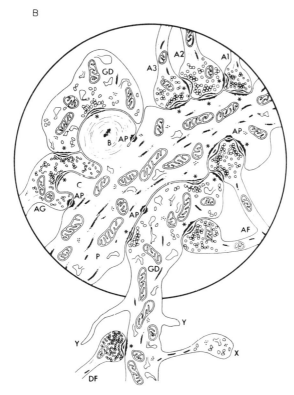

B. Synaptic contracts in the synaptic nest between the afferent fibre (AF), dendrite of the principal cell (running across the middle of the diagram), and a dendrite of a Golgi type II cell (GD). DF: Descending (centrifugal) fibre from cortex. From Morest (1975), Fig. 22.

body. David *et al.* (1977) and Keidel (1974) have shown cells in the medial geniculate of the unanaesthetized cat apparently sensitive only to specific speech parameters or to other complex features. It is obvious that such experiments designed to uncover either specific transformations in a nucleus or specific feature detectors face enormous difficulties. It will be recalled that even as early as the dorsal cochlear nucleus there are neurones that will respond to broadband stimuli but not to tones (Young and Brownell, 1976). Such neurones may have led to reports of neurones in the cochlear nucleus responding only to 'complex' stimuli. A great deal of care is needed to distinguish the different types of complex response, and this may be beyond the limits of our present techniques, in a nucleus as high in the system as the medial geniculate. It is also obvious that the central state of the animal influences the responses. Thus Whitfield and Purser (1972) noted that in the freely moving animal the responses in the medial geniculate body were labile, with say, bands of excitation and inhibition appearing and disappearing over time.

In the medial division, which projects generally to the auditory cortex, Aitkin (1973) in the unanaesthetized cat, showed very wide and complex response areas, many onset responses, and much habituation. Three-quarters of the units were binaural. We expect there to be multimodal interactions in the nucleus, and Aitkin suggested that the wide response

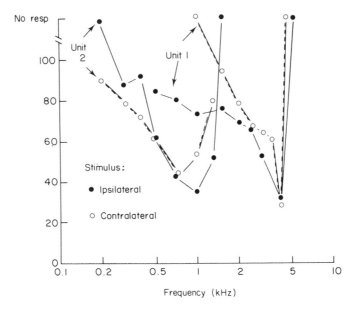

Fig. 6.19 Tuning curves in the medial geniculate body to ipsilateral and contralateral stimuli. From Aitkin and Webster (1972), Fig. 5.

areas were a reflection of this nonspecificity. Units in the dorsal division did not appear to respond to sound at all in the barbiturate-anaesthetized cat, although they may respond to clicks in the chloralose-anaesthetized animal (Altman *et al.*, 1970).

G. Brain Stem Reflexes

The brain stem is the main auditory reflex centre of lower vertebrates, and it would be surprising if some of these functions were not retained in man and other mammals.

1. Unlearned Reflexes

One of the most elementary auditory reflexes is the middle ear muscle reflex. The tensor tympani and stapedius muscle contract reflexly to loud sounds. Borg (1973) showed that an arc of three to four neurones was involved, consisting of a projection from the ventral cochlear nucleus to the MSO and then to the motor nuclei of the facial and trigeminal nerves. But in addition to this short-latency pathway, he presented evidence for a slower pathway, perhaps projecting via the red nucleus or the reticular formation, both of which receive an auditory input.

At a rather higher level, the inferior colliculus has also been implicated in many auditory reflexes. It has been implicated in a reaction known as the auditory startle response, in which a sudden sound produces a characteristic and widespread muscular contraction. Fox (1979) showed that the reaction persisted in rats decerebrated above the inferior colliculus, but that additional lesions of the colliculi abolished the response. While the nervous pathways involved are not known, it was suggested by Willott *et al.* (1979) that the pericentral and external nuclei, rather than the central nucleus were involved, because in unanaesthetized animals the neurones there habituated in the same way as did the startle reflex. Audiogenic seizures also seem to require structures up to the level of the inferior colliculus, but not beyond. In certain susceptible strains of animals, early deprivation of auditory input leads to a hypersensitivity of the central nervous system, so that a later auditory stimulus produces a motor seizure (Saunders *et al.*, 1972). Lesion of the inferior colliculus, or structures below it, reduces the susceptibility to seizure, whereas lesion of higher centres does not (Koenig, 1957; Kesner, 1966). Similarly, auditory influences on spinal reflexes require an intact inferior colliculus (Wright and Barnes, 1972). Wright and Barnes suggested that, of all the brain stem auditory nuclei, the inferior colliculus had the richest projection to the reticular formation. Thompson and Masterton (1978) have also shown that structures in the region of the colliculus were necessary for the initial reflex turning of the head towards a sound source.

The inferior colliculus also seems important for directing the animal's attention to auditory stimuli. Jane *et al.* (1965) trained cats to avoid an electric shock, with a combined tone and light as a warning stimulus. In later testing, the efficacy of the two stimuli separately was measured in unreinforced trials in which only one or the other stimulus was presented; normal animals responded mainly to the tone rather than the light. However, animals in whom the inferior colliculus had been lesioned before training responded primarily to the light. By contrast, lesions in other auditory structures did not have this effect. It seems, therefore, that the inferior colliculus was necessary for establishing the importance of sound in governing the animals' normal behaviour.

One of the reasons for the experimental emphasis on the inferior colliculus as a reflex centre was Cajal's (1909) view that the inferior colliculus in the auditory system had a role comparable to that of the superior colliculus in the visual system. The superior colliculus receives collaterals from the main visual projection which bypasses the colliculus. In accordance with this view, he had described the main ascending auditory pathway as bypassing the inferior colliculus. It is now known that the central nucleus is an essential relay of the ascending pathway to the medial geniculate. The external, pericentral and intercollicular nuclei (Robards *et al.*, 1976) may, however, play some integrative part in auditory reflexes. The anatomical projections for many of these reflexes are not known. Although the early authors described rich interconnections in the brain stem, these have not always been confirmed by modern techniques (e.g. Elverland, 1978).

2. Learned Reflexes

Oakley and Russell (1977) showed that rabbits retained differential conditioned reflexes to light and tone after total ablation of the neocortex. This suggests that the conditioning was *normally* stored outside the neocortex. Taking such experiments further, and analysing the role of the brain stem in normal conditioning, has proved very difficult. For instance, analysing the level of the brain stem at which transection *abolishes* learning, is open to the objection that the lesion could have abolished what might be called the 'performance' aspect of the task. Therefore our best evidence arises from experiments in which some learning is *preserved* after low transections of the brain stem. Evidently, some modifiability exists in the low levels of the central nervous system. In the auditory system, decerebrate rats can learn classical auditory conditioned reflexes (Lovick and Zbrozyna, 1975). While such experiments show that plasticity exists in low levels of the nervous system, and that the reflex connections must therefore also exist, they unfortunately indicate very little about the structures involved in normal learning. Such animals only show conditioned reflexes after very long periods of training, far longer than necessary to establish conditioning in normal animals. And the modifying influence of the upper parts of the nervous system on the remaining lower parts is missing.

In an attempt to show the lowest levels of the nervous system at which modifability occurs during normal learning in the intact animal, many electrophysiological records have been made of neuronal responses during the process of conditioning. Thus, modifiability of auditory responses during training has been seen in the inferior colliculus (e.g. Ryan and Miller, 1977; Birt *et al.*, 1979) and in the medial geniculate body (e.g. Birt *et al.*, 1979; Ryugo and Weinberger, 1978). The interpretation of these interesting experiments is fraught with difficulties, not only because of the difficulty of stimulus control during the measurements, but also because of the influence of pathways descending from the higher levels of the nervous system. Thus it is possible that descending pathways from the cortex affect the responses of the earlier stages of the auditory system according to their significance for the animal. In Chapter 8 some results will be described which suggest that such modulation occurs even at the level of the hair cells, by means of the olivocochlear bundle. The descending or centrifugal pathways may have still more important functions in learning. It is for instance possible that some learning, even if it requires the presence of the auditory cortex, is stored subcortically. It is possible that the closure of many auditory reflexes occurs not in the cortex, but rather subcortically, and under the influence of descending pathways from the cortex.

H. Summary

1. The electrophysiological analysis of the auditory brain stem is faced with difficulties, because we do not have good ideas of the sensory features to which the auditory system is particularly responsive. It is also quite possible that many of the features extracted are represented not in the activity of single cells, but only in a pattern of activity over many cells.

2. The cochlear nucleus has three divisions, known as the anteroventral, the posteroventral, and the dorsal cochlear nuclei. Each division of the cochlear nucleus is, like all other auditory nuclei, tonotopically organized, and the best frequencies of the neurones make a spatially ordered map. In the anteroventral division, the neuronal responses are rather similar to those of auditory nerve fibres, with simple tuning curves, no inhibitory sidebands, and monotonic rate-intensity functions. In the dorsal cochlear nucleus, the tuning curves are very complex, with strong bands of inhibition, and rate-intensity functions that are nonmonotonic. Responses in the posteroventral cochlear nucleus have an intermediate form. This is correlated with the form of the poststimulus–time histograms to tone bursts: those in the anteroventral cochlear nucleus are similar to those of auditory nerve fibres, whereas those more dorsally in the nucleus tend to show inhibitory pauses. It is reasonable to suppose that neurones in the anteroventral nucleus relay the auditory information to the next nucleus with very little transformation, whereas those in the dorsal cochlear nucleus have already begun some complex sensory analysis. Some neurones in the dorsal cochlear nucleus appear particularly responsive to tones which are amplitude and frequency

modulated. In addition, inhibitory sidebands may serve to extract signals from background noise over a wide range of stimulus intensity.

3. The anteroventral and posteroventral cochlear nuclei project mainly to the superior olivary complex, which receives an input from the cochlear nuclei of both sides. The superior olivary complex has several component nuclei. The largest, known as the lateral superior olivary nucleus (or S-segment) receives an input from both sides, the ipsilateral input being predominantly excitatory, and the contralateral input predominantly inhibitory. The nucleus is therefore responsive to interaural intensity disparities, and may use these to code the direction of a sound in space. Another component nucleus, the medial superior olivary nucleus, is responsive to disparities in interaural timing, and therefore can be said to code the direction of a sound in space on the basis of timing differences.

4. The next major nucleus of the auditory pathway is the inferior colliculus, which receives afferents bilaterally from the superior olivary complex and contralaterally from the cochlear nucleus, mainly the dorsal division. The inferior colliculus therefore combines the spatially coded input from the superior olivary complex with the results of the complex sensory analysis of the dorsal cochlear nucleus.

    The inferior colliculus is tonotopically organized, with cells arranged in iso-frequency sheets across the nucleus. Within each sheet, there seems to be a functional organization, with cells having different binaural sensitivities located in different regions. The inferior colliculus seems to play an important part in many auditory reflexes.

5. The medial geniculate body receives its input from the inferior colliculus and projects to the auditory cortex. It has three divisions, only one of which, the ventral division, is a specific auditory relay. Neuronal responses are complex, although it is difficult to judge the extent to which they are in advance of those in the inferior colliculus.

6. Many auditory reflexes are established at the brain stem level, although our knowledge is sketchy. One of the most elementary reflexes is that by which the middle ear muscles contract in response to loud sounds. It involves an arc of three to four neurones, running from the ventral cochlear nucleus to the medial superior olive and then to the motor nuclei of the facial and trigeminal nerves. The inferior colliculus has also been implicated in many auditory reflexes. It seems important for the startle response to loud sounds, and for the development of audiogenic seizures, a motor response resulting from a central hypersensitivity of

the auditory system following early deprivation of auditory input. Auditory influences on spinal reflexes also seem to require an intact inferior colliculus. The inferior colliculus further affects the animal's attention to auditory stimuli.

Learning has been shown to produce modification of neuronal responses in the inferior colliculus and medial geniculate body, but we do not know if the modification resulted fron neuronal plasticity at those levels, or was due to descending influences from, say, the cortex. Nevertheless, there is some plasticity at these levels, because decerebrate animals can form auditory conditioned reflexes.

I. Further Reading

The cochlear nucleus is reviewed by Brugge and Geisler (1978), Evans (1975a), and Webster and Aitkin (1975).

The superior olivary complex is reviewed by Brugge and Geisler (1978), and Goldberg (1975).

The inferior colliculus and medial geniculate bodies are reviewed by Erulkar (1975), and Webster and Aitkin (1975).

Harrison (1978) and Kiang (1975) give general accounts of auditory processing in the brain stem.

VII. The Auditory Cortex

The anatomical definition of auditory cortex has recently been simplified by the introduction of axonal transport techniques, which allow a definition of the cortical areas on the basis of their thalamic connections. The anatomical and physiological organization of the auditory cortex will be described, together with what is known of the neuronal responses. The auditory cortex has been a favourite target for behavioural scientists: unfortunately the behaviour-ablation method has in recent years proved to be less powerful for analysing the function of the auditory cortex than it seemed to be 20 years ago. The general functions of the auditory cortex are still not certain, and some hypotheses are listed.

A. Organization

1. Anatomy and Projections

The auditory cortex has been most commonly studied in the cat, where it displayed on the surface of the brain. Until recently, much less work has been done in primates, where the auditory cortex lies on the superior temporal plane hidden in the lateral or Sylvian fissure.

A framework for analysing the areas of the cat auditory cortex can be built on Rose's (1949) delimitation of the cytoarchitectural areas of the temporal cortex (Fig. 7.1). By defining areas with constant cellular characteristics as seen with the Nissl stain, he described primary auditory cortex (AI), secondary cortex (AII), and a further auditory area on the posterior ectosylvian gyrus (Ep). Primary auditory cortex was described as being cytoarchitecturally similar to other primary sensory cortex, with six layers and a high density of pyramidal and granule cells in layers II, III and IV, but with sparse staining in layer V. The high density of granule cells leads to the term

194

koniocortex, or 'dust cortex'. Later, Rose and Woolsey (1958) showed that the secondary somatosensory area (SII) and the insulo-temporal area (I–T) were also auditory areas.

The projection from the thalamus to the auditory cortex has recently been worked out with the horseradish peroxidase technique by Winer *et al.* (1977) and Niimi and Matsuoka (1979). The conclusions of these studies are shown in Fig. 7.2, although some of the minor projections have been omitted. The major part of the ventral division of the medial geniculate, the section that is the specific auditory relay, projects almost entirely to AI. The medial division projects to almost all the areas of the auditory cortex, and the dorsal division, as defined in Chapter 6, projects to the insulo-temporal area and Ep, together with lesser projections to AII. Thus we can define a 'core' system, running from the specific thalamic auditory relay, namely the ventral division of the medial geniculate body, to the primary auditory cortex. The 'belt' system, surrounding AI, receives projections from the other divisions of the medial geniculate. The belt area also receives projections from other thalamic groups, and in particular the posterior group of thalamic nuclei. There are intense reciprocal connections between the cortical areas, and back from the cortex to the thalamic projecting nuclei (Diamond *et al.*, 1969).

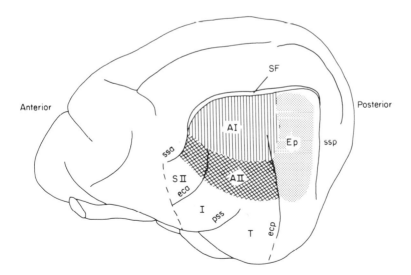

Fig. 7.1 The divisions of the cat's auditory cortex described by Rose (1949) are indicated by shaded areas, together with the other auditory cortical areas now recognized. Cortical areas: AI: primary auditory cortex; AII: secondary auditory cortex; Ep: posterior ectosylvian gyrus; SII: secondary somatosensory area; I: insular area; T: temporal area; SF: suprasylvian fringe area, buried on the upper surface of the suprasylvian sulcus; Sulci: ssa and ssp: anterior and posterior suprasylvian sulci; eca and ecp: anterior and posterior ectosylvian sulci; pss: pseudosylvian sulcus. Adapted from Rose (1949).

The afferent fibres from the ventral division of the medial geniculate end mainly in layer IV but also in layer III. The constituent cells of AI, especially in layer IV, appear to be organized in vertical columns. The cells appear to be situated around the periphery of small vertical cylinders, of diameter 50–60 μm, oriented with their axes at right angles to the cortical surface (Sousa-Pinto, 1973). Smith and Moskowitz (1979) have also described vertical columns in layer IV of the monkey. Many of the cells showed direct soma-to-soma contacts with other cells in the column. Smith and Moskowitz suggest these may represent gap junctions between the cells in one column.

The cell types of the primary auditory cortex appear to be similar to those of other cortical areas, including for instance pyramidal cells (with axons extending into the white matter) and fusiform cells (with two tufts of dendrites) (Sousa–Pinto, 1973). It appears that dendrites and axons ramify horizontally more than is typical of sensory cortex (Sousa–Pinto, 1973), especially along the iso-frequency lines running across the cortex (Glasser *et al.*, 1979). However the synaptic organization of the auditory cortex has not been described in as much detail as in other auditory structures.

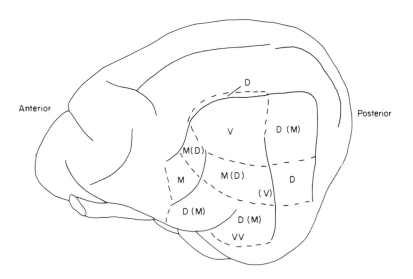

Fig. 7.2 Divisions of the medial geniculate body projecting to the auditory cortex are indicated on a map of the cat auditory cortex. The smaller projections are indicated in brackets. V: from ventral division; M: from medial division; D: from dorsal division; VV: from extreme ventral (non-laminar) division. Many still smaller contributions are now shown.

Primary auditory cortex (AI) receives projections only from the ventral division. The surrounding areas receive their projections from the dorsal and medial divisions. Adapted from Ravizza the Belmore to incorporate the results of Niimi and Matsuoka (1979).

2. Tonotopic Organization

The tonotopic organization of the afferent projections was worked out with gross evoked potentials by Woolsey (1960). His plan (Fig. 7.3A) shows that auditory evoked potentials were recordable in many auditory areas. Tonotopic organization was shown for some of these areas and is indicated by the representation of the base of the cochlea (B) or the apex (A). Tunturi (1952) in the dog showed that between these two extremes there was a complete representation of stimulus frequency, with areas having the same frequency lying in strips at right angles to the line of frequency progression (Fig. 7.3B).

Merzenich *et al.* (1975) and Reale and Imig (1980) have more recently shown that the tonotopic organization of the cortex is preserved at the single cell level (Fig. 7.4). In AI, cells were sufficiently sharply tuned for best frequencies to be definable, and tonotopic organization and iso-frequency strips as described above were found. In an area running just above the Sylvian fissure, known as the suprasylvian fringe, and in the area just anterior to AI, best frequencies could also be defined with some certainty. Interestingly, Knight (1977) and Reale and Imig (1980) have suggested that the region just anterior to AI, which Woolsey (1960) had suggested was the low frequency continuation of the suprasylvian fringe area, was in fact a separate area of its own with a complete frequency map in its own right. In AII, by contrast, the degree of tonotopicity appears to be poor, with cells in the same region having a wide range of characteristic frequencies (Reale and Imig, 1980).

The map of frequency therefore seems to undergo a series of transformations up the auditory pathway. A sound of one frequency is represented by a single point in the cochlea, by two-dimensional sheets of cells in the intervening auditory nuclei, and by a one-dimensional strip of cells in the primary cortex.

Tonotopicity may be less obvious in unanaesthetized cats (Evans *et al.*, 1965).

The cortical areas have been investigated less extensively in primates. The primary area is situated on the superior temporal plane within the Sylvian fissure (Fig. 7.5A). Again, there is a tonotopic orgaization of AI, with low frequencies represented rostrally and high frequencies caudally (Merzenich and Brugge, 1973; Imig *et al.*, 1977). As in the cat, AI is surrounded on all sides by other auditory areas (Fig. 7.5B), some of which are tonotopically organized, although the terminology differs between investigators, and the apparent details of the fields differ between the different species of primate. In man, in which the limits of the auditory cortex have to be defined on cytoarchitectonic rather than electrophysiological grounds, the auditory cortex appears to be in a similar position (Economo and Horn, 1930).

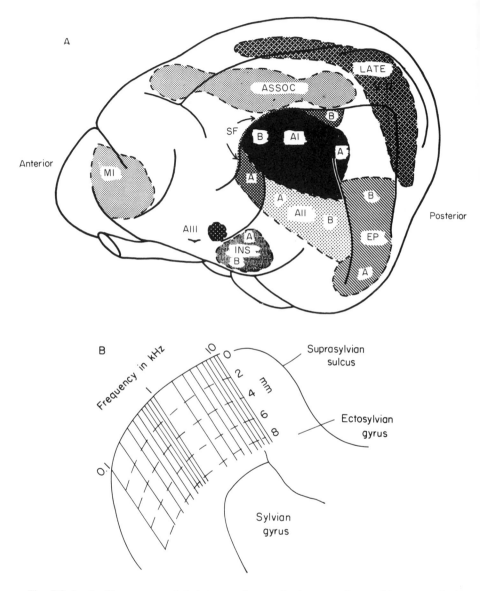

Fig. 7.3 A. Auditory areas and their tonotopic organization were shown with gross evoked potentials by Woolsey (1960) in the cat. Where the areas are organized tonotopically, the representation of the high frequency base of the cochlea (B), and of the low frequency apex (A), are indicated. MI: precentral motor area. AIII is now called SII. Other abbreviations as in Fig. 7.1. From Woolsey (1960), *Neural Mechanisms of the Auditory and Vestibular Systems* (G. L. Rasmussen and W. F. Windle, eds) Courtesy of Charles C. Thomas, Publisher, Springfield, Illinois.
B. Isofrequency strips in the dog auditory cortex. From Tunturi (1952), Fig. 2.

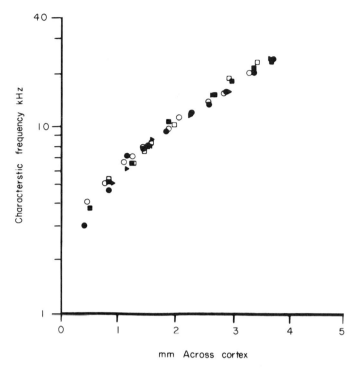

Fig. 7.4 Best frequencies of neurones in a single cat's auditory cortex are plotted as a function of distance across the cortex. The neurones were located on five parallel lines across the cortex, and different symbols are used for each line. From Merzenich *et al.* (1975), Fig. 6.

3. 'Columns' in the Auditory Cortex?

Within AI, many attempts have been made to identify the functional columns of cells described in somatosensory and visual cortices (e.g. Mountcastle, 1957; Hubel and Wiesel, 1963). In these studies it had been found that cells in a single radial column in the cortex had similarities in their optimal stimulus characteristics. Neighbouring columns may have different stimulus characteristics, and there would be a sharp jump in the characteristics measured as a sampling electrode left one column and entered another. In the auditory cortex, the possibility of frequency specific columns within the overall tonotopic organization was first investigated. Thus Merzenich *et al.* (1975) reported that cells in a single radial electrode penetration of the cortex had the same frequency, and that stepwise changes in frequency were often observed in oblique penetrations. In a systematic analysis, Abeles and Goldstein (1970) showed that units close together had similar best frequencies. However there was no sign of discrete transitions between adjacent columns. Either there are smooth transitions in frequency across the iso-frequency contours, or the frequency columns are too small (100 μm or less) to be detectable by the technique. Sousa-Pinto's (1973) anatomical cylinders of cells were 50 μm across. He did not think they could be associated with discretely different frequencies, because the separation of the columns was less than the lateral spread of the incoming axonal arborization.

With an analysis of binaural sensitivity, however, there appears to have been more success in identifying functional columns. Thus Imig and Adrian (1977) showed that in AI, cells which were excited by both ipsilateral and

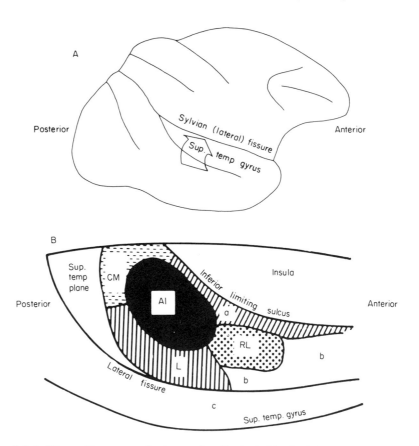

Fig. 7.5 A. The auditory cortex in the monkey lies buried in the Sylvian or lateral fissure (arrow). If the cortex above the fissure is removed, the areas or cortex on the lower surface of the fissure, the superior temporal plane on the upper surface of the superior temporal gyrus, become visible.
B. The superior temporal plane seen from above, after removal of the overlying cortex. AI: primary auditory area; RL: rostrolateral field; L: lateral field; CM: caudomedian field; a,b,c: additional auditory areas. From Merzenich and Brugge (1973), Fig. 14.

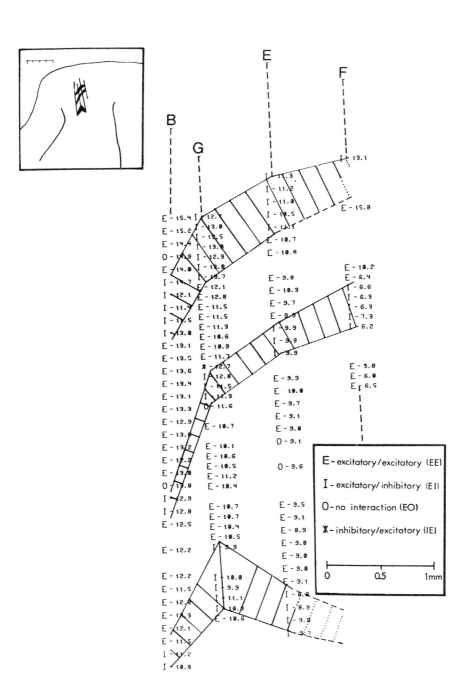

Fig. 7.6 Columns of cells that are excited by one ear and inhibited by the other (EI cells, shown in crosshatched areas) are segregated from columns of cells that are excited by both ears (EE cells). The cell CFs are indicated by numbers along the electrode tracks. Inset shows the cortical area sampled. From Middlebrooks *et al.* (1980), Fig. 4.

contralateral stimuli (EE cells) were located in discrete radial columns separate from cells which were excited by one ear and inhibited by the other (EI cells). In a surface view, the EE or EI cells formed patches wandering over the surface of the cortex. Middlebrooks *et al.* (1980) suggested that these patches were organized in strips running roughly at right angles to the iso-frequency contours (Fig. 7.6). Thus the two-dimensional sheet of the auditory cortex seems to be organized in both directions. In one direction, it is organized in frequency, although probably with smooth rather than step-wise transitions in frequency between the iso-frequency strips. At approximately right angles to this, the cortex is organized in terms or binaural dominance; the strips in this direction seem to have discrete borders.

B. The Responses of Single Neurones

1. Response Types

In the early stages of the auditory pathway there seemed to be some hope that an objective classification into discrete response types might be possible, and that the classes might correspond to anatomically separable classes of cells. However in the auditory cortex there seems such a diversity of response types, and such a degree of dependence on the behavioural state of the animal, that this does not at the moment seem possible. In addition, even in the unanaesthetized, paralysed animal, a certain proportion of the units (20% according to Goldstein and Abeles, 1975) do not seem to respond in a determinate way.

Only a certain proportion of neurones seem responsive to sound at all. In the anaesthetized cat, Erulkar *et al.* (1956) found that only 66% of neurones in AI were responsive to sound. In the unanaesthetized and freely moving, or unanaesthetized and paralysed, cat this proportion seems higher, being 77% according to Evans and Whitfield (1964), and 95% according to Goldstein *et al.* (1968).

Oonishi and Katsuki (1965) described a wide variety of tuning curve shapes in the barbiturate-anaesthetized cat. Some cells were sharply tuned, with the V-shaped tuning curves of units in the lower stages of the auditory system. Others had more than one dip, and were termed multipeaked units. Some had broad tuning curves (Fig. 7.7). The thresholds at the tip of the tuning curve have been reported by some to be as low as in earlier stages of the auditory system (e.g. Goldstein *et al.*, 1968), although others have found best thresholds to be at 50–60 dB SPL (Evans and Whitfield, 1964).

Different temporal patterns of response can be seen for different cells. For the cells which respond in a determinate way, Abeles and Goldstein (1972) in the unanaesthetized paralysed cat described 'through' (i.e. sus-

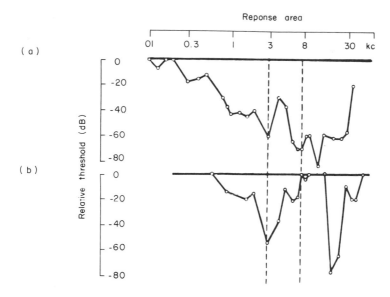

Fig. 7.7 Broad (a) and multipeaked (b) tuning curves are seen in the auditory cortex. Single peaked tuning curves are also present. From Oonishi and Katsuki (1965), Fig. 1.

tained), 'on', 'on–off' and 'off' responses (Fig. 7.8). The same unit may show different temporal patterns for different frequencies of stimulation. A similar variety of response patterns has been described earlier in the auditory system, and it is by no means certain that such an analysis indicates any significant increase in response complexity.

In multipeaked units, responses to excitatory stimuli in one range could only be inhibited by stimuli in the same frequency range (Abeles and Goldstein, 1972). In broadly tuned units the inhibitory range of frequencies varied with the frequency of the exciting tone. Some of these properties can be explained by the convergence, onto single units, of the projections of cells with different best frequencies, where each of the projecting cells has inhibitory sidebands.

In their rate-intensity functions, many neurones showed very sharp non-monotonicity, with the firing rate falling by perhaps 50% for deviations of stimulus intensity by 10 dB or so from the optimum (Fig. 7.9; Brugge and Merzenich, 1973; Benson and Teas, 1976).

2. Sound Localization

Many neurones in AI show binaural interactions (e.g. Brugge *et al.*, 1969; Brugge and Merzenich, 1973; Benson and Teas, 1976). Many cells were

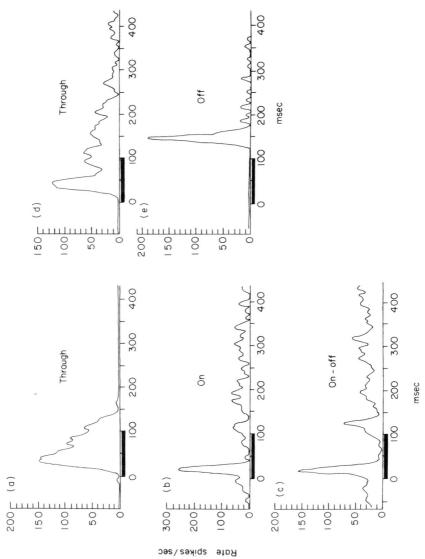

Fig. 7.8 Temporal response patterns in primary auditory cortex, according to Abeles and Goldstein (1972), Fig. 2.

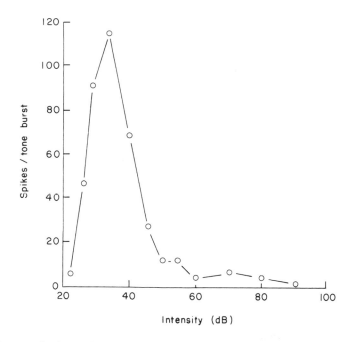

Fig. 7.9 Neurones in the auditory cortex can have very sharply nonmonotonic rate-intensity functions. From Brugge and Merzenich (1973).

sensitive to interaural phase or intensity differences. For unilateral stimuli, stimulation of the contralateral ear was generally the more potent, and this had a correlate in the binaural case where the interaural intensity and phase responses were such that each cortex predominantly responded to stimuli on the contralateral side. It further seems that different cells in a single cortical column may be sensitive to different types of sound from the same direction (Brugge and Merzenich, 1973).

When interaural phase was varied, the firing of many units showed cyclic functions similar to those obtained at the lower stages of the auditory pathway (Fig. 7.10). In some cases the optimal time disparity was independent of stimulus frequency (Fig. 7.10A), indicating that it was appropriate to think in terms of a characteristic delay. In others, this was not the case (Fig. 7.10B). For such a unit, if it is appropriate to think in terms of sound localization at all, we would expect the optimal location of the sound source to vary with stimulus frequency. Time disparities for click stimuli have been measured as well (Benson and Teas, 1976; Brugge and Merzenich, 1973). In some cases the functions relating the two measures of interaural time disparities matched (Fig. 7.11A) and in some cases they did not (Fig. 7.11B). An explanation in terms of sound localizing ability therefore does not always seem appropriate. In general the functions for clicks were broader than for tones, and were monotonic rather than coming to a peak at any one time disparity. This suggests that phases of inhibition from previous cycles of the waveform helped to produce the peaks seen in the cyclic function for tones.

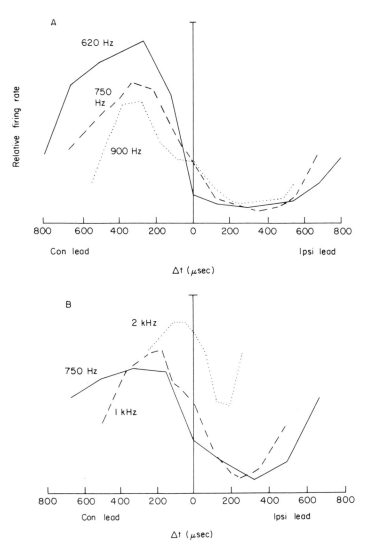

Fig. 7.10 The cyclic dependence of firing rate on interaural time delay indicates in A a neurone with an optimal time disparity which is independent of stimulus frequency, and in B one with a disparity which is dependent on stimulus frequency. From Benson and Teas (1976), Fig. 4.

A sound source in space can give rise to differences in intensity at the two ears, as well as to differences in phase. In a corresponding way, some neurones gave their optimal response for specific intensity differences between the two ears (Brugge and Merzenich, 1973).

In the experiments described so far, a direction for the sound source was simulated by varying the interaural phase and intensity differences. However some units are able to code the *real* direction of sound sources (Eisenman, 1974; Evans and Whitfield, 1964). Eisenman in the paralysed cat found that 33% of units responded most strongly to contralateral sources, 16% to ipsilateral sources, and 28% to both equally. Similar proportions were obtained by Evans (1968). Most neurones showed a rather broad directional tuning of responsiveness (Fig. 7.12). Generally, but not always, the direction giving the maximal response was independent of the type of stimulus and its intensity.

Sovijärvi and Hyvärinen (1974) have described units specifically responsive to the direction of *movement* of a sound source. In response to stationary stimuli such cells gave a complex on–off response, indicating that this particular sensitivity arose from multiple excitatory and inhibitory inputs onto the cell.

3. The Detection of Other Features

Whitfield and Evans (1965) in the unanaesthetized, unrestrained cat described cells apparently specifically responsive to frequency-modulated tones. In some of these units, and particularly those with complex temporal patterns of discharge, the response to frequency-modulated tones could not be predicted from the response to steady tones (see also Funkenstein and Winter, 1973). As was described above, some such units have been described as early as the dorsal cochlear nucleus (Britt and Starr, 1976b). However, the FM sensitivity of cells in the cortex showed a significant advance over that in the cochlear nucleus. It appeared that cells in the cortex tended to show a greater specificity in their sensitivity to sweep direction than did cells in the dorsal cochlear nucleus. And the effective range of frequency modulation found by Whitfield and Evans, sometimes ± 2.5% or less, was much smaller than that necessary in the dorsal cochlear nucleus. In some cases Whitfield and Evans found responses to small modulations, when the modulated frequency range lay entirely within the steady tone response area. Sometimes small sweeps in different regions of the response area all gave similar responses. In some cases responses to FM-stimuli were obtained with stimuli entirely *outside* the steady tone response area. This was in accordance with the observation that FM stimuli were in general the more effective stimuli for cortical cells, as was the observation that some units could be driven by FM stimuli but not steady tones at all.

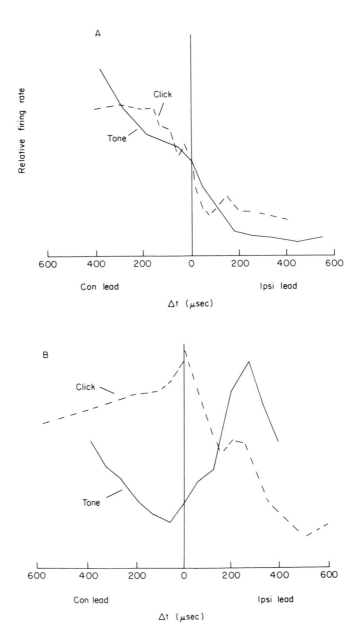

Fig. 7.11 The relations between firing rate and interaural time delay are compared for click and tone stimuli. In A the functions are consistent, in B they disagree. From Benson and Teas (1976), Fig. 8.

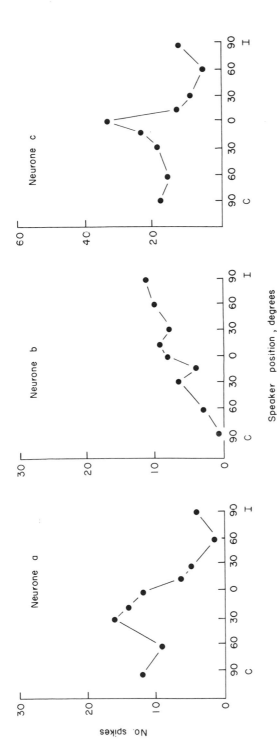

Fig. 7.12 The broad directional selectivity of cortical neurones. C: contralateral; I: ipsilateral. From Eisenman (1974), Fig. 1.

Such studies show that a degree of response specificity for feature extraction exists in the cortex. But the extent to which we are able to divide such cells into separate classes of specific feature detectors, analogous to, say, simple or complex cells in the visual system, is doubtful. Thus, while Goldstein and Abeles (1975) report that FM stimuli were very effective stimuli for cortical cells, the FM-sensitive cells were situated on a continuum of cells responding to a range of complex features.

If we wanted to pursue the idea of a hierarchy of specific feature detectors, we might expect neurones at the highest levels of the nervous system to respond only to stimuli of particular significance for the animal concerned. Attempts have been made to measure the responses of cortical cells to the vocalizations of the species, or to other sounds of presumed biological significance. Thus Newman and Wollberg (1973) and Sovijärvi (1975) recorded the responses of cells in the auditory cortex to animal calls. Ninety percent of the cells responded to one or more of the calls. In many cases the responses to the calls could not be predicted from the response to tones. It was concluded that the calls must therefore have been responding to some of the more complex features of the cells. But evidence was not presented to show that animal calls in general were more effective stimuli than were other complex sounds. Although these experiments suggest that the cortex is indeed involved in the handling of complex sounds, there is no evidence to suggest that animal calls, or indeed other stimuli of presumed biological significance when not incorporated in a behavioural task, form special classes which are specifically represented in the cortex.

Although some cells respond to auditory stimuli in a repeatable, if complex, way, there are others which do not. For instance, Manley and Müller-Preuss (1978) found that 50% of cells in AI, and 62% of cells in AII spontaneously varied their response to a constant vocalization. Evans and Whitfield (1964) noted that the responses of many units habituated rapidly. In these units, the apparent novelty of the stimulus was an important factor in governing their response. Some cells responded only when the attention of the animal was drawn to the source of the sound, perhaps by visual means, and in some cases the response to sound disappeared when the animal was induced to shut its eyes (Evans, 1968). These may be the 'attention' units described in auditory cortex by Hubel *et al.* (1959). Such units responded only to novel stimuli, and once the response to one stimulus had habituated, a new stimulus would again evoke a response. It is apparent that the animal's behavioural relation with the stimulus is an important factor in governing the response of such neurones. Some studies have attempted to control this by recording responses under different conditions of arousal, or by using the auditory stimulus in a behavioural task.

Thus a greater number of action potentials are found to auditory stimuli in the awake than in the drowsy or sleeping animal (Brugge and Merzenich,

1973; Pfingst *et al.*, 1977). The labile responses seen in the naive animal became more discrete, stable and generally enhanced in animals which had been trained to use the auditory stimulus in a reaction time task; they were further enhanced when the animal was performing a frequency discrimination (Beaton and Miller, 1975). Selective attention can also increase responsiveness (Benson and Heinz, 1978). These studies suggest that the function of neurones in the auditory cortex can be more satisfactorily assessed while the stimuli are being used as cues in a behavioural task. It further implies that the greatest increase of all might be obtained if the task is one for which the cortex has been shown to be necessary. In studying the function of a high level structure such as the auditory cortex, behavioural studies therefore become paramount.

C. Behavioural Studies of the Auditory Cortex

1. Introduction

A considerable effort has been put into analysing the function of the auditory cortex, by testing performance on various auditory tasks before and after cortical lesions. In spite of a great deal of progress, and some intriguing leads, we are still uncertain about the cortical function, or functions, underlying many of the discovered deficits. Ablation of the auditory cortex does not lead to a near-complete loss of function, as is the case in the visual system. Indeed, with many simple tests it is difficult to show any effects at all. Absolute thresholds and differential intensity thresholds are only slightly, if at all, affected (e.g. Kryter and Ades, 1943; Oesterreich *et al.*, 1971). Tests have therefore been aimed at higher level functions for the auditory cortex. In spite of many attempts to suggest a unifying function for the auditory cortex, it is most likely that there will be several different functions underlying the deficits seen in the different tasks. And it is unfortunately likely too, that apparently small differences in the training and testing procedures, perhaps so small that they were unreported in the original papers, will turn out to have had a decisive influence on the results. Thus in frequency discrimination, for instance, we are still not sure of the role of the auditory cortex even after nearly 40 years of work.

2. Frequency Discrimination

Allen (1945) trained dogs to lift a foreleg to a sound of one frequency, produced by tapping a bell, but not to a sound of another frequency, produced by tapping a tin cup. He showed that the discrimination was lost after large lesions of the auditory cortex. Meyer and Woolsey (1952) later trained cats in a rotating cage to remain still to a short series of 1.0 kHz tone pipes but to rotate the cage when the series was terminated by a pip at 1.1 kHz (Fig. 7.13A). The discrimination could be relearned if any portion of the auditory field (e.g. AI, AII, Ep, SII) remained intact, but not if all areas were ablated bilaterally. Thus at this time it seemed that the auditory cortex was necessary for frequency discrimination, and that any sector of the auditory cortex remaining could mediate the discrimination. However only a few years later Butler *et al.* (1957) showed that after similar lesions frequency discrimination was still possible. They used a different method of training, in which a neutral series of tone pips at 800 Hz was presented continuously. The cats had to cross the cage only when alternating pips at 1 kHz were interposed (Fig. 7.13B). Not only was performance intact after the lesion, but frequency discrimination limens were nearly as good as before. The apparent conflict between the two sets of results was solved by Thompson (1960) who showed that it depended on the differences between the two tasks used. Thompson pointed out that in the tasks in which a deficit had been found after cortical lesions, namely those of Allen (1945) and Meyer and Woolsey (1952), both the positive and negative stimuli had been presented against a neutral background of silence. The animals therefore had to make responses to one stimulus but withhold responses to the other. On the other hand, in the study in which no deficits had been found, the negative stimulus was presented continuously and itself formed the neutral background, and the animal had to respond to the change to a new stimulus. That the task was critical was shown by training cats with the negative stimulus presented either as a continuous background (Fig. 7.14A), or presented only on discrete trials with silence in between (Fig. 7.14B). The lesioned cats were able to perform on the first test but not on the second. Thompson suggested that after lesions of the auditory cortex cats were unable to withhold responses to stimuli, whether positive or negative, when they were presented against a neutral background. This agreed with his observation that such animals tended to respond to *all* stimuli, both positive and negative. The function of the auditory cortex might therefore be to withold responses to irrelevant stimuli, and so be more closely related to the response rather than the sensory system.

It is indeed a common observation that after ablation of the auditory cortex cats tend to make too many false positive responses in a shuttle box. But there are some important exceptions which make it unlikely that Thompson's hypothesis forms a complete explanation. It was shown in Thompson's own data that, if in training, animals were given *countershock* for false positive responses, being shocked whenever they crossed to a neutral stimulus, lesions reduced both false positives and correct crossings together. Similarly, other experiments incorporating some form of punishment for false positives in initial training, have generally shown a reduction

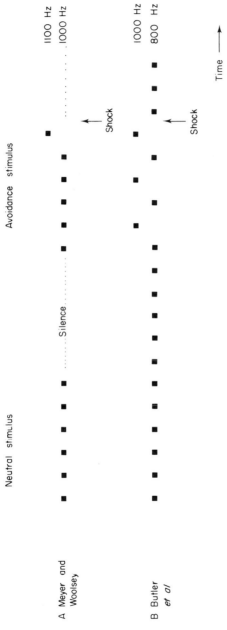

Fig. 7.13 The sequences of stimuli used by Meyer and Woolsey (A) and Butler *et al*. (B) in tests of frequency discrimination.

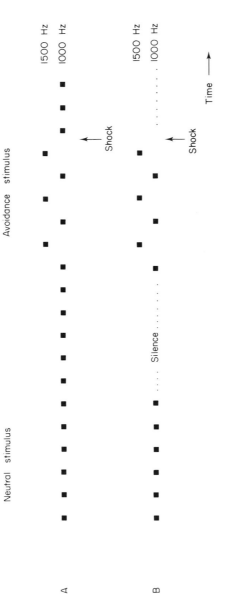

Fig. 7.14 Two sequences of stimuli used by Thompson (1960) in tests of frequency discrimination. After cortical lesions cats could perform successfully on task A but not B.

in responses to the 'nogo' stimuli after lesions (e.g. Cranford *et al.*, 1976 a,b). Other explanations must therefore be sought for at least some of the uncoupling of stimulus and response found after cortical lesions.

Such an alternative hypothesis had been produced by Neff (1960, 1961), who suggested that after cortical lesions, cats were only able to respond to change, or in other words to the activation of new neural channels, and were not able to identify which ones. Once it is realized that the nervous system will habituate to repeated stimuli, this can be thought of as an ability to detect a net increase in total neural activation. Thus in the study of Butler *et al.* (1957), the positive stimulus activated neural channels not activated by the ongoing neutral background (Fig. 7.13B). But in Meyer and Woolsey's experiment, and indeed any experiment where both the positive and negative stimuli were presented against a silent background, both types of stimuli activated new neural channels and the cats would respond to both indiscriminately; in other words, after lesions cats were able to *detect* the stimuli, but were not able to *identify* them on any absolute basis (Elliot and Trahiotis, 1970). This becomes a versatile hypothesis, if the activation of a neural channel includes the activation of any subcortical feature detectors which might be present (e.g. for sliding tones; Kelly and Whitfield, 1971).

Although Neff's hypothesis has been successful in predicting the results of many experiments, there are again some exceptions which mean that it is not likely to represent the whole truth. Cranford *et al.* (1976a) have shown that cats were able to perform one form of an absolute recognition task after large cortical lesions. In the experiment of Cranford *et al.* (1976a), cats were trained to cross a shuttle-box when a background series of 1 kHz tone pulses was changed to an alternating 1.0 and 0.8 kHz series, and were then trained to inhibit responding to an alternating 1.0 and 1.2 kHz series. After bilateral ablation of all cortical auditory areas the cats were able to relearn the discrimination in about the same number of trials as normal animals. And rather more surprisingly, when the neutral background of 1 kHz tone pulses was omitted, the cats were able to cross to the positive 0.8 kHz tone pulses and withhold responses to the negative 1.2 kHz pulses. They were therefore able to perform satisfactorily in a task containing two elements which had previously been thought to make performance impossible, namely an absolute frequency discrimination without a reference signal, and a go–nogo task where they had to withhold responses to a negative signal presented against a silent background. In explaining the discrepancy between these results and the previous ones, we are forced to appeal to differences in the training procedure. In the experiments of Cranford *et al.* (1976a), the animals were initially trained on a change-from-background task and then transferred to an absolute discrimination. The transfer was immediate; but in for instance Thompson's (1960) experiment where some cats were initially trained on an absolute discrimination task, learning was very slow. It appears that when the task was arranged so that it was easy, cortical lesions had no effect, but when it was difficult, they did. This is in accordance with the suggestion of Weiskrantz and Mishkin (1958) that cortical lesions are more likely to upset difficult tasks than easy ones. It may be that lesions produce a generalized interference with behaviour. Alternatively, it may be that when cats have to learn tasks that turn out to be difficult, they have to use strategies which require the operation of the part of the cortex in question. The function of the cortex should then be related to strategies rather than tasks.

If Neff's (1960, 1961) hypothesis is nevertheless correct, and animals after auditory cortex ablation can only detect differences in the total amount of neural activity, it is appropriate to ask the complementary question: what does the cortex do to make such discriminations possible in the normal animal? One answer might be that of keeping the stimulus elements separate, perhaps along the time dimension. It therefore becomes appropriate to test the animals on tasks which can only be solved by utilizing the temporal sequence of the elements. Such tests are provided by tests of auditory pattern recognition. Such tests were used by Diamond and Neff (1957), with the intention of producing in the auditory modality, at least one possible aspect of the deficits in pattern perception that had already been found in the visual modality.

3. Patterns, Memory and Time

Diamond and Neff (1957) tested the ability of cats to discriminate changes in an ongoing pattern of tone pips, shown in Fig. 7.15. They found that the pattern could be relearned if any part of AI were preserved, but there was complete loss and no relearning if the lesions included AI, AII, Ep and I–T. Clearly, these areas are then necessary for distinguishing sequences that differ in their temporal ordering but are otherwise identical. Interestingly, the I–T area seems to have a particularly important function in this task, since Goldberg *et al.* (1957) have shown that such discriminations are lost after lesions of the I–T area alone. It seems probable that the I–T area in the cat has in fact a supramodal role in temporal pattern perception, since Colativa has shown that lesions of I–T upset the perception of visual and somatosensory as well as auditory temporal patterns (Colativa, 1972, 1974; Colativa *et al.*, 1974). In man, there seems a correlate, since subjects with temporal lobe lesions have difficulty in perceiving temporal patterns of auditory stimuli (Milner, 1962; Karaseva, 1972). Lesions of the auditory cortex also upset tasks in animals where the subject has to indicate whether two successive sounds are the same or different by having to make a response when they are the same but not when they are different. In cats, dogs and monkeys, lesions of the primary auditory cortex or the belt area

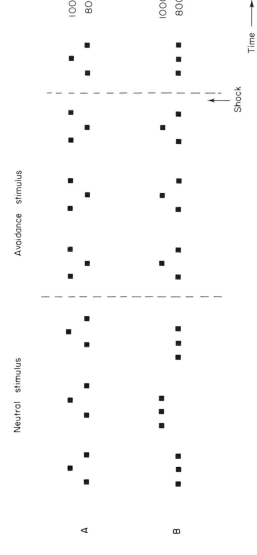

Fig. 7.15 Two sequences of stimuli used by Diamond and Neff (1957) in tests of pattern discrimination. Performance on neither test survived complete lesions of the auditory cortex.

prevented the task from being relearned (Cornwell, 1967; Chorazyna and Stepien, 1963; Stepien *et al.*, 1960). These animals therefore had some difficulty in relating the trace left by one auditory stimulus with the next auditory stimulus, or translating this into response terms, or both.

The same point was investigated by Dewson *et al.* (1970) who trained rhesus monkeys to reproduce a two-element pattern of tone and noise bursts on two panels, one corresponding to each stimulus. The intervals between the two stimuli and the duration of the stimuli were systematically varied by means of a rule that maintained performance around 79% correct. After lesions of the auditory cortex, performance was only possible for a much more limited set of time relations than before, either for shorter stimuli or for shorter silent intervals between them. This then suggests that the monkeys had difficulty relating one stimulus to another if the two are separated in time. However, the deficit is not one of short term memory in general. Forcing the monkeys to wait before making a response did not produce further deficits (Cowey and Weiskrantz, 1976). These subjects therefore had a specific difficulty in relating one auditory stimulus to a later one, and could be said to have a deficit in 'auditory memory'.

Such a deficit may be one aspect of a general deficit in coding or utilizing the temporal dimension of auditory stimuli. One of the most elementary of such deficits was described by Gershuni *et al.* (1967) and Baru and Karaseva

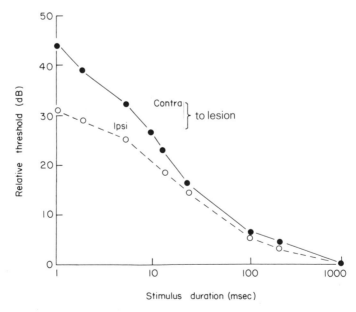

Fig. 7.16 Lesions of the auditory cortex selectively affect the thresholds of short stimuli in the contralateral ear. From Gershuni *et al.* (1967).

(1972) who showed that in man and dogs unilateral lesions of the auditory cortex resulted in a loss of sensitivity to short tones in the opposite ear, but not to long ones, nor to either type of stimulus in the ipsilateral ear (Fig. 7.16). Presumably the cortex plays some role in extending the effect of brief stimuli so that they can influence other neural events. Note however that the deficit only appeared for very short stimuli, lasting 10 ms or so. This is an order of magnitude less than the time intervals over which the deficit appeared in Dewson *et al.*'s (1970) pattern discrimination task, and so presumably reflects a completely different mechanism. Their subjects appeared to have a general difficulty with short stimuli, because frequency discrimination limens were raised for short but not long stimuli (Gershuni *et al.*, 1967), as has also been found in the cat (Cranford, 1979b).

An example of another temporal task, which used time intervals in the range of the temporal pattern tests described above, was that of duration discrimination. Scharlock *et al.* (1965) trained cats to respond when the duration of tone pips increased from 1 s to 4 s. Lesions of AI, AII, Ep and I–T allowed relearning, but if SII was included relearning was not possible.

4. Sound Localization

A very different task, with very different implications for the function of the auditory cortex, is that of sound localization. Although sound localization depends in part on the utilization of timing information, it is *not* likely that the whole of the deficits obtained can be related to the temporal functions described above.

Neff (1968) trained cats to approach the source of a sound, as in Fig. 7.17. He showed that after bilateral lesions of AI, AII, Ep, I–T, SII and the suprasylvian gyrus, the cats were unable to approach the correct box. If the suprasylvian gyrus was spared, performance was still poor postoperatively, although better than chance (Neff, 1968; Strominger, 1969). Wegener (1973) found analogous effects in the monkey, and some effects have also been reported in man (e.g. Jerger *et al.*, 1969).

These experiments indicated that sound localizing tasks, in which an animal has to approach the sound source, require the presence of an intact auditory cortex. But some further experiments have shown that under certain circumstances lesioned animals were able to localize sounds after all, and indicate that the deficit must have a more complex basis than a simple sensory one. Ravizza and Masterton (1972) showed that opossums trained to drink from a water spout when sounds came from the right, but to stop when sounds came from the left, were still able to localize after nearly complete removal of the neocortex. Similar positive results have been found in the cats in a 'lateralization' task, in which signals differing in phase and intensity were presented separately to the two ears through headphones. In these conditions, in man at least, the sound appears to be coming from one side or the other. Cranford (1979a) showed that after bilateral ablations of AI, AII, Ep, SII and I–T, cats could be trained to use a change in the intensity or phase disparity of the signals to the two ears, as a signal to move across a shuttle box. Moreover, the threshold disparities detectable were little greater than those of normal animals. Now both these tasks differed from those giving deficits after lesions, in that the information about sound locus was merely used as a sign that a response was needed, while the response was unrelated to sound locus itself. By contrast, in the experiments of Neff (1968) the animals had to approach the source of the sound. This raises the possibility that we are not dealing with a deficit in analysing the direction of a sound source, but rather with deficits in making a motor response which has to be oriented in auditory space.

Heffner and Masterton (1975) tested this point directly. They showed that lesions of the primary auditory cortex upset the ability of monkeys to locomote towards the source of a brief sound, but not their ability to indicate the source of the sound by lever pressing. The animals therefore had not lost their ability on the sensory side of the task, but only on the locomotor side, or perhaps on the connection between the two. It is however unfortunate that in this study different conditions were used for the two aspects of the testing. In the locomotor task the speakers were twice as far away as in the lever pressing task, and Heffner (1978) later showed that dogs with cortical lesions were able to locate near sources but not far ones. And whereas testing in the lever-pressing task was performed in a soundproofed room,

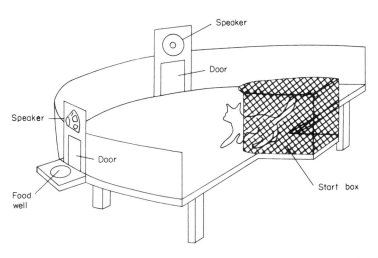

Fig. 7.17 In an apparatus for testing sound localization, one speaker sounds, the cat is released, and has to push open the door under the correct speaker.

that in the locomotor task was performed in a normal room, perhaps with echoes present. It is known that the confusing effect of echoes increases after cortical lesions (Whitfield *et al.*, 1972). These differences may have been critical. Leaving these doubts aside for the moment, the possible explanations are that the lesioned monkeys had a deficit in motor performance, or in some aspect such as attention, or in relating the sensory and motor sides of the task. In order to decide between these possibilities, Heffner (1978) trained dogs to approach one of two goal boxes not on the basis of the position of a sound source, but on the basis of the rate of a brief train of clicks presented through a *central* speaker. After bilateral removal of primary and secondary auditory cortices the dogs were able to use this cue to approach one goal box or the other. But if the very same stimuli, presented now through one of two speakers over the goal boxes, were used in the localization task, the animals failed. Thus under these conditions, neither making a motor reaction, nor remembering the correct response, nor attending to a brief stimulus, were the critical factors. It appears that the dogs had a specific deficit in connecting the location of a sound source with the necessary movement towards it. As Neff *et al.* (1975) say: "Perhaps, in the absence of auditory cortex, organization of a 'spatial world' based on acoustic information is no longer possible'.

We should, however, end with a word of caution. Although hypotheses of complex functions for the cortex are attractive, we should not be seduced away from simpler, if less interesting, hypotheses. Thus Jerger *et al.* (1969) found that a patient with unilateral damage to the temporal lobe had deficits in sound localization and also abnormal thresholds for short stimuli. Plainly, abnormal temporal integration of brief stimuli, if unilateral, could lead to a *distortion* of auditory space, with the result that the subject might not be able to walk to or point to the source of a sound, while still being able to discriminate changes in source position. He would still have the concept of auditory space; it merely no longer matches real space, due to a comparatively simple sensory deficit.

5. Ear Selection

Following the complex interpretations of the previous section, we now turn to experiments where a simpler explanation of one aspect of auditory cortex function is at least possible.

It appears that if a cat is trained to respond to auditory signals in one ear, and to ignore competing signals in the other ear, its performance is reduced by lesions of the auditory cortex contralateral to the attended ear. Kaas *et al.* (1967) trained cats to respond to changes in the pattern of tone pulses, when the elements of the pattern were presented separately to the two ears through headphones. Figure 7.18 shows the paradigm. Although the task can be learned on the basis of the binaural pattern, it is simpler to attend to one ear only, the one in which the pattern changes from L–L–L–L for the neutral stimulus to L–H–L–H for the warning stimulus. Transfer tests showed that this is in fact what the cats did. When the auditory cortex (AI, AII, Ep, SII, I–T) was ablated unilaterally, there were severe initial deficits with lesions contralateral to the attended ear, but not ones ipsilateral to it. It appears therefore that each cortex relates specifically to the contralateral ear. It will be recalled that this was also suggested by the electrophysiological evidence; neurones in one auditory cortex are most strongly excited by stimuli in the contralateral ear.

	Neutral stimulus	Avoidance stimulus
Attending ear	L – L – L – L – L – L	L – H – L – H – L – H –
Ignoring ear	– L – H – L – H – L –	– L – H – L – H – L – H
Binaural pattern	L L L H L L L H L L L	L L H H L L H H L L H H

Fig. 7.18 In a test of ear selection used by Kaas *et al.* (1967), binaural stimuli were presented through headphones. Cats learned the task by responding to the stimuli in the 'attending ear' Attention to one ear was upset by lesions of the contralateral cortex.

Analogous deficits can be found if the cat has to detect tone pips in one ear in the face of a particular effective masker in the other. Cranford (1975) used as a contralateral masker, a continuous train of noise bursts, synchronized with the tone pips in the signal ear. He showed that unilateral lesions of the cortex, contralateral to the signal ear, increased the amount of contralateral masking. The effect, as we might expect, only appeared with lesions contralateral to the attended ear. It appears therefore that unilateral cortical lesions can alter the effective *balance* of excitation arriving from the two ears. Such an interpretation was supported by the further lesioning of the second auditory cortex. Once the cortices on both sides were ablated, the degree of contralateral masking returned to normal.

The above tasks are reminiscent of those that have been used in the analysis of interaural attention in man. A stimulus, such as spoken text, might be presented to one ear, and a competing stimulus to the opposite ear (e.g. Cherry, 1953; Broadbent, 1958). The subjects have to respond to one stimulus or another. Not surprisingly, such tests reveal deficits with unilateral cortical damage (e.g. Berlin and McNeil, 1976).

D. Hypotheses as to the Function of the Auditory Cortex

1. The Analysis of Complex Sounds

Electrophysiological experiments have shown the stimuli to which neurones in the auditory cortex are specially responsive. However it is very difficult to decide any specific role for the cortex from such experiments. The stimuli to which neurones in the cortex seem specifically responsive, which may include frequency-modulated tones and vocalizations, are in themselves so complex and on close analysis produce such complex responses, that it is generally very difficult to decide the extent to which the cortex shows any significant advance in processing over the lower stages of the auditory system. Lesion experiments have at least the virtue of indicating whether or not a structure is essential for a particular task; but again pinning down the exact role in complex tasks is also often difficult. Leaving those difficulties aside, there is one possible link between the electrophysiological observation of responses to complex sounds (whether or not this represents specific feature detection) and behavioural experiments. The discrimination of complex sounds, such as speech sounds, is upset after cortical lesions. This has been shown in the cat (Dewson, 1964), and the monkey (Dewson *et al.*, 1969), and agrees with the extensive literature in man showing deficits in speech perception after lesions of the temporal cortex.

2. Response Inhibition

A hypothesis which related the auditory cortex to a motor function rather than a sensory function was that of Thompson (1960). He suggested that the auditory cortex was necessary for the inhibition of inappropriate responses. This can no longer be held in its simple form because in some experiments lesioned animals tended to make too few rather than too many responses (e.g. Cranford *et al.*, 1976a, b). The appearance of this particular deficit depends on the method of training, but the hypothesis still seems valid under certain circumstances.

3. Identification Versus Detection

A hypothesis, derived from Neff's (1961) hypothesis of the abilities that *survive* cortical damage, is that the cortex is necessary for the *identification* of stimuli on an absolute basis, but not for their *detection*, nor for the detection of change (Elliot and Trahiotis, 1970). Again, this hypothesis cannot be held in its simple form, because in some experiments lesioned animals could still identify stimuli by their absolute attributes, rather than only by their relative ones (e.g. Cranford *et al.*, 1976a,b; Cranford, 1979a).

4. Ear Selection

The cortex may govern interaural attention, the cortex on one side potentiating the effect of stimuli in the opposite ear (Kaas *et al.*, 1967; Cranford, 1975). It is possible that this hypothesis can be extended to stimuli reaching both ears but originating in space on one side or the other (Whitfield *et al.*, 1972).

5. Pattern Discrimination

Deficits have been found in many tasks where animals have to relate one stimulus to another, when the stimuli are separated in time (e.g. Diamond and Neff, 1957; Dawson *et al.*, 1970; Chorazyna and Stepien, 1963). The I–T cortex may play a particularly important role in this, and may govern the utilization of the temporal relations of stimuli in the visual and somatosensory as well as the auditory modalities (Colativa, 1972, 1974). When the time dimension is critical, many auditory tasks have been disrupted, and the cortex may well have a role in prolonging and utilizing the trace left by an auditory stimulus. The deficit may not be in memory generally, but in relating one element of an auditory stimulus to a later one.

6. Auditory Space

The deficit in sound localization seems not to be in the purely sensory aspect of the task, but in relating the direction of the source to a spatial schema (Diamond and Ravizza, 1974; Heffner and Masterton, 1975; Heffner, 1978; Cranford, 1979a). The deficit may be in the formation of the concept of 'auditory space', and the cortex may be necessary for performing manipulations within such a space.

7. Concept Formation

Whitfield (1979) has suggested that the role of the cortex in forming the concept of auditory space was a reflection of a general phenomenon, that of forming concepts generally. More specifically, he suggested that the auditory cortex posits the real objects to which auditory stimuli relate. These posited real objects form the concepts unifying the different auditory stimuli. Transfer tests, such as performed by Masterton and Diamond (1964), in which dichotic click pairs were treated as equivalent to stimuli on one side or the other, only before and not after cortical lesions, form part of the evidence.

8. Task Difficulty

It has been a general finding that difficult tasks tend to be most frequently disrupted by cortical lesions. The difficulty of a task may depend on details of the training technique use by the experimenter. It will vary with the strategy used by the animal in finding a solution. The function of the auditory cortex should therefore be thought of in terms of strategies rather than the tasks themselves. It has been suggested, for instance, that where the training procedure makes absolute frequency discrimination difficult for cats, cortical lesions produce deficits, but where they are such as to make the task easy, cortical lesions do not (Cranford *et al.*, 1976a). It is quite possible that where the task is arranged so as to be difficult, the auditory cortex becomes involved in establishing or maintaining performance. The function of the cortex would therefore be that of helping store or utilize strategies. The analysis of the strategies actually used by the individual animals in behavioural experiments would therefore be an essential, though forbidding, requirement.

It is obvious that present electrophysiological techniques would have great difficulty in uncovering the single neurone correlates of the more complex of these hypotheses.

E. Summary

1. The auditory cortex consists of a 'core' area, surrounded by a 'belt'. The core, which is the primary auditory cortex or AI, receives its input from the main specific auditory relay of the thalamus, the ventral division of the medial geniculate body. The belt receives its input mainly from the other divisions of the medial geniculate.

2. The primary auditory cortex, and some of the divisions of the belt area, are tonotopically organized. Iso-frequency strips lie at right angles to the line of frequency progression.

3. A discrete columnar organization of frequency is not obvious in the auditory cortex; although cells in the same radial direction have similar characteristic frequencies, there do not appear to be sudden jumps in frequency as an electrode is moved tangentially in the cortex. Binaural dominance, on the other hand, does seem to be related to the existence of discrete columns. Cells of the same binaural dominance (e.g. ipsilateral ear excitatory, contralateral one inhibitory) lie in the same radial direction in the cortex, and are segregated into discrete strips, running

along the cortical surface at roughly right angles to the iso-frequency strips.

4. Not all neurones in the primary auditory cortex show responses to sound. In those that do, a variety of shapes of tuning curve, including broad and multipeaked ones, can be found. Many neurones show complex temporal patterns of response. Many neurones show binaural interactions suggesting that they code sound direction. Each cortex predominantly represents sound sources on the contralateral side.

5. Many neurones show particular sensitivity to the features of complex sounds. Some cells seem specifically responsive to frequency-modulated stimuli. Others respond only to complex sounds such as animal calls: but there is no evidence that such cells can be regarded as specific detectors for those features.

6. Behavioural studies of the auditory cortex, in which auditory performance is tested before and after cortical lesions, have shown that the auditory cortex is implicated in many tasks. It is often however very difficult to work out the functions underlying the deficits. Frequency discrimination, for instance, was once thought to be impossible after complete lesions of the auditory cortex. Later it was shown that frequency discrimination was possible after cortical lesions if the animals had to detect *changes* in the frequency of an ongoing series of tone pips, and this led to hypotheses either that lesioned animals were only able to respond to stimuli on the basis of change, or that they had difficulty in inhibiting inappropriate responses. Now however, lesioned animals have been shown to respond in ways which contradict both theories, and we have to resort to explaining the results in terms of task difficulty. Cortical lesions upset performance on these tasks only if the initial learning was difficult.

7. Cortical lesions upset tasks where the animals have to utilize the temporal dimension of auditory stimuli. This suggests that the auditory cortex may be necessary for auditory short-term memory.

8. The auditory cortex seems to be necessary for normal sound localization. The difficulty may be in relating the results of the sensory spatial analysis with the motor response.

9. The auditory cortex seems to affect the ability to attend to sounds in the opposite ear.

10. Hypotheses as to the function of the auditory cortex suggest:
      (i) that it may be necessary for the analysis of complex sounds;
      (ii) that it serves to inhibit inappropriate motor responses;
      (iii) that it serves to identify stimuli on an absolute basis;
      (iv) that it is necessary for the formation of concepts about auditory stimuli;
      (v) that it is necessary for short-term memory when one auditory stimulus has to be related to another later in time;
      (vi) that it is necessary for the formation of an 'auditory space';
      (vii) that it is necessary for selective attention to auditory stimuli on the basis of source position;
      (viii) that it is necessary for auditory tasks that are difficult.

F. Further Reading

The anatomy of the auditory cortex is reviewed by Ravizza and Belmore (1978) and Harrison and Howe (1974a).

Neuronal responses are reviewed by Goldstein and Abeles (1975).

Behavioural studies are reviewed by Neff *et al.* (1975) and Ravizza and Belmore (1978).

VIII. The Centrifugal Pathways

The centrifugal auditory pathways run from the higher stages of the auditory system to the lower. One pathway, the olivocochlear bundle, runs from the superior olivary complex to the hair cells of the cochlea. The central auditory nuclei are targets for other centrifugal pathways. It has been suggested that the pathways are organized into a chain, running from the cortex to the cochlea. In this chapter, electrophysiological and behavioural experiments on centrifugal pathways will be described, and some hypotheses as to the function of the pathways discussed.

A. Introduction

So far we have considered the auditory pathway as one in which information is handed exclusively from the lower to the higher levels of the nervous system. Such a view is, however, far from that of the whole picture. In particular the auditory system posesses a large number of nerve fibres running in the reverse direction, from the higher levels of the nervous system to the lower. The fibres run close to, but not generally within, the tracts carrying the ascending information. In this way the activity of the lower levels of the nervous system can be influenced by the complex responses of the highest. We might also expect the central state of the animal to affect the sensory responses of the early stages of the auditory pathway. Centrifugal pathways have been known since the end of the nineteenth century (e.g. Held, 1893); however recent interest in centrifugal pathways was triggered by Rasmussen's description in 1946 of the olivocochlear bundle, running from the superior olive to the hair cells. Interest was also triggered by the possibility that the centrifugal pathways could modify the sensory input during processes such as attention (Hernandez–Peon *et al.*, 1956).

B. The Olivocochlear Bundle

1. Anatomy

The cochlea receives a centrifugal, commonly called 'efferent', innervation from the superior olivary complex. The innervation is bilateral, the fibres from the opposite side running over the dorsal surface of the brain stem just below the floor of the fourth ventricle (Rasmussen, 1946; Fig. 8.1). The fibres are then joined by ipsilateral fibres, and a few branch off to enter the cochlear nucleus. The others leave the brain stem by way of the vestibular nerve, cross over into the auditory nerve, and enter the cochlea. Within the cochlea, the fibres terminate in two ways. Some fibres terminate with large, granulated, synaptic terminals around the lower ends of the outer hair cells. They appear to envelope both the base of the outer hair cells and the afferent terminals (Fig. 3.5B). They therefore appear to be able to control not only the state of the hair cells but possibly also synaptic transmission to the afferent pathway. A rather greater proportion of the fibres end in the region of the inner hair cells; they make axodendritic synapses *en passant* with the afferent fibres under the inner hair cells and also make contact with the afferent terminals on the base of the inner hair cells. Only rarely, however, do they make contact with the inner hair cells themselves (Smith, 1961). The density of efferent terminals is greatest towards the basal or high frequency end of the cochlea, although they are missing at the extreme base.

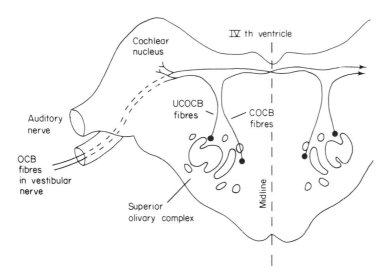

Fig. 8.1 The paths of the uncrossed olivocochlear bundle (UCOCB) and crossed olivocochlear bundle (COCB) are shown on a schematic cross-section of the cat's brain stem.

The details of the sites of origin in the brain stem have been worked out by means of axonal transport techniques by Warr (1975) and Warr and Guinan (1979). They showed that in the cat there were about 1800 fibres in all, of which about 1200 were uncrossed. Their cell bodies lay in the superior olive, not in the divisions associated with the ascending pathway, such as the lateral and medial olivary nuclei, but around their borders and in many of the surrounding pre- and periolivary nuclei (Fig. 8.2). Such an association of the centrifugal system with the areas surrounding, but not identical with, the ascending pathway seems to be reproduced at many levels of the auditory system. The cells projecting to the region of the inner hair cells seemed to be morphologically distinct from those projecting to the outer hair cells. The projection to the region of the inner hair cells appeared to arise from small cells situated laterally in the superior olivary nucleus (LSO). This projection was almost exclusively ipsilateral (Fig. 8.3). The projection to the outer hair cells appeared to arise almost entirely from cells with larger bodies situated more medially in the superior olivary complex. Three-quarters of the fibres

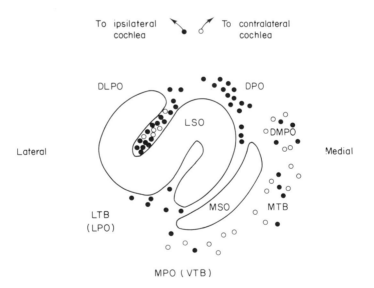

Fig. 8.2 The cells of origin of the crossed and uncrossed olivocochlear bundles were shown by applying horseradish peroxidase to either the contralateral or ipsilateral cochleae. The cells of origin, represented here schematically, lie in the pre- and periolivary cell groups, and on the dorsal border of the LSO.
LSO: lateral superior olivary nucleus; MSO: medial superior olivary nucleus; DLPO: dorsal periolivary nucleus; DMPO: dorsomedial periolivary nucleus; DPO: dorsal periolivary nucleus; LTB: lateral nucleus of the trapezoid body, or lateral preolivary nucleus (LPO); MPO: medial preolivary nucleus, or ventral nucleus of the trapezoid body (VTB); MTB: medial nucleus of the trapezoid body. Data from Warr (1975).

to the outer hair cells originated contralaterally. This separation into two systems, one to the region of the inner hair cells and one to the outer hair cells, may well be associated with a functional separation, associated with the different roles of the inner and outer hair cells in transduction.

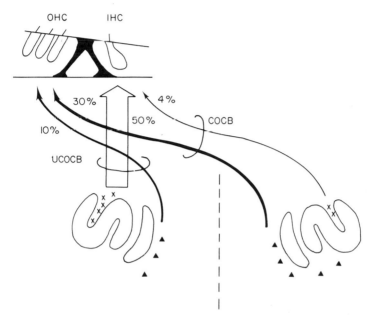

Fig. 8.3 The distribution of fibres of the olivocochlear bundle to inner and outer hair cells in the cat. Large cells (▲) project mainly to outer hair cells, small cells (+) project mainly to the region of inner hair cells. The indicated proportions do not add up to 100% because the other fibres add a few percent (e.g. from ipsilateral large cells to the region of the inner hair cells). COCB: crossed olivocochlear bundle; UCOCB: uncrossed bundle. Adapted from Warr (1978), to incorporate the results of Warr and Guinan (1980).

2. Pharmacology

The transmitters in many of the centrifugal pathways, in contrast to those in the centripetal, or afferent, pathways, are known. There is clear evidence that the transmitter of the olivocochlear bundle is acetylcholine (for review, see Klinke and Galley, 1974). Acetylcholine can be collected when the cochlea is perfused during stimulation of the olivocochlear bundle. Furthermore, the efferent terminals, axons, and cell bodies contain acetyl-cholinesterase. In addition, the effects of stimulating the olivocochlear bundle can be reproduced by the infusion of cholinomimetics, and can be blocked by both muscarinic and nicotinic cholinergic blockers. Unusually for a cholinergic system, however, strychnine is also a powerful blocker.

3. Physiology

(a) Effect on the ascending system

(i) Effect on the gross cochlear potentials. The crossed olivocochlear bundle (COCB) can be stimulated electrically, where it crosses the floor of the fourth ventricle. Galambos (1956) showed that such stimulation reduced the gross neural response of the cochlea, the N_1 potential. The effect has a comparatively long latency, the inhibitory effect appearing some 15 ms after the onset of stimulation, and increasing over a further 50 ms. The reduction was greatest at low intensities (Fig. 8.4). Under the most favourable circumstances the effect was equivalent to reducing the stimulus intensity by 20–25 dB, although 15 dB was a more common figure. In one way, however, the changes were different from a reduction in the stimulus intensity: the latency of the N_1 potential was unchanged, whereas reducing the stimulus intensity increases the latency. Later Fex (1959) showed that the decrease in N_1 was accompanied by an increase of a few dB in the cochlear microphonic (CM). There were also effects on the standing potentials: stimulation of the COCB made the scala media more negative and the organ

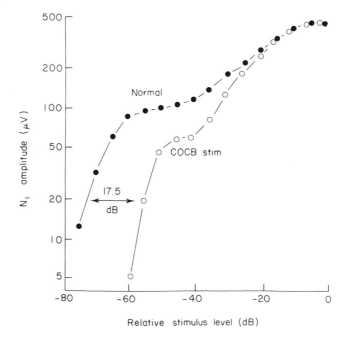

Fig. 8.4 Electrical stimulation of the crossed olivocochlear bundle reduces the amplitude of the N_1 action potential. At the lowest intensities, the effect shown here was equivalent to attenuating the stimulus by 17.5 dB. From Wiederhold (1970), Fig. 9.

of Corti (that is, below the reticular lamina, but outside the hair cells) more positive (Fex, 1967). These results are consistent with the simple scheme illustrated in Fig. 8.5. It is known that the COCB is directed almost exclusively to outer hair cells. The hypothesis suggests that activation of the efferent synapses at the base of the outer hair cells raises the permeability to ions such as K^+ and Cl^-. The demonstration of Desmedt and Robertson (1975) that perfusing the cochlea with solutions of altered Cl^- concentration affected the potentials induced by COCB stimulation, suggests that Cl^- ions at least are involved. We expect hair cells to become hyperpolarized because their interiors are dragged towards the equilibrium potentials for K^+ and Cl^- defined across the basal membrane. This agrees with the observation of Fex (1973) that activation of the olivocochlear bundle hyperpolarizes cells,

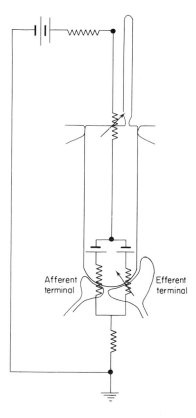

Afferent terminal

Efferent terminal

Fig. 8.5 In the theory of action of the olivocochlear bundle on outer hair cells, the efferent terminals reduce the resistance of the adjacent basal membrane, hyperpolarizing the cell, and shunting current away from the afferent terminal. The CM is thereby increased. Adapted from Klinke and Galley (1974).

perhaps hair cells, in the organ of Corti. The battery so developed pulls the scala media more negative, and the fluid in the organ of Corti more positive. The decreased membrane resistance associated with the increased permeability decreases the local resistance of the pathway through which the microphonic currents flow. Such decreases in the impedance of the scala media were measured by Geisler *et al.* (1980). In addition, the cochlear microphonic produces greater current flows, and greater voltages are produced across the other resistances in the circuit. The measured CM is therefore increased. Current is shunted away from the afferent synapses at the base of the hair cells and so neural activation is decreased. The hyperpolarization also means that the afferent synapses are less likely to be activated.

Although this scheme explains many phenomena, it does not explain how changes in the activation of the afferent synapses on outer hair cells can affect the afferent auditory nerve fibres. All, or nearly all, auditory nerve fibres make contact with inner rather than outer hair cells. This is related to our problem in understanding how outer hair cells contribute to neural excitation anyway (see Chapter 5), and is one of the lines of evidence suggesting that outer hair cells must affect afferent activity, although by unknown mechanisms.

Leaving aside the problems associated with neural activation, it is also possible that the olivocochlear bundle may be able to affect even the mechanics of the hair cells. Mountain (1980) showed that activation of the olivocochlear bundle could affect the acoustic f_2-f_1 distortion product reflected back into the ear canal by the cochlea. Could the mechanical properties of the cochlear partition, perhaps including the stereocilia, be affected by the intracellular potential of the hair cell? One possibility is that the intracellular potential alters the extent of actin–myosin interactions in the stereocilia, perhaps as a result of altered Ca^{2+} influx (Macartney *et al.*, 1980).

Stimulation of the uncrossed OCB, which sends 80% of its fibres to the region of the inner hair cells, reduces the N_1 potential of the cochlea, but has no effect on the CM (Sohmer, 1966). The latter effect is consistent with the idea that most of the CM is generated by the outer rather than the inner hair cells.

(ii) *Effect on single auditory nerve fibres*. As might be expected from the effect on the gross neural potential N_1, the responses of single auditory nerve fibres are reduced by stimulation of the crossed olivocochlear bundle. Wiederhold (1970) showed that the inhibition reduced the effective intensity of the sound stimulus, so that the rate-intensity function was shifted to one side (Fig. 8.6A). The greatest reduction in firing was therefore seen at the steepest part of the rate-intensity function. Presumably the effective intensity of the stimulus was also reduced at the highest intensities; but that was not visible because the firing was saturated.

The inhibition was greatest at the tip, rather than the tail, of the tuning curve (Fig. 8.6B). The effect at the tip was greatest for fibres with characteristic frequencies in the 5–10 kHz range (in the cat) where the efferent innervation is most dense (Fig. 8.6C).

Stimulation of the crossed olivocochlear bundle does not affect the spontaneous activity of auditory nerve fibres. However stimulation of the uncrossed bundle seems to do so (Comis, 1970). This is understandable, since the uncrossed bundle ends directly on the afferent nerve fibres.

(b) What normally activates the olivocochlear bundle?

The fibres of the olivocochlear bundle are responsive to sound. It is also likely that the fibres are affected by the more central neural activity of the animal, since the bundle can be activated by the electrical stimulation of certain sites higher in the central nervous system.

Fex (1962) showed that fibres of the olivocochlear bundle fired spontaneously with a particularly regular firing pattern. Sound drove the olivocochlear fibres with a latency of 10 to 30 ms. The thresholds were 50 dB SPL or greater. Some fibres had V-shaped excitatory tuning curves like afferent fibres: others had broad tuning curves, and some had bands of excitation and inhibition.

The maximum rate at which sound could drive fibres of the olivocochlear bundle was 100/s; yet the maximal olivocochlear effect on the cochlea is attained with electrical stimulation at 400/s. This has suggested to many workers that there is an additional central facilitation of the olivocochlear bundle, facilitating the reflex effects when required. One such influence was shown by Desmedt (1975). He showed that the olivocochlear bundle could also be activated by electrical stimulation of the insulo-temporal cortex.

(c) How does the olivocochlear bundle affect afferent activity in normal hearing?

Although it has not so far been possible to record the effect on the afferent pathway of natural stimulation of the olivocochlear bundle in intact, unanaesthetized animals, some suggestive effects have been produced in anaesthetized or decerebrate animals, by recording the response of afferent auditory nerve fibres from one ear, while stimulating the opposite ear with sound. If care is taken to exclude crosstalk and contractions of the middle ear muscles, then the effect of one cochlea on the other must be due to the olivocochlear bundle. Buño (1978) showed that stimulation of one ear reduced the response of auditory nerve fibres running from the other ear, with a latency of some 100 ms. When the frequency of the contralateral

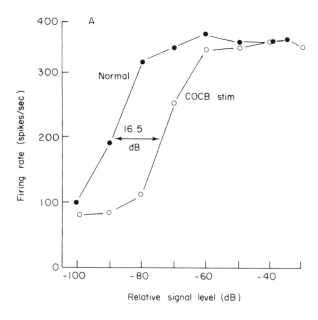

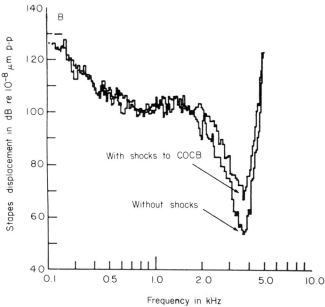

Fig. 8.6 A. Effect of stimulation of the crossed olivocochlear bundle (COCB) on the rate-intensity function of an auditory nerve fibre. From Wiederhold (1970).
B. Effect of stimulation of the COCB on the tuning curve. From Kiang *et al*. (1970), Fig. 16.

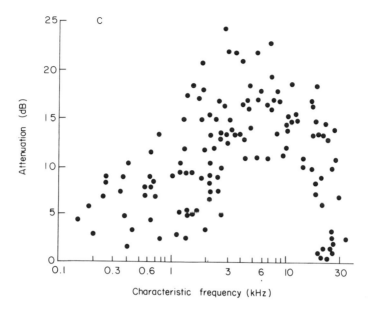

C. Equivalent attenuation of the signal (in dB), measured at the tip of the tuning curve, for fibres of different characteristic frequencies, after COCB stimulation. From Wiederhold (1970), Fig. 12.

stimulus was plotted against the effectiveness of its action on the ipsilateral response, the resulting frequency response curves were usually V-shaped and centred on the characteristic frequency of the fibre being inhibited (Fig. 8.7). Occasionally W-shaped crossed inhibitory effects were found, with the dips of the W on either side of the characteristic frequency. There seems therefore to be an approximate point-to-point frequency correlation in the projection of the olivocochlear bundle, such that a sound of one frequency will tend to give reflex effects on fibres responding to that, or adjacent, frequencies. In the rarer types with W-shaped frequency relations, the effect would be to sharpen the contrast in the sensory pattern.

(d) Functional significance of the olivocochlear bundle

In spite of a large number of experiments, we are still unsure of the importance of the olivocochlear bundle in hearing. It is not known whether it produces a dramatic or a trivial modification of the auditory input in normal behaviour. It has, for instance, often been difficult to show any difference in the auditory performance after cutting the olivocochlear bundle. However, in such experiments, only the crossed olivocochlear bundle was cut. When the experiments were done it was believed that three-quarters of all olivocochlear fibres would be cut by such a procedure. Now it is known that the uncrossed olivocochlear bundle is larger than was previously thought, and that two-thirds of the total fibres would have been intact. The null results may not be as decisive as they once appeared to be.

Borg (1971) showed that normally the olivocochlear bundle has a tonic inhibitory effect on the input. He measured the strength of reflex middle ear muscle contractions as an indication of the activity reaching the central nervous system. He showed that the reflex was increased after section of the olivocochlear bundle. The effect at the optimal intensity was equivalent to 12 dB.

Buño *et al.* (1966) suggested that the degree of olivocochlear tone could vary in an unpredictable way. They bypassed the middle ear apparatus by disarticulating the middle ear bones and introducing the sound directly into the middle ear cavity through a tube. This ensured that the input to the cochlea was constant, although the impedance mismatch meant that the effective stimulus level was reduced. They showed that there was a continual fluctuation in the size of N_1, with a tendency for CM to vary in the opposite direction. The effect was reduced by cutting the crossed olivocochlear bundle.

What could the role of the olivocochlear bundle be under such circumstances? One possibility can be suggested by analogy with the lateral line organ of fishes. The hair cells of the lateral line are embedded in pits or canals in the skin of fishes, and detect flow of water by deflection of their

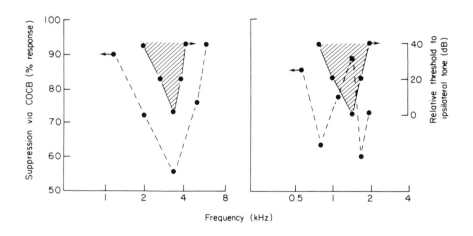

Fig. 8.7 Interactions of ipsilateral and contralateral stimuli in the auditory nerve reveal the effects of acoustic stimulation of the olivocochlear fibres on afferent activity. Tuning curves for ipsilateral stimuli are shown by shaded areas, frequency functions for the contralateral effect by the dotted lines. The contralateral effect (via the OCB) is tuned to the same frequency region as the ipsilateral activation. From Buño (1978), Fig. 4.

hairs. They are direct evolutionary analogues of the hair cells of the organ of Corti, and, like the latter, have a centrifugal innervation. Russell and Roberts (1974) showed that when dogfish made violent escape swimming movements, the sensitivity of the lateral line cells was reduced. They suggested that the efferents to the lateral line served to protect the system from overstimulation by self-produced movements. In the auditory system, the middle ear muscles seem to have a similar function, since they contract during active bodily movements and vocalizations (Carmel and Starr, 1963). Unfortunately for this story, the olivocochlear bundle does not seem to have a similar role: the activity of crossed olivocochlear fibres in unanaesthetized animals does not show any correlation with body movement or vocalization (Banks *et al.*, 1979).

4. Behavioural Experiments

A different approach to discovering a function for the olivocochlear bundle is that of testing auditory discrimination behaviourally before and after lesions of the olivocochlear bundle. Absolute and masked tonal thresholds and frequency discrimination limens were unaffected in cats by transection of the olivocochlear bundle (Galambos, 1960; Trahiotis and Elliott, 1970). Capps and Ades (1968) however found positive results with frequency discrimination in the squirrel monkey. Transection of the crossed olivocochlear bundle increased frequency discrimination limens from 150 Hz to 450 Hz at 1 kHz. The preoperative frequency discrimination limens were unusually large, and the monkeys may not have been performing a frequency discrimination as it is commonly understood. The true basis of the deficit is not known.

Dewson (1968) suggested that the olivocochlear bundle aided the discrimination of signals in noise. He trained rhesus monkeys to discriminate between two vowel sounds in the presence of masking noise. After cutting the crossed olivocochlear bundle, the noise had to be reduced in intensity to allow the discrimination to be performed as well as it was previously. In other words, the animals' signal-to-noise ratio had altered. Thus, when animals had to discriminate *between* two sounds in a noise there seemed to be an effect, although where they had to *detect* a *single* sound in a noise there was not, as described in the previous paragraph. It is not known whether this difference is the significant one. The neural basis of the effect is not known, since the influence of the olivocochlear bundle on the responses of auditory nerve fibres to complex stimuli has not been described.

A hypothesis that has generated a great deal of interest is that the olivocochlear bundle is involved in attention, attenuating the auditory input when it is judged to be irrelevant. Such a hypothesis could explain the common experience of fluctuations in the awareness of auditory stimuli.

Hernández–Peón *et al.* (1956) published a seminal experiment, in which they implanted electrodes in a cat's cochlear nucleus, and measured click-evoked responses both when the cat was relaxed, and when it was alert, attending to a mouse in a bottle. The auditory evoked potentials were smaller in the latter case, and the authors suggested that when the cat was attending to the visual modality the auditory input was attenuated. Disappointingly, many attempts made to repeat the experiment failed. Worden and Marsh (1963) showed that the experiment was lacking in necessary controls. The variation in the evoked potentials could have been due, for instance, to variation in the intensity of the acoustic input when the cat moved to look at the mouse, and to contraction of the middle ear muscles. Even the interpretation that the cat switched its attention from audition to vision when it saw the mouse, is open to an alternative, which is that the cat was generally inattentive when relaxed, and listening to as well as looking at the mouse when alert. These experiments triggered an interest in centrifugal pathways which has not delivered all it promised: however the succeeding experiments did define the controls necessary for a rigorous experiment.

Although the recent consensus has been that the olivocochlear bundle does *not* gate the sensory input in attention, there is one positive report, in a nevertheless apparently well controlled study. Oatman (1976) trained cats, with middle ear muscles cut, to make a visual discrimination for a food reward. Clicks were continuously delivered at 1/s through ear tubes. When the cat was performing the visual discrimination, the N_1 potential of the cochlea was smaller, and the CM larger, than when the cat was relaxed. The effect on N_1 was greatest at low intensities. The pattern of changes therefore exactly paralleled those expected with the olivocochlear bundle. This was important corroborative evidence that the olivocochlear bundle was activated. However, the important control, of showing that the effect disappeared when the olivocochlear bundle was cut, was not done.

C. Centrifugal Pathways to the Cochlear Nuclei

1. Anatomy

The cochlear nuclei receive centrifugal fibres from several sources. By far the largest innervation appears to arise in the superior olivary complex. Centrifugal fibres from the dorsal and ventral nuclei of the lateral lemniscus, the inferior colliculus, and the reticular formation have also been described.

Some of the centrifugal fibres from the superior olivary complex consist of branches of the olivocochlear bundle. Others run ipsilaterally by rather more direct paths in the dorsal and intermediate acoustic striae, and, from superior olives on both sides, in the trapezoid body (Fig. 8.8). As with the olivocochlear bundle, the centrifugal innervation does not arise in the main nuclei associated with the ascending system, but in some of the surrounding pre- and periolivary nuclei (Elverland, 1977; Adams and Warr, 1976). These nuclei, of course, receive an auditory input, so the centrifugal pathways can be activated by sound as well as by central influences.

The centrifugal innervation from the inferior colliculus arises laterally in the colliculus, and descends and runs along the ventral surface of the brain stem, where it turns and ascends dorsally into the middle layers of the DCN (Rasmussen, 1960). The fibres from the nuclei of the lateral lemniscus have been the least well described and not all authors agree on the details. Both the dorsal and ventral nuclei of the lateral lemniscus on both the ipsilateral and contralateral sides have been suggested as sites of origin. The reticular formation also sends a projection to the cochlear nucleus (Adams and Warr, 1976).

All divisions of the cochlear nuclei receive centrifugal fibres in different degrees from the different sources. There is considerable detail in the projections — for instance, Cant and Morest (1978) described six groups of centrifugal axons ending in different ways in the anteroventral nucleus alone.

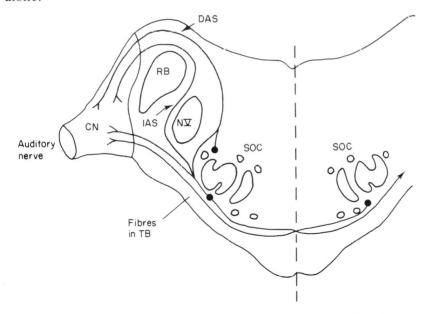

Fig. 8.8 A schematic representation of some of the centrifugal pathways from the superior olivary complex (SOC) to the cochlear nucleus (CN). Branches of the olivocochlear bundle also run from the SOC to the CN but are not shown here. The fibres run by three routes: the dorsal acoustic stria (DAS), the intermediate acoustic stria (IAS) and in the trapezoid body (TB). RB: restiform body (inferior cerebellar peduncle); NV: fifth nerve nucleus. Data from Elverland (1977).

2. Pharmacology

As in the cochlea, the neurotransmitters associated with the centrifugal system are known rather better than those associated with the centripetal system. Moreover, knowledge of their pharmacology has been useful in discovering the function of the centrifugal pathways.

There is evidence that some of the centrifugal pathways to the cochlear nucleus are cholinergic. Many of the terminals in the cochlear nucleus and the cells of origin, particularly in the superior olive, react positively for acetylcholinesterase. Osen and Roth (1969) ascribe the reaction exclusively to the olivocochlear bundle, which of course sends branches to the cochlear nucleus. They disagree with Rasmussen (1954), who described the tracts running directly from the ipsilateral superior olive in the intermediate acoustic stria as also reacting positively.

Whatever the pathways involved, Comis and Whitfield (1968) produced strong evidence that an excitatory centrifugal pathway running from the superior olive used acetylcholine as a transmitter. The excitation produced by electrical stimulation of the pathway could be blocked by cholinergic blockers such as atropine and dihydro-β-erythroidine applied to target cells of the cochlear nucleus. The effects of stimulating the pathway could be mimicked by applying acetylcholine to cells of the cochlear nucleus. And Comis and Davies (1969) showed that electrical stimulation of the superior olive could release acetylcholine from the cochlear nucleus.

A second centrifugal neurotransmitter in the cochlear nucleus seems to be noradrenaline. Noradrenaline-containing terminals have been demonstrated in the cochlear nucleus by an immunofluorescence technique, and the noradrenaline-containing fibres traced to cell bodies in, at least, the dorsal nucleus of the lateral lemniscus (Swanson and Hartman, 1975). Comis and Whitfield (1968) showed that stimulation of the nuclei of the lateral lemniscus could give inhibition in the cochlear nucleus. The effects were similar to those of noradrenaline applied to single cells of the cochlear nucleus, which was always inhibitory.

It is very likely, of course, that there are centrifugal neurotransmitters to the cochlear nucleus in addition to acetylcholine and noradrenaline.

In contrast to noradrenaline which was associated with inhibitory centrifugal pathways, it appears that at least some of the inhibition intrinsic to the nucleus may be mediated by γ-amino-butyric acid and glycine (Godfrey *et al.*, 1977).

3. Physiology

Comis and Whitfield (1968) electrically stimulated the superior olive and recorded the activity of cells in the cochlear nucleus. Stimulation of most of the superior olive excited cells of the ipsilateral anteroventral cochlear nucleus. There was evidence of 'gating' of the auditory input by the centrifugal pathway, since electrical stimulation could lower the threshold of neurones in the nucleus by as much as 15 dB. On the other hand, stimulation of the extreme lateral region of the superior olive, in the region of the dorsolateral periolivary and the lateral preolivary nuclei, inhibited cells in the cochlear nucleus (Comis, 1970). In some cases this inhibition occurred because the olivocochlear bundle had been activated, reducing the responses of the cochlea. In such cases the inhibition could be released by the application of strychnine, a powerful blocker of the olivocochlear bundle in the cochlea, to the round window. In other cases this could not be done, and it is possible that direct inhibitory pathways were being activated. It is not known to what extent such effects can be explained by the activation of the branches of the olivocochlear bundle which run directly to the cochlear nucleus. There is evidence that such branches can be both excitatory and inhibitory. Starr and Wernick (1968) found that with the cochlea destroyed, stimulation of the crossed olivocochlear bundle increased the spontaneous activity of 42%, and decreased the activity of 16%, of cells recorded in the cochlear nucleus. Of course, some of these effects may have been indirect, mediated by the activity of inhibitory interneurones.

A pathway which was generally inhibitory, but sometimes excitatory, ran from the contralateral nuclei of the lateral lemniscus (Comis and Whitfield, 1968).

Some effects of natural stimulation of the centrifugal pathways can be shown by stimulation of the contralateral ear. There are no direct afferent auditory nerve fibres from one cochlea to the contralateral cochlear nucleus: all influences must be by centrifugal pathways, via the superior olivary complex, or perhaps via higher nuclei such as the nuclei of the lateral lemniscus and the inferior colliculus.

Mast (1970, 1973) showed that some cells in the dorsal cochlear nucleus could be excited or inhibited by contralateral sound. Tuning curves for the direct ipsilateral and the centrifugal contralateral effects were generally very similar in threshold, best frequency, and shape. Klinke *et al.* (1969) showed that the contralateral stimulus could sometimes produce a W-shaped tuning curve, with two inhibitory sidebands. The latter effect is reminiscent of the effects obtained in a minority of cases via the olivocochlear bundle (Buño, 1978).

4. Behavioural Experiments

The behavioural analysis of the olivocochlear bundle was comparatively straightforward, because the crossed component of the bundle can be cut in the midline, without danger of damage to other auditory structures. In contrast, most centrifugal pathways to the cochlear nucleus run inter-mingled with the afferent pathways, so an analogous approach is not avail-able. However, the centrifugal system uses acetylcholine and noradrenaline as neurotransmitters. Since these are not used by the centripetal system, pharmacological methods can be used to affect the centrifugal system selec-tively.

Pickles and Comis (1973) chronically implanted a cannula over the coch-lear nucleus in cats, so that drugs could be applied to the nucleus in the unanaesthetized animals. There is, as described above, good evidence that some of the centrifugal pathways from the superior olive to the cochlear nucleus are cholinergic and that their action can be blocked by atropine. The cats were trained to detect tone pips both in silence and against masking noise. In such behavioural tests, atropine applied to the cochlear nucleus raised the absolute thresholds for tone pips by a few dB, but raised masked thresholds significantly more (Fig. 8.9). This suggests that atropine might have been blocking a system whose normal action was to *help* the animal hear signals in masking noise.

The psychophysics of the atropine effect was investigated in further experiments. It is known, that if we are detecting a tone against masking noise, most of the masking is due to noise components which are near to the signal in frequency. By systematically varying the frequency relations of the masker and signal, it is possible to define a function relating the extent to

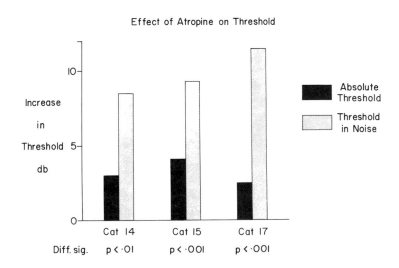

Fig. 8.9 Atropine applied to the cochlear nucleus in unanaesthetized cats raised masked thresholds to a greater extent than absolute thresholds. Thresholds were determined beha-viourally. Data from Pickles and Comis (1973).

which different frequency components contribute to masking. The results of such experiments show that it is as though we hear the tone through a bandpass filter, and it is the noise that gets through the filter that masks the tone. The filter has a well-defined bandwidth for each test tone frequency. The filter is known as the critical band, and will be discussed further in Chapter 9. The experiments with atropine suggested that the critical band filter had been increased in width. Accordingly, Pickles (1976a) measured critical bands behaviourally in the cat before and after the application of atropine to the cochlear nucleus.

Critical bands were measured by masking a 1 kHz tone with bands of noise of variable bandwidth but constant total power. If all the noise were concentrated within the same critical band filter as the signal, it would all contribute to the masking of the signal, with the result that the signal threshold would be high. If it were widened beyond the critical band filter, a smaller proportion would contribute to masking, and the masked threshold would be lower. As the masker bandwidth is increased, therefore, we would expect the signal threshold to be constant for masker bandwidths less than the critical bandwidth, and to start falling in inverse proportion to masker bandwidths for wider bands. The latter would be represented by a straight line of slope −10 on log–log scales, if the threshold in dB is plotted against log masker bandwidth. The point of transition between this function and the constancy observed for narrower bandwidths measures the critical bandwidth. Such functions were indeed observed in normal animals (Fig. 8.10, curve c).

After atropine, however, the function became significantly flatter (Fig. 8.10, curves a and b). For the larger doses of atropine the masked threshold became independent of masker bandwidth, and this indicated that noise over the whole 4 kHz band contributed to masking. In other words, the critical band had been widened enormously, or indeed its mechanism had been abolished completely. Intermediate doses produced intermediate effects, indicating that the critical band was wider than normal, with shallow slopes. These results indicate that the integrity of the cholinergic, and hence probably centrifugal, neuronal system of the cochlear nucleus was necessary for normal frequency resolution as indicated by the critical band. They suggest that the centrifugal pathway aided the detection of signals in noise by determining the extent to which background stimuli were filtered out.

Noradrenaline, a transmitter in a second centrifugal system to the cochlear nuclei, has also been applied through the cannula to block the normal operation of the noradrenergic system by the blanket activation of the receptors (Pickles, 1976b). Both absolute and masked thresholds were affected. The loss in masked threshold depended on the bandwidth of the masking noise, again suggesting that the critical bandwidth had been affected.

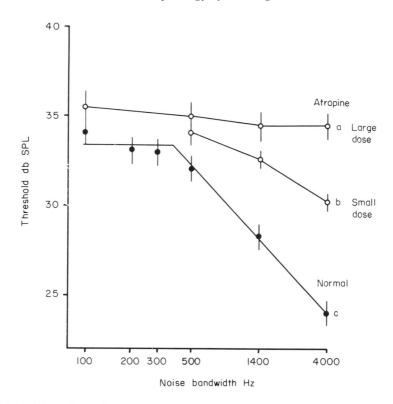

Fig. 8.10 Effect of atropine on the critical bandwidth. In the normal cat wideband noise produced a lower masked tone threshold than did narrowband noise of the same total power (curve c). Atropine applied to the cochlear nucleus abolished the relation (curve a). Smaller effective doses of atropine had an intermediate effect (curve b). From Pickles (1976), Fig. 2.

D. Centrifugal Pathways in Higher Centres

1. Anatomy

Two descending systems have been described as originating in the auditory cortex. Firstly, it appears as though each cortical area sends a descending projection to the division of the medial geniculate from which it receives an ascending projection (Diamond *et al.*, 1969). The descending fibres terminate on the very cells that project back to the cortex (Morest, 1975). Such a terminal of a descending fibre is shown by the ending 'DF' in Fig. 6.18B. There seems therefore a close coupling in the loop of afferent and efferent fibres, suggesting that, within each functional division, the thalamus and cortex act as one unit. Secondly, the cortex also sends descending projections to a wide range of diencephalic and midbrain nuclei, including other nuclei of the thalamus, the tegmentum, the inferior colliculus and two areas connected to the motor system, namely the corpus striatum and the pontine nuclei (Diamond *et al.*, 1969).

The inferior colliculus receives a descending innervation from both the auditory cortex and the medial geniculate body. The axons terminate in the pericentral nucleus and the dorsomedial division of the central nucleus (Fig. 8.11; Rockel and Jones, 1973a,b). These areas do not receive the main ascending supply. A similar picture was produced in electrophysiological experiments by Massopust and Ordy (1962). Stimulation of the auditory cortex produced evoked potentials in the 'rind' of the inferior colliculus, whereas sound produced evoked potentials in the central region. There seems therefore some separation between the ascending and descending auditory systems, already noted in the superior olivary complex.

Harrison and Howe (1974b) suggest that the collicular areas receiving a descending centrifugal innervation from the cortex might in turn give rise to centrifugal axons descending further down the auditory system. These might end on the pre- and periolivary nuclei of the superior olivary complex, which themselves are known to give rise to centrifugal axons. Other centrifugal fibres run directly from the inferior colliculus to the dorsal cochlear nucleus (Rasmussen, 1965). In this way, a complete chain of descending pathways, running from the cortex to the periphery, could exist.

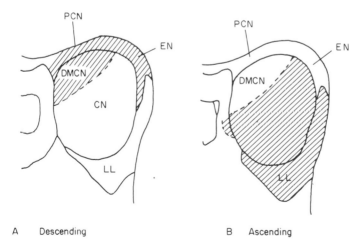

A   Descending   B   Ascending

Fig. 8.11 Descending and ascending fibres to the interior colliculus end in predominantly different parts of the nucleus. Here, patterns of terminal degeneration are shown, as they appear after lesions of the descending (A) and ascending (B) innervation. CN: central nucleus of the IC; DMCN: dorsomedial division of the central nucleus of the IC; EN: external nucleus of the IC; LL: lateral lemniscus; PCN: pericentral nucleus of the IC. From Rockel and Jones (1973a), Fig. 21, Rockel and Jones (1973b), Fig. 1.

2. Physiology and Function

There have been very few studies of the physiology of the more central of the centrifugal pathways. There have been reports that electrical stimulation of the cortex can produce both excitation and inhibition in single units of the medial geniculate body (Watanabe *et al.*, 1966; Andersen *et al.*, 1972). Ryugo and Weinberger (1976) suggested that the closed corticogeniculate loops could be responsible for the reverberations seen in the firing of many geniculate neurones. Many such neurones show a reverberatory after discharge, lasting 100 ms or more after an auditory stimulus. Cooling the cortex reduced the response.

Dewson *et al.* (1966) detected the influence of the I–T (insulo-temporal) area of the auditory cortex on the cochlear nucleus by recording recovery functions to paired clicks in the cochlear nucleus. In this technique, the responsiveness of the nucleus after one click was tested by measuring the size of the response to a second click. In unanaesthetized cats, after lesion of the I–T area, the responsiveness recovered particularly rapidly after each click, and Dewson *et al.* interpreted this as suggesting that normally the I–T cortex, by means of the centrifugal pathways, was prolonging the effect of stimuli in the cochlear nucleus. Beyond that, they did not speculate on the significance of the finding.

Desmedt (1975) and Desmedt and Mechelse (1958) presented physiological evidence for a train of centrifugal pathways descending from the cortex to the cochlea. Electrical stimulation of many stages of the brain, generally close to but not within the ascending tracts, altered auditory evoked potentials earlier in the system. Desmedt suggested that the centrifugal pathways formed one system, which he called CERACS (Centrifugal Extrareticular Activating System), the extrareticular to indicate that the system was not part of the reticular formation, which also can have a modifying effect on the sensory input.

We should not, however, think of the centrifugal system as affecting only the periphery. It is very likely that it produces changes in neuronal processing in the intermediate nuclei. Examples have already been given where the cholinergic efferent supply seems to alter the detection of signals in noise in the cochlear nucleus as well as at the periphery. There is also evidence that centrifugal pathways must be involved in more complex behaviour. It was described in the previous chapters how some learned auditory tasks survive complete ablation of the neocortex. The reflexes may therefore have been established subcortically. Furthermore, it is likely that in the intact animal the cortex would have been able to influence the reflexes. This influence must therefore occur through the centrifugal pathways. We therefore have a system, in which reflexes can be established at many levels, and in which the cortex controls the reflexes through descending influences, and not one in which all sensory activity is relayed to the cerebral cortex, where learned connections are made, and then relayed down the effector pathways. In this way it is possible that the centrifugal pathways from the cortex can be thought of as being some of its principal output pathways.

E. Summary

1. Centrifugal (efferent) auditory pathways parallel the centripetal (afferent) auditory pathways along the entire length of the system, forming a chain which runs from the cortex to the hair cells. In many stages of the auditory pathway, they run adjacent to, but not actually within, the tracts and nuclei principally associated with the ascending system.

2. The hair cells are innervated by the olivocochlear bundle, which arises bilaterally in the superior olivary complex. About one third of olivo-cochlear fibres give rise to synaptic terminals on the base of outer hair cells; these fibres are mainly crossed. The others give rise to terminals on the afferent nerve fibres and their synaptic terminals below inner hair cells; these fibres are almost exclusively uncrossed. The transmitter is acetylcholine.

3. Electrical activation of the crossed olivocochlear bundle reduces the response of auditory nerve fibres to sound. Fibres of the olivocochlear bundle are themselves responsive to sound and often have complex tuning curves. Olivocochlear fibres terminate in areas of the cochlea corresponding to the frequency of the sound that drives them best, and so make closed frequency specific feedback loops. Central influences also affect the activity of the olivocochlear fibres.

4. The function of the olivocochlear bundle in auditory performance is uncertain. There is some evidence that it reduces the auditory input when the subject is attending to stimuli in another modality. The olivo-cochlear bundle also seems to affect auditory discriminations in the presence of noise.

5. The cochlear nucleus receives branches of the olivocochlear bundle, together with other centrifugal fibres from the superior olivary complex, and from higher auditory nuclei, including the nuclei of the lateral lemniscus and the inferior colliculus. Some of the transmitters seem to be acetylcholine and noradrenaline.

6. Centrifugal fibres to the cochlear nucleus are both inhibitory and excitatory. The cholinergic innervation affects the animal's ability to detect signals in noise. The innervation affects the critical bandwidth, which is the bandwidth of noise that contributes to masking.

7. There have been comparatively few studies of the physiology of centrifugal fibres at higher levels of the auditory system. There is evidence that the fibres are organized into a functional chain, so that the cerebral cortex can affect the activity of the lower stages of the auditory system. There significance is not known: they may for instance serve to control auditory reflexes established at lower levels of the auditory system.

F. Further Reading

Harrison and Howe (1974b) describe the anatomy of the centrifugal auditory system.

Klinke and Galley (1974) give an account of the anatomy, physiology and pharmacology of the olivocochlear bundle. Desmedt (1975) reviews some of the physiology of the centrifugal auditory pathways. Behavioural experiments are described by Neff *et al.* (1975).

Physiological Correlates of Auditory Psychophysics and Performance

There has been a tendency for auditory psychophysicists to seek correlates of psychophysical phenomena in the neuronal responses of the earliest stages of the auditory system for which we have definite information. Thus, for instance, the factors governing our handling of frequency and intensity information have been sought in the responses of single fibres of the auditory nerve. The validity of such correlations will be examined here. The relation of the absolute threshold to the best thresholds of auditory nerve fibres, together with the possible aspects of auditory nerve firing used as cues by the subject, will be discussed first. The physiological correlates of psychophysical frequency resolution and discrimination will be examined, followed by the coding of auditory stimuli as a function of intensity and the determinant of the sensation of loudness. The relation of sound localization to neuronal binaural interaction will be examined. Finally, neuronal responses to speech will be described. This chapter requires knowledge of the information contained in Chapters 1 to 4. In addition, there are some specific referrals back to Chapters 6 and 7.

A. Introduction

In this chapter we shall try to analyse the extent to which some aspects of auditory performance can be explained in terms of known physiological processes. The chapter by no means attempts to be a balanced review of the psychology or psychophysics of hearing, but to deal with certain phenomena whose explanation has, or seems to have, a close correlate with physiology.

B. The Absolute Threshold

The absolute threshold seems to be a reasonably close match to the minimum thresholds of auditory nerve fibres (Fig. 4.4, p. 77). The behavioural audiogram is near, or is about 10 dB below, the lowest neural thresholds. A small discrepancy is not surprising. Even if the subject uses only mean neural firing rates, he may be able to do better than suggested by the tuning curves of individual fibres, because he is able to average activity over many fibres.

The discrepancy between the neural and behavioural data is more serious at high frequencies. The reason for this is not clear; the surgical preparation for the electrophysiological experiment may have had an influence.

Is phase-locking rather than an increase in mean firing rate used as a cue at threshold? In electrophysiological recordings of auditory nerve fibres the first indication of activation by a tone of low frequencies can be a phase-locking of the spontaneous activity to the stimulus, rather than a net increase in firing. The threshold for phase-locking may be 10–20 dB below that for an increase in mean firing rate. How this happens may be understood from the membrane potential of inner hair cells. At low intenstities the depolarizing phases of the intracellular potential will add just as many spikes as the hyperpolarizing phase subtracts, and phase-locking will increase without any net increase in firing rate. In order to see whether phase-locking is used as a cue, we might think of seeing whether the behavioural threshold falls below the neural mean rate threshold to a greater extent at low, than at high frequencies, where phase-locking does not occur. Unfortunately, there are so many uncertainties in the comparison that it turns out not to be practicable. There are such large interindividual differences in both the neural and electrophysiological sets of data that comparisons have to be made in the same animals. The anaesthetic and the surgical preparation for recording will produce unknown and uncertain effects. At the moment, the comparison has not been possible at the required level of certainty.

There is however some psychophysical evidence that phase-locking is not used as a detection cue at threshold. A beating sensation can be produced between two sinusoids with slightly different frequencies presented to the two ears. The beats are likely to arise from an interaction of phase-locked action potentials in the central nervous system. Groen (1964) showed that binaural beats could be detected when one of the stimuli was as low as 20 dB below its absolute threshold. This suggests that phase information could be transmitted by the auditory nerve when the stimulus was below threshold, and has the corollary that the phase information itself did not determine the absolute threshold.

C. Frequency Resolution

1. A Review of the Psychophysics of Frequency Resolution

(a) Frequency resolution and frequency discrimination

One of the most fundamental properties of the auditory nerve system is its frequency selectivity. Psychophysically, we distinguish two phenomena of frequency selectivity. One is that known as frequency discrimination. Two tones are presented one after the other, and we have to tell whether there is a difference between them. Frequency difference limens in this case can be very small, perhaps as small as 0.2% or 0.3% of the stimulus frequency. The fine resolution comes from our ability to compare two neural patterns that are separated in time. The other phenomenon is known as frequency resolution, and corresponds more closely to the physiological mechanisms of frequency selectivity studied by the electrophysiologist. In this case the subject has to detect one frequency component of a complex stimulus in the presence of other frequency components, all presented simultaneously. It measures the extent to which the subject is able to filter one stimulus out from others on the basis of frequency. In an analogy, we can think of tuning a radio receiver so that the filter in the input circuit receives the desired station and rejects all others. The resolution of the filter tells us how good it is at passing one station while rejecting others that are close to it in frequency. In the auditory system such resolution bandwidths are a measure of the fundamental frequency filtering properties of the auditory system. These resolution bandwidths are much larger than frequency difference limens, and are perhaps 15–20% of the stimulus frequency. It is the latter case of frequency resolution that will be dealt with in this section; frequency discrimination will be dealt with later.

(b) Masking patterns as an indication of frequency resolution

One of the most immediate demonstrations of psychophysical frequency resolution is provided by the masking pattern produced by a narrowband stimulus, such as a narrow band of noise (Fig. 9.1). The masker is presented continuously, and the threshold of a tonal signal, called the probe, is plotted as a function of probe frequency. It is assumed that the threshold of the probe is a measure of the amount of activity produced by the masker in neurones with characteristic frequencies equal to the probe's frequency. The logic is that the probe is detected only if it produces more activity than the masker alone. The masking pattern becomes therefore a correlate of the iso-intensity curves of Fig 4.7, B–D. The masked threshold is greatest near the masker frequency, and at high masker levels the pattern spreads more to high than to low frequencies. The asymmetry has an obvious correlate in the asymmetry of tuning curves, which in the cat for neurones above 1 kHz extend further below than above the characteristic frequency. The reversal of the pattern of asymmetry between the psychophysical and neural cases stems simply from the method of measurement. An electrophysiologist plots the response of *one* neurone to stimuli of many different frequencies. In contrast, the psychophysicist measures the response in *many* different frequency regions to a masker of *one* frequency. Viewed in another way, a masker is able to activate the low frequency tails of the tuning curves of neurones of much higher characteristic frequency, and so mask probes of much higher frequency. But a masker is comparatively ineffective at activating neurones of lower characteristic frequency, because the high frequency cutoffs of their tuning curves are so sharp. Maskers are therefore not effective at masking probes of much lower frequency. This accounts for the predominantly upwards spread of masking at higher masking levels.

A technique which might give a close psychophysical correlate of neural tuning curves is that known as the 'psychophysical tuning curve' (Zwicker, 1974). In this case, the probe is fixed in frequency and is presented at a low constant intensity, such as 10 dB above threshold. Presumably, such a

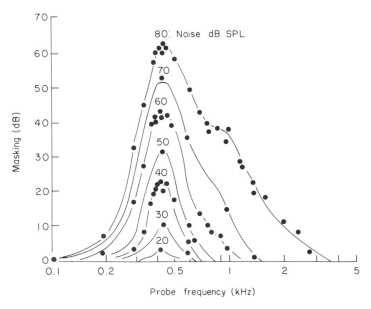

Fig. 9.1 The masking pattern produced by a narrow band of noise. The elevation in threshold of a probe tone was plotted as a function of the probe frequency. At high intensities, the masking pattern spreads more to high to than low frequencies. Masker width 90 Hz, centred at 410 Hz. From Egan and Hake (1950), Fig. 8.

low-level probe will activate only a few neurones and will provide a near approximation to the electrophysiologist's measurement of single neurones. The *masker* is varied in frequency, and is adjusted in intensity to keep the *probe* at threshold. Again we presume that the probe is detected if it produces more activity in any neurones than the masker alone. We might therefore expect the probe to stay at threshold as the masker is moved in frequency and intensity around the edges of the tuning curves of the neurones at the probe frequency. The resulting psychophysical tuning curves indeed appear very similar to the tuning curves of auditory nerve fibres (Fig. 9.2).

The masking patterns of Figs 9.1 and 9.2 appear to be similar to the frequency responses of bandpass filters. This suggests that we can think of the frequency resolving power of the auditory system as being due to a set of bandpass filters. Such filters have been measured extensively, and have given us the phenomenon known as the critical band.

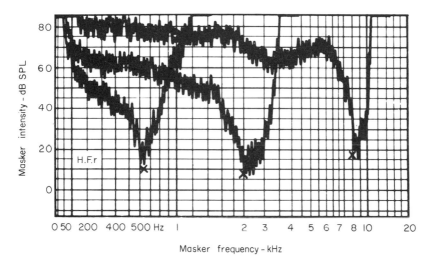

Fig. 9.2 Psychophysical tuning curves are produced by plotting the locus of frequency and intensity necessary to just mask a constant low level probe (shown by crosses). The curves were determined with a Békésy audiometer, in which the subject continuously adjusted the masker intensity as its frequency was swept, in order to keep the probe at threshold. From Zwicker (1974), Fig. 2.

(c) Critical bands

Fletcher (1940) introduced the concept of the critical band to deal with the masking of a narrowband stimulus by wideband noise. He found that he could electronically filter out noise components remote in frequency from the signal without affecting the signal's threshold. However, there was a critical frequency region around the signal in which noise was essential for masking. He called this range the critical bandwidth. We can think of critical bands as a series of bandpass filters situated early in the auditory system. Only noise which falls in the same critical band filter as the signal will mask it. The filters correspond to the filters underlying the masking patterns of Figs 9.1 and 9.2, the bandwidth of the filters being known as the critical bandwidth. The effective bandwidth is about 15–20% of the stimulus frequency. Stimuli will interact to different extents depending on whether or not they lie within the same critical band filter. Critical bands in this way affect a wide variety of auditory tasks, including frequency masking patterns, sensitivity to phase relations, tonal dissonance and roughness (e.g. Scharf, 1970).

An important demonstration of the critical band in masking was made by Zwicker (1954). The signal was a narrowband of noise masked by two tones, one above and the other below it in frequency. As the tones were moved apart in frequency, the signal threshold at first was constant, and then fell precipitously (Fig. 9.3).

It is difficult to tell the exact shape of the psychophysical filter from such experiments, because the probe threshold is affected by factors such as temporal interactions between the masker and probe, and by the detection

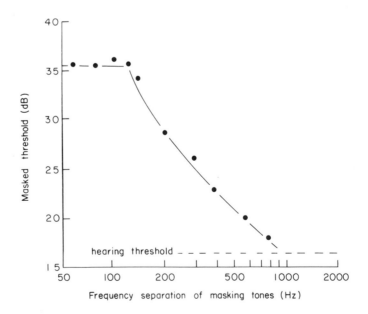

Fig. 9.3 The masked threshold of a narrowband probe, masked by two tones, is shown as a function of tone separation. The masked threshold shows a sudden fall as the maskers are moved outside the critical bandwidth. From Zwicker (1954), Fig. 5.

of combination tones produced between the masker and probe. One task which is probably affected less than most is the masking of a tone by bandstop noise, that is, by noise with a gap in its spectrum. Psychophysical filters determined with such a masker have an approximately Gaussian shape, that is, with a rounded tip, rather like the tuning curves of auditory nerve fibres (Patterson, 1976).

(d) Nonsimultaneous masking techniques

A technique for measuring frequency resolution that has produced a great deal of interest depends on nonsimultaneous, rather than direct or simultaneous, masking (Houtgast, 1972, 1977). One example is forward masking. The masker is pulsed, each pulse being followed by a brief probe, lasting only 10 or 20 ms. The stimuli are ramped on and off to reduce the effects of spectral splatter. The masker will, of course, raise the threshold of the probe. If the critical band measurements are repeated with nonsimultanous masking a surprising difference emerges: the calculated psychophysical filters necessary to explain the results are now rather narrower, and are now surrounded, particularly on the high frequency side, by areas of *negative* transmission. The negative areas can be explained by supposing that they are areas of lateral inhibition or suppression (Fig. 9.4; Houtgast, 1977).

Lateral inhibition or suppression is of course widespread in the auditory system, but had not hitherto been demonstrated convincingly by simultaneous masking techniques. Houtgast pointed out an obvious reason. We

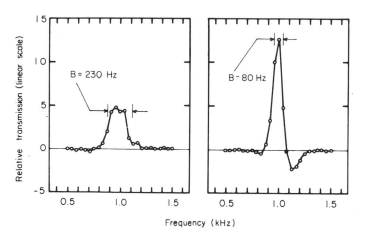

Fig. 9.4 Calculated psychophysical filter shapes derived by direct masking techniques (left) are broader than those determined by nonsimultaneous masking (right). That determined by nonsimultaneous masking also has an inhibitory sideband. 'B' indicates the effective bandwidth of the filter, or the bandwidth of the equivalent rectangular filter. From Houtgast (1974), Fig. 9.5.

calculate the internal representation of a masker by measuring the threshold of a probe superimposed on the masker. If the elements of a complex masker interact and suppress the masker in some frequency regions, a simultaneously presented probe will be suppressed as well and to a similar extent. Because the signal-to-noise ratio is in effect unchanged, the probe threshold will be unchanged, and the suppression areas will not be reflected in the probe threshold. Forward masking acts rather differently. A complex masker will produce regions of high activity, and, as a result of lateral suppression or inhibition, some regions of low activity. When the masker is turned off, the thresholds of neurones of some later stage in the auditory system will be raised, to an extent which depends on the amount of previous activity produced by the masker. If a probe is now presented, its threshold will reflect the influence of the inhibitory bands as well as the excitatory ones.

Nonsimultaneous masking techniques have generated interest because they reveal the effects of lateral inhibition. This has suggested that nonsimultaneous masking might provide a more accurate picture of the neural representation of auditory stimuli than does simultaneous masking. On the other hand, the detection cues have not been investigated as thoroughly as in simultaneous masking, and the errors they introduce are not as well known (Moore, 1980).

2. Relating Psychophysics to Physiology in Frequency Resolution

Having accumulated the information needed on the psychophysics of frequency resolution, we are now in a position to see how psychophysical frequency resolution relates to the physiology of the auditory system. Simultaneous or direct masking will be discussed first.

Fletcher (1940) suggested that the critical bandwidth was equal to the resolution bandwidth of the pattern of mechanical excitation on the basilar membrane. We are still not in a position to confirm or refute that opinion. Because the adequacy of the measurement of basilar membrane motion is at the moment uncertain, it is better to compare the psychophysical results with the responses of the neurones of the auditory pathway. The latter can at least be measured with certainty and over the whole of the psychophysical intensity range, even if not necessarily in alert animals.

Firstly it is obvious that the direct masking patterns of Figs 9.1 and 9.2 are generally similar to the tuning curves, or iso-response curves, of Figs 4.3 and 4.7A. It is not currently doubted that, in broad terms at least, these functions are all reflections of the basic frequency resolving power of the auditory system, so we can therefore use the results of the psychophysical tests described above to measure some aspects of the physiological frequency resolution of the auditory system.

How precise and close are the analogies between neural tuning curves and the psychophysical masking functions of Figs 9.1 and 9.2? Detailed analysis shows that the relation is not as precise as it might seem at first sight. There are three lines of evidence suggesting that the two types of function may reflect different processes:

(i)   We have supposed that the masking patterns of Figs 9.1 and 9.2 provided direct measurements of the amount of excitation produced by the masker. The logic was that the probe would be detected if it produced more excitation in any neurone than the masker alone. But it is likely that two-tone suppression, or lateral inhibition in auditory nuclei, also contributes to masking. The masker may reduce the response to the probe by suppressing or inhibiting it, and not only by swamping it with its own excitation. Therefore in generating the psychophysical tuning curve of Fig. 9.2 the masker may have been following the outer edges of the neural two-tone suppression areas. The two-tone suppression areas are of course more broadly tuned than the central excitatory region of the neural tuning curve. The psychophysical tuning curves therefore could be significantly wider than excitatory neural tuning curves.

Note that this explanation of the role of suppression or inhibition in simultaneous masking differs in an important way from that given by Houtgast. Houtgast suggested that suppression would not itself affect masked thresholds, because it would always affect the masker and probe to the same extent. However, we have just seen a case where this is not true. A stimulus in the two-tone suppression areas of an auditory nerve fibre can reduce the response to an excitatory tone. Here, suppression by itself does the masking. It is therefore possible that, with simultaneous masking, probe thresholds *do* sometimes reflect the action of two-tone suppression, or lateral inhibition in auditory nuclei.

(ii) Psychophysical resolution bandwidths measured behaviourally by direct masking in the cat, when compared with the excitatory bandwidths of single auditory nerve fibres in the same animals, suggest that psychophysical bandwidths are wider by a factor of two or three (Fig. 9.5; Pickles, 1975, 1979a, 1980).

(iii) It was suggested above that nonsimultaneous masking techniques might provide the more accurate picture of the neural representation of auditory stimuli. This suggestion arose because nonsimultaneous masking revealed lateral inhibitory or suppressive sidebands. As was indicated by Fig. 9.4, nonsimultaneous masking techniques gave bandwidths of frequency resolution that were narrower than those given by direct masking. Direct masking may therefore give bandwidths that are wider than neural tuning curves.

While three lines of evidence suggest that psychophysical resolution band-widths or critical bandwidths as measured by direct masking, may be wider than neural tuning curves, the position is not entirely clearcut. Comparable psychophysical resolution bandwidths can also be demonstrated with signals of variable bandwidth. Gässler (1954) for instance asked subjects to detect a multitone complex. The total power of the signal at threshold was found to be independent of the signal bandwidth up to the critical bandwidth, showing perfect integration of energy over frequency in this range. The most direct model to account for the results supposes that neurones in the auditory system were also able to integrate energy over the critical bandwidth, with the result that neural excitatory bandwidths would be the same as the critical bandwidth.

A second problem arises from the suggestion made in paragraph (i) above, that two-tone suppression in the auditory nerve is responsible for the difference between the bandwidth of the neural tuning curve and the bandwidth of psychophysical frequency resolution. If the psychophysical tests are imitated electrophysiologically on single fibres of the auditory nerve, the

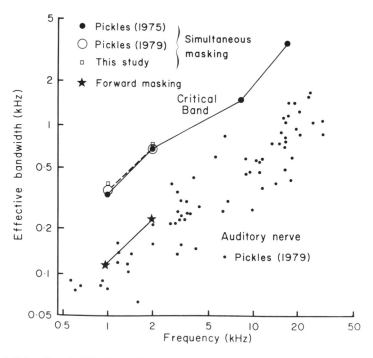

Fig. 9.5 Critical bandwidths determined by simultaneous masking, and bandwidths determined by forward masking, compared with the bandwidths of auditory nerve fibres in the same animals. In all cases effective bandwidths, i.e. bandwidths of the equivalent rectangular filter, are plotted. From Pickles (1980), Fig. 2.

resolution bandwidths so obtained should then agree with the psychophysical bandwidths rather than the excitatory bandwidths of the neural tuning curves. This however is not always the case. Pickles and Comis (1976) measured the responses of auditory nerve fibres to tones, when their responses were masked by a band of noise of variable width, centred on the characteristic frequency. The masked threshold of a tone at the characteristic frequency was plotted as a function of the bandwidth of the masking noise — an exact analogue of a psychophysical test used for measuring the critical bandwidth. The variation of the tone threshold with masker bandwidth showed the bandwidth over which the auditory nerve fibres integrated the masking noise. The integration bandwidths so obtained were identical to those expected from the excitatory neural tuning curve. They were clearly different from critical bandwidths obtained by simultaneous masking in behavioural psychophysical tests using the very same stimuli in the same animals. This suggests that two-tone suppression in the auditory nerve is *not* responsible for the difference seen between the bandwidths of auditory nerve fibres and the critical bandwidth, at least as determined by simultaneous masking techniques.

In view of these contradictory results, we cannot be sure of the neural correlates of psychophysical frequency resolution as measured by simultaneous masking. Do then nonsimultaneous masking techniques provide a more direct measure of neural frequency resolution? The answer at the moment seems to be that they do, but because nonsimultaneous masking techniques are newer, possible probems with the correlation have not been analysed in detail.

Pickles (1980) measured resolution bandwidths behaviourally by forward masking in the cat, and showed that the bandwidths so obtained were similar to the resolution bandwidths of cat auditory nerve fibres (Fig. 9.5).

Nonsimultaneous masking techniques can also be used to plot out suppression areas similar to the two-tone suppression areas of auditory nerve fibres of Fig. 4.16. Houtgast (1972, 1973) performed the psychophysical analogue of measuring neural two-tone suppression. With nonsimultaneous masking, he used not one, but two, tones during the masking periods. One tone provided the masking, and the other suppressed the first tone. The net amount of excitation was assessed from the threshold of a third, or probe, tone. He was able to plot the contours of intensity and frequency within which the suppressing tone, or unmasker, provided 3 dB or more of release from masking. The resulting two-tone suppression areas appear very similar to the two-tone suppression areas of auditory nerve fibres (Fig. 9.6).

As with simultaneous masking, we can turn the full circle and use psychophysical tests in electrophysiological experiments to see whether the psychophysics and electrophysiology agree as we would expect. Harris and Dallos (1979) obtained 'psychophysical' tuning curves by forward masking in single auditory nerve fibres. They masked the response to a tone burst at the fibre's characteristic frequency by preceding it with a masking tone burst. As in the psychophysical test, the masker was varied in frequency and adjusted in intensity to keep the probe tone at threshold. Tuning curves made in this way exactly followed the excitatory tuning curve determined in the conventional way with single tones. Similarly, unmasking the forward masker by a suppressing tone revealed two-tone suppression areas which agreed substantially with the two-tone suppression areas determined in the conventional way (Harris, 1979). As far as the evidence goes at the moment, it seems that nonsimultaneous masking techniques do provide a reasonable measure of the neural representation of auditory stimuli.

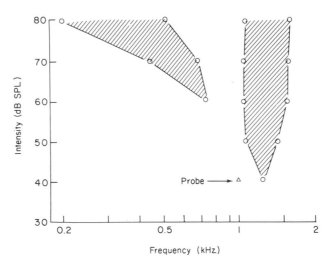

Fig. 9.6 Two-tone suppression areas (shaded) can be revealed by psychophysical nonsimultaneous masking techniques. From Houtgast (1974), Fig. 5.3.

3. Influence of Lateral Inhibition on Frequency Resolution

The mechanical frequency resolving power of the cochlea, as shown by von Békésy (1960), was rather poor, and he suggested that the greater frequency resolution of the whole organism was produced by neurally-mediated lateral inhibition. He suggested that the pattern of excitation in the cochlea was sharpened up by neural inhibitory networks in the cochlea and elsewhere. We now know that this view was wrong; neural lateral inhibition does not occur in the cochlea. Nevertheless, von Békésy's ideas both about the existence of neural lateral inhibition in the cochlea, and the role of inhibition in sharpening frequency resolution, often continue to be reproduced.

As was pointed out in Chapter 4, there is no evidence that there is any lateral inhibition in the cochlea mediated by inhibitory synapses (this is discounting effects produced by the olivocochlear fibres, but these act too slowly to account for the psychophysical results). The usually rather weak phenomenon of two-tone suppression depends on the nonlinearity of the cochlea. Two-tone suppression itself does not serve to increase frequency resolution; stimuli which activate both excitatory and suppressive areas do not produce noticeably sharper tuning than do single tones. This is shown by the agreement between the tuning curves produced with single tones, and those produced with broadband noise as a stimulus, calculated by the reverse correlation technique (Fig. 4.13A). Two-tone suppression does not make a substantial contribution to frequency resolution because the suppressive effect is not only rather weak, but is broadly tuned (Fig. 4.15).

Nor docs neural lateral inhibition in, say, the dorsal cochlear nucleus serve to sharpen neural tuning curves, at least near the tip. Cells of the dorsal cochlear nucleus have strong inhibitory sidebands (Chapter 6), but the sharpness of their tuning curves, as shown by the 10 dB bandwidths, is comparable to that of auditory nerve fibres (Goldberg and Brownell, 1973). It is only well above threshold that lateral inhibition in the dorsal cochlear nucleus affects frequency resolution, by stopping thc tuning curves from widening with intensity as much as they would othcrwise have done (Fig. 6.5B and C).

This discussion is relevant to thc prcvious discussion of the differences in bandwidths of frequency resolution found with simultaneous and non-simultaneous masking techniques. Nonsimultaneous masking techniques give much smaller 10 dB bandwidths than do simultaneous masking techniques (Fig. 9.4), and one hypothesis to explain the difference is that suppressive or inhibitory sidebands, by overlapping the excitatory response area, serve to decrease its bandwidth. Nonsimultaneous masking techniques, which reveal the effects of suppression or inhibition on the neural representation, will show this narrower bandwidth. That hypothesis however cannot be held, if suppression and inhibition do not serve to decrease the 10 dB bandwidths of auditory neurones (Goldberg and Brownell, 1973).

So far the evidence has been presented as though thc tips of tuning curves do not become any sharper at later stages of the auditory pathway, and that any sharpening produced by inhibition is confined to the region well above threshold. In one nucleus, however, this may not be the case. Erulkar (1959) originally, and Aitkin *et al.* (1975) later, reported unusually sharp tuning curves in the inferior colliculus. Aitkin *et al.* (1975) found seven out of 92 neurones in the central nucleus that had tuning curve tips a little narrower than auditory nerve fibres, and four out of the 92 with tips that were substantially narrower. One had a Q_{10} with the extraordinarily high value of 38, as against a maximum of 10 for auditory nerve fibres. This very sharp tuning has so far been seen only for a very small proportion of the neurones in only one nucleus. At the moment, we do not know its significance for psychophysical tasks.

D. Frequency Discrimination

1. Introduction

Frequency discrimination refers to our ability to distinguish two tones, on the basis of frequency, when they are separated in time. Frequency difference limens are very much smaller than critical bands. Two mechanisms are possible. For instance, the subject may detect shifts in the place of maximum excitation in the cochlea. This is called the 'place theory'. Or he may use temporal information. We know that the firing in the auditory nerve is phase-locked to the stimulus waveform up to 5 kHz. On this theory, called the 'temporal' or 'frequency' theory, the subject discriminates the two tones by using the time intervals between the neural firings. It is not certain which of the two mechanisms is used. Indeed the controversy has been active for nearly 100 years, and the fact that it is not yet settled shows that we still do not have adequate evidence. Auditory physiologists divide into three groups, namely those that think only temporal information is used, those that think only place or spectral information is used, and an eclectic group who suppose that temporal or frequency information is used at low frequencies, and place information at high.

In one of the most explicit formulations of the place theory, Zwicker (1970) suggested that frequency discrimination depended on detecting shifts in the place of excitation of the nerve fibre array (Fig. 9.7).

The most extreme form of the temporal, or frequency, theory was put forward by Rutherford (1886) who said that each hair cell in the cochlea responded to every tone, and that frequency information was carried only in the frequency of the nerve impulses. Auditory nerve fibres do not fire continuously faster than about 300/s, and Wever (1949) formulated the principle of volleying by supposing that different fibres were activated on different cycles, so that the summed response was able to follow each cycle of the stimulus waveform up to much higher frequencies. A modern formulation would be, that in the frequency range below 5 kHz in which phase-locking is possible, it is the timing of the nerve action potentials that conveys frequency information.

There are several lines of evidence for and against these two theories, none of which is conclusive.

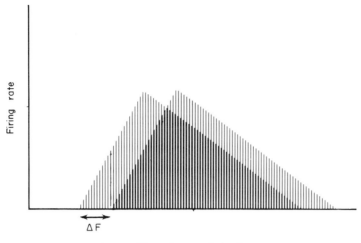

Nerve fibre characteristic frequency

Fig. 9.7 The place theory of frequency discrimination. The pattern of activity in the nerve fibre array is represented schematically by a series of vertical lines, each line representing the firing rate of one neurone to the stimulus. The neurones are arranged in order of ascending characteristic frequency. Shifts in the place of excitation are detected.

2. Evidence on Place Versus Time Coding of Frequency

(a) Small size of limits

Protagonists of both place and time theories point out how small the detectable limits have to be when translated into the terms of the other theory. Temporal theorists point out that a frequency discrimination limen of 3 Hz at 1 kHz corresponds to a shift in the pattern of excitation on the basilar membrane of 18 μm, or the width of two hair cells. Frequency theorists point out that the same limen corresponds to a time discrimination of 3 μs, as against some 1000μs for the width of the nerve action potential, and a possible jitter of 100μs in its initiation. In both cases averaging over many neurones would be able to reduce the limens below those of the individual neurones.

(b) Differences above and below 5 kHz

Because phase-locking is lost in the auditory nerve above 5 kHz, only place theories must operate above that limit. If auditory perception is qualitatively different above and below that limit, the implication is that temporal information might be used. It seems that there are some important differences in the perception of tones above and below this limit, so that for instance tunes cannot be recognized.

(c) Frequency discrimination with short stimuli

In a quasi-linear spectral analyser such as the cochlea the physical limits of frequency resolution are limited by the duration of the stimulus, as a result of spectral splatter: stimulus duration × spectral line width ≈ 1. In other words, with spectral cues, very short stimuli can only be poorly resolved. Temporal theories are not so limited; indeed, given a sufficiently good signal-to-noise ratio, good discrimination is possible by measuring between two similar points only one cycle apart. On the hypothesis that place and not spectral cues are used, we can calculate a lower limit for the frequency discrimination limen as a function of the length of the stimulus. Moore (1973) showed that below 5 kHz frequency discrimination for short stimuli was up to an order of magnitude better than expected on a spectral basis. This again suggests that temporal information may be used below 5 kHz.

(d) The missing fundamental

If tones such as 1000 Hz, 1200 Hz, and 1400 Hz are sounded together, a pitch corresponding to the fundamental of 200 Hz, which is not present in the stimulus, is also heard. The phenomenon was for a long time used as an argument for temporal processes in perception, because the resulting complex waveform has a periodicity of 200 Hz. Indeed, the phenomenon was once called 'periodicity pitch'. Alternative explanations are known as 'pattern' theories. They suppose that the auditory system, by recognizing that the tones sounded are the upper harmonics of a low tone, supplies the missing fundamental that would have generated them. This is again an area which is controversial, and over the years opinions have swayed in favour of one hypothesis or the other. At the moment pattern theories are dominant, for the following reason: suppose high harmonics generate a low pitch. They will be relatively closely spaced and will not be resolved by the auditory system. Recognition of the spectral pattern will not therefore be possible, but the harmonics will be able to interact in the nervous system to produce a periodically varying waveform. Temporal theories are therefore supported. On the other hand, low harmonics will be resolved spectrally, and if they generate the low pitch, pattern models are possible. The harmonics will not be able to interact to produce a periodically varying waveform and temporal models become unlikely. Plomp (1967) and Ritsma (1967) showed that the low, resolved, harmonics were dominant in generating the low pitch. Pattern models are therefore favoured, and the phenomenon is not now used to support temporal coding as much as it was before.

It is however recognized that a weak sensation of pitch can be conveyed by pure temporal information, for instance by the unresolved high harmonics, by regularly chopped noise or by certain binaural stimuli. Some have suggested that the mechanisms involved in binaural time analysis are also used for pitch discrimination (e.g. Nordmark, 1970). However the sensation of tonality is so much weaker than that evoked by real tones that it probably reflects a different mechanism.

(e) Electrical stimulation of the cochlea or auditory nerve

Electrodes have been placed in the cochlea or auditory nerve, in an attempt to restore some hearing in otherwise deaf patients. Because of current spread, only the crudest of place information should be possible. On the other hand, the temporal relations of the nerve firings should be unaffected, so that if correct timing is sufficient, discrimination should be perfect. Different reports of the tonality of the sensation emerge: in some cases the stimuli appeared to be clearly tonal, in others completely atonal, like a noise. Similarly, the discrimination of frequency is in many cases poor or absent. The lack of success in many patients has therefore been taken as indicating that temporal information is by itself not sufficient for frequency discrimination or for the sensation of pitch.

Closer examination, however, shows that the evidence is not as strong as it appears to be. Periodic electrical stimuli will, if they activate a fibre at all, activate it on every cycle. The upper limits of phase-locking to electrical stimuli will be set by the refractory period of the nerve membrane, giving limits of 1 kHz and below. By contrast, tones do not generally activate a fibre on every cycle of the stimulus, and this means that some phase-locking will be preserved at frequencies well beyond those set by the refractory period. This explains why electrical stimuli above a few hundred Hz are poor at conveying temporal information.

Secondly, electrodes in the cochlea are usually inserted at the basal end, which normally transduces high frequency stimuli. Now it is known from psychophysical experiments that high frequency fibres are particularly poor at generating a low sensation of pitch when periodically activated at a low frequency. In the phenomenon of the missing fundamental a sinsoidal high frequency sound wave can be modulated in amplitude by a low frequency waveform, and a low pitch corresponding to the low modulating frequency can be heard. This however does not occur if the high frequency 'carrier' sinusoid is above about 5 kHz, even though the modulation may be at 500 Hz or below. It is fibres in just this high frequency region that will have been stimulated by the implanted electrodes. It is not therefore surprising that they are poor at producing a sensation of pitch to periodic activation at low frequency.

The conclusion is that the poor pitch sensations and frequency discrimination limens often shown by patients with cochlear implants cannot be taken as evidence that timing information is not used in frequency discrimination. Indeed, the fact that it sometimes *is* possible supports the idea that timing information can be so used.

(g) Harmonic consonance

It might be thought that the pleasant consonance of simple musical intervals depends on the simple relations between their periods, resulting in synchronous nerve firing. However, once it is realized that most musical notes are rich in overtones, and that consonance might depend on a lack of beats between the harmonics, the argument cannot be used to support the importance of time information.

(h) A model for the analysis of temporal information

One of the greatest problems facing temporal theories of frequency discrimination is that of finding a realistic mechanism for analysing the information.

When we discriminate a tone of 1000 Hz from one of 1010 Hz, we can activate our muscles to one stimulus and not to the other. We do not transmit nerve impulses to our muscles at 1000 Hz in one case and at 1010 Hz in the other! Temporal information must therefore be transformed into place information at *some* point in the nervous system. In fact, since timing information is degraded by synapses, the earlier the information is transformed the better.

The 'on' cells of the cochlear nucleus, among which are the octopus cells of the posteroventral cochlear nucleus, are responsive to the periodicity of auditory stimuli. They are able to follow every click in a series up to a certain rate, above which the response drops sharply (Godfrey *et al.*, 1975a). Figure 9.8 shows a cell that at 10 dB stimulus attenuation could discriminate between stimuli at 700 and 800 Hz on the basis of temporal information. Such a cell might be able to respond to a complex waveform or a tone on the basis of its overall periodicity. But we do not have enough information to tell whether these cells are reasonable candidates for the analysis of temporal information in the ways suggested by psychophysical data. Moreover, the frequency limits of the cells are typically below 800 Hz, well below the 5 kHz that has been suggested as the limit of temporal processing.

(i) Conclusions

It is not possible to decide between the temporal and spectral theories of frequency discrimination. The eclectic view, which is that temporal information is used at low frequencies and spectral information at high, does not conflict with most of the evidence. In any case, the best support for the eclectic view is the rather negative one that the evidence in favour of either of the other two theories is not conclusive, and this may be a function of the quality of the evidence available rather than of the actual operation of the auditory system.

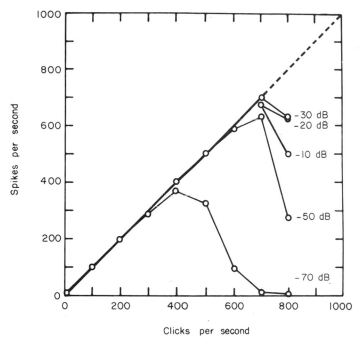

Fig. 9.8 Firing rate of an 'on' cell of the cochlear nucleus, as a function of click rate. The drop in firing at high stimulus rates may be able to signal the periodicity of auditory stimuli. From Godfrey *et al*. (1975a), Fig. 14.

E. Intensity

1. Stimulus Coding as a Function of Intensity

As the stimulus intensity is raised, the tuning curves of auditory nerve fibres become wider and wider (e.g. Fig. 4.3). This in itself does not necessarily mean that frequency resolution deteriorates, because iso-rate functions determined at different rates above threshold show that resolution is practically unchanged as long as the firing is not saturated (Fig. 4.7A). When the firing is saturated, however, frequency resolution deteriorates sharply. This is indicated by the diagrams of the nerve fibre array in Fig. 9.9A and B. Below saturation, the elements of a complex stimulus are resolved. Once the fibres are driven into saturation, resolution is no longer possible. But in cells with strong inhibitory sidebands, as in cells of the dorsal cochlear nucleus, frequency resolution is preserved (e.g. Evans, 1977). We can understand how. The strong inhibitory sidebands will serve to keep the neural firing near the middle of the range irrespective of overall stimulus intensity, so that the details of the stimulus pattern can be transmitted (Fig. 9.9C). Put in other terms, the inhibitory sidebands stop the tuning curve from becoming as wide as it would otherwise have been (Fig. 6.5B and C). The picture will also hold for cells with similar response characteristics at higher levels of the auditory system. Such responses can explain the great dynamic range of 80 to 100 dB over which psychophysical frequency resolution is preserved practically unchanged (Scharf and Meiselman, 1977).

What is unexplained is how the information is transmitted by the auditory nerve in the first place, when the intensity is so high as to saturate the firing of the great majority of its fibres. The psychophysical dynamic range may be contrasted with a dynamic range of only 30 to 50 dB in the firing of auditory nerve fibres. The great majority of auditory nerve fibres have thresholds in the bottom 10 dB of the range, and we would therefore expect nearly all fibres to be saturated at 50–60 dB above threshold.

Several hypotheses have been advanced to account for the wide psychophysical range of hearing, compared to the restricted dynamic range of auditory nerve fibres.

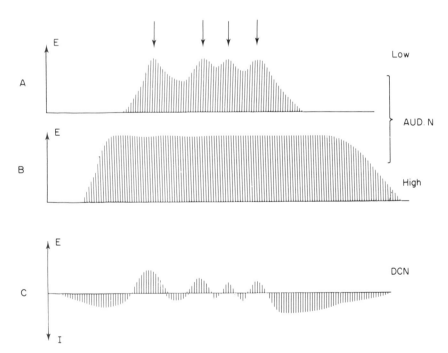

Fig. 9.9 The response of the auditory nerve fibre array is shown to a complex acoustic stimulus at low (A) and high (B) intensities. At high intensities resolution is lost in the auditory nerve (B), but not in the dorsal cochlear nucleus (C). Arrows mark peaks of energy in the stimulus. E: excitation; I: inhibition.

(a) Range of thresholds

As described in Chapter 4, the great majority of auditory nerve fibres have thresholds in the bottom 10–15 dB of the range. Liberman and Kiang (1978) have shown that there is also a significant proportion of fibres with higher thresholds (Fig. 4.4). It is not known whether these fibres are found in the normal state. The cats were raised in a soundproofed room and would have been free from noise trauma before the experiment was begun. Nevertheless there is always the possibility that noise from opening the bone during the surgical preparation could have been traumatic, and that the powers of recovery of the cochlea were reduced under anaesthetic. Even if high threshold fibres exist in the normal animal, we still have to explain how the comparatively few fibres of high threshold are able to convey information as accurately at high intensities as the much larger number of low threshold fibres at medium intensities. It is difficult to escape the conclusion that the low threshold fibres must also have been contributing to some extent.

(b) Sloping saturation of rate-intensity functions

Sachs and Abbas (1974) showed that the firing of some auditory nerve fibres did not saturate in a sharply defined manner, but went on increasing gradually at high intensities (Fig. 9.10). These fibres also tend to have higher thresholds than the others. However the proportion of fibres still unsaturated at high intensities is only a few percent (Palmer and Evans, 1980). Again, we have a problem in explaining how psychophysical abilities do not

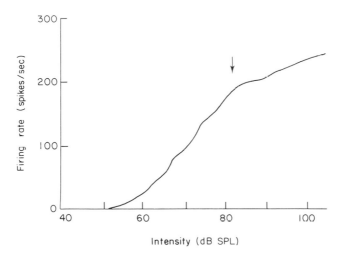

Fig. 9.10 In auditory nerve fibres exhibiting sloping saturation, the rate-intensity function shows a knee (arrow), and then goes on increasing. Such neurones may partly explain the wide dynamic range of hearing. From Sachs and Abbas (1974), Fig. 6.

fall markedly at high intensities. We would, for instance, expect the detection thresholds for tones in wideband noise to deteriorate substantially. Not only would fewer fibres be able to convey information, but those fibres still unsaturated would be stimulated in a flatter part of their rate-intensity functions.

(c) Edge detection

The rate-intensity functions of Fig. 4.6 show that although a fibre may be saturated by stimuli at the characteristic frequency, it may not be saturated by stimuli of other frequencies. Figure 9.11 shows how at high intensities information can be conveyed by fibres at the edges of the active array of nerve fibres. Such mechanisms might explain how, for instance, frequency discrimination is possible at high intensities. The mechanisms will only operate for narrow band stimuli. The explanation will not work with wideband stimuli, where fibres of the whole frequency range are saturated.

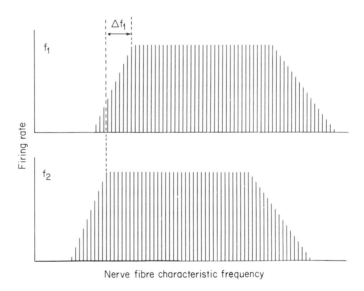

Fig. 9.11 The place theory of frequency discrimination, for stimuli of high intensity. Changes on the edge of the active nerve fibre array are detected.

(d) Two-tone suppression

Other sense organs, such as the retina, preserve a wide dynamic range by lateral inhibition, so that the response to a pattern is relatively independent of the overall intensity. In the auditory system, cells with strong inhibitory sidebands in for instance the dorsal cochlear nucleus behave in the same way. Could two-tone suppression in the auditory nerve function similarly? Two-tone suppression is after all maintained in saturation. However, the effects are far weaker than neural lateral inhibition. Gilbert and Pickles (1980) found that the suppression produced by wideband noise was on average only 8% of the evoked firing rate. So we might expect two-tone suppression to preserve spectral contrasts to some extent, and for some sorts of stimuli, but only to a very small extent. For other sorts of stimuli, two-tone suppression seems to *reduce* spectral contrasts. For vowel sounds some of the peaks of activity in the nerve fibre array seem to be suppressed more than the troughs so that the pattern of activity in the nerve fibre array becomes flatter (Sachs and Young 1979).

(e) Temporal information

Auditory nerve fibres show phase-locking to stimuli below 5 kHz. The phase-locking is preserved at high intensities in spite of a saturation of the firing rate. Indeed, in spite of a loss of frequency selectivity in mean firing rate terms, the frequency selectivity indicated by temporal information deteriorates only slightly or not at all at high intensities. This is shown by the tuning curves determined from the time pattern of the nerve firings by the reverse correlation technique (Fig. 4.13). Consider the following example showing how frequency resolution may be preserved. At low intensities a fibre may fire phase-locked to a tone at its characteristic frequency of 1.0 kHz, but not fire at all to one of 1.5 kHz. At high intensities, either one of the two tones will saturate the fibre. The two tones will therefore activate the fibre to the same extent if presented separately. This occurs because the 1.5 kHz tone will drive the fibre as fast as it can fire, and the 1.0 kHz tone alone cannot produce more activity. But if the two tones are presented together, the 1.0 kHz tone will again show itself to be more effective in driving the fibre, and the nerve firings will be predominantly phase-locked to 1.0 kHz. Corresponding results have been shown for a complex stimulus, namely a vowel sound (Fig. 9.12). At low intensities, both mean firing rates and phase-locking showed that the formants were resolved. At high intensities, the firing of the majority of fibres was saturated, and the formants were not discriminated by a mean rate analysis. Phase-locking to the formants was however preserved, so that if the temporal information was used, frequency resolution could be maintained (Sachs *et al.*, 1980).

Psychophysical frequency resolution, as shown by the wideband masking of tones, deteriorates more with increasing intensity above than below the 5 kHz limit for phase-locking (Scharf and Meiselman, 1977; Moore, 1975). The implication is that below 5 kHz temporal information had been used at high intensities, when the nerve firing was saturated.

The problem is to find a physiological mechanism to extract the timing information. The only possibility seems to be the 'on' cells of the postero-ventral cochlear nucleus, which respond to the periodicity of auditory stimuli, as explained above (Fig. 9.8). However, cells of the dorsal cochlear nucleus seem to be able to resolve spectral components when the firing of auditory nerve fibres is saturated, and we have absolutely no indication that this results from a decoding of temporal information, either directly in the dorsal cochlear nucleus, or as transmitted from the 'on' cells.

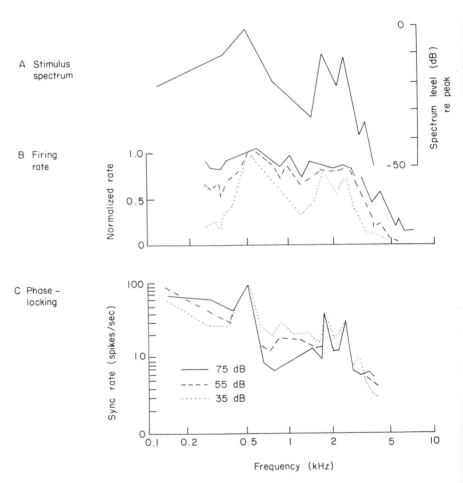

Fig. 9.12 Neurograms of auditory nerve fibre activity to the vowel sound 'e' (spectrum on top trace). The activity of a large number of auditory nerve fibres was sampled in response to the one stimulus, and the activity of each fibre plotted against its characteristic frequency. The curves shown in B and C are running means, in B of firing rate, and C of phase-locking. At high intensities the formants were discriminated by phase-locking but not by mean rate critera. From Sachs *et al.* (1980), Figs 6 and 7.

(f) The middle ear muscle reflex

Sound-elicited contractions of the middle ear muscles may attenuate the sound input by as much as 20 dB. Wever and Vernon (1955) showed that the middle ear muscle reflex could act as an automatic gain-control, keeping the input approximately constant when the stimulus intensity was varied over a range of 20 dB above the reflex threshold, which was usually about 80 dB SPL. Such powerful control will only be expected to occur for sound frequencies in the range where transmission is strongly affected by the middle ear muscle reflex, well below 1 kHz. It will not explain the wide dynamic range of hearing for frequencies of 1 kHz and above.

(g) Conclusions

No one mechanism seems entirely satisfactory to explain the transmission of spectral information by the auditory nerve at high intensities. Hypotheses suggesting that small variations in mean firing rates are used (based on a range of thresholds in auditory nerve fibres, sloping saturations of the rate-intensity functions, and two-tone suppression) have the advantage that no unknown mechanism is needed to translate the variations into mean rate terms in a nucleus such as the dorsal cochlear nucleus, where a wide dynamic range can be measured for wideband stimuli. In such a nucleus, variations around the mean rate of firing could be extracted by lateral inhibition, and then amplified by steep rate-intensity functions. But we have to explain why incremental thresholds and signal-to-noise ratios do not fall when detection depends on small changes in firing rates in the auditory nerve. On the other hand, temporal information is preserved over a wide intensity range in the auditory nerve, but we do not know how this could be translated into mean rate terms in a nucleus such as the dorsal cochlear nucleus.

2. *Loudness*

The sensation of loudness seems to depend on the total sum of activity transmitted by auditory nerve fibres. When some auditory nerve fibres are destroyed unilaterally, as for instance by a tumour of the brainstem, the loudness of a stimulus can grow more slowly than normal. This can be measured by requiring the subject to match the loudness of a stimulus in the abnormal ear to one in the normal ear (Citron *et al.*, 1963).

In a different type of experiment, Zwicker *et al.* (1957) asked normal subjects to match the loudness of tone complexes with the loudness of a standard stimulus. The bandwidth of the test stimulus was varied but its total power was kept constant. As the bandwidth of the stimulus increased up to and beyond the critical band, the loudness at first stayed constant and then, beyond the critical bandwidth, increased (Fig. 9.13A). We can explain this if

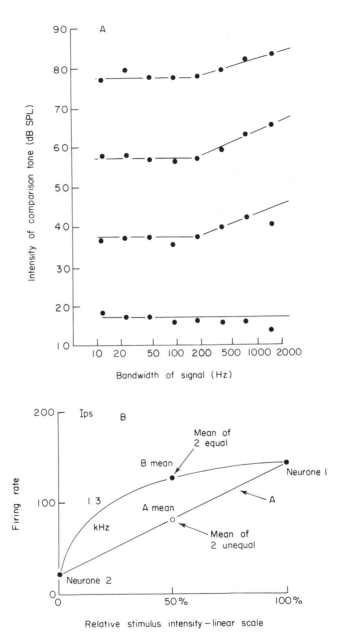

Fig. 9.13 A. The loudness of a four-tone complex is plotted as a function of overall tone spacing. Stimuli centred on 1 kHz. From Zwicker *et al.* (1957), Fig. 3.
B. The rate-intensity function of an auditory nerve fibre (curved line) is plotted on a linear, rather than a logarithmic, scale of intensity. The greatest mean firing rate taken over two neurones is produced if both are stimulated equally (B mean), rather than one maximally and the other not at all (A mean). See text for explanation.

we assume that critical bands correspond to the bandwidths of auditory nerve fibres. As was mentioned above, this correspondence may not be true in detail. Leaving that aside for the moment, we can show that the total amount of activity in the auditory nerve increases as a stimulus of constant total power is spread beyond the integration bandwidth of the individual neurones. Figure 9.13B shows one of the rate-intensity functions for the auditory nerve fibre of Fig. 4.6 replotted on a linear, rather than logarithmic or dB, scale of acoustic power. Over practically all of the dynamic range the curve is a negatively accelerating function, becoming shallower and shallower as the stimulus power is increased. Such functions have the property that the greatest *mean* output is obtained if the stimulation is spread as equally as possible over all the input channels. Figure 9.13B illustrates this for the case of two neurones. In one case, marked 'A', the power is concentrated in one neurone, which is stimulated at relative power 100, while the other is unstimulated. 'A mean' indicates the mean firing rate, averaged over the two neurones. In the other case the same total power is spread evenly over the two neurones, each of which is stimulated with a relative power of 50. The mean firing rate, indicated by the letter 'B', is now greater. This follows simply from the negatively-accelerated shape of the function, and the same argument applies over any number of neurones. This shows, in agreement with Fig. 9.13A, that the greatest sum of activity is produced by spreading the input power over as many channels as possible. On the other hand, the very foot of the function, if drawn on an expanded scale, will be seen not to be negatively accelerated to the same extent, and this may explain why the increase in loudness does not occur at the very lowest intensity.

Two-tone suppression will also affect the results: as a signal is widened onto the neural suppression areas, the total number of action potentials will be reduced below the number that would otherwise have been possible. This will delay the increase in net activity as a signal is widened, so that the critical bandwidth determined by loudness summation will tend to be wider than the effective bandwidths of the auditory nerve fibres. This agrees with previous results on the relation between auditory nerve fibre bandwidths and the critical bandwidth, as determined by other methods (p. 259).

F. Sound Localization

A real sound source in space will stimulate both ears. Experiments with headphones have suggested that the side on which a source is heard depends on timing and intensity differences at the two ears. The sensation of the sound as arising 'out there' in space depends on the coloration added by resonances and reflections arising from the head, pinna and concha (Chapter

2). The latter have not been investigated by electrophysiological means. However the responses of neurones in the auditory system to stimuli differing in timing and intensity at the two ears have been investigated extensively.

As was pointed out in Chapters 6 and 7, a large proportion of the neurones at and beyond the superior olivary complex are responsive to timing or intensity differences at the two ears. This is good *a priori* evidence that the cells are involved in sound localization and in some cases the results seem to agree with the results obtained with real sound sources in space. In the owl, and perhaps in other species, the neurones can be organized in a spatial map. One of the problems is that many cells, and indeed the majority, seem optimally responsive to timing and intensity disparities that are greater than could be produced by any real sound source in space. Figure 9.14 shows for instance that in the medial superior olive the characteristic delays of most neurones are greater than the maximum delay calculated from the separation of the ears. The same point has been made for the cortex by Benson and Teas (1976). Benson and Teas also showed that the same was true for intensity differences: direct measurements have shown that the maximum interaural intensity difference expected in the chinchilla for stimuli below 2 kHz is 4–5 dB, yet cortical neurones of these characteristic frequencies were optimally sensitive to intensity differences as great as 20 dB. Such neurones may have a role, not in representing the direction of a sound

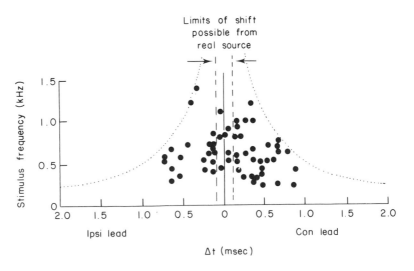

Fig. 9.14 The characteristic delays in neurones of the kangaroo rat MSO are compared with the maximum interaural delay possible for a real signal source stimulating the two ears (dashed lines). Because phase delays greater than half a cycle give ambiguous results, the characteristic frequencies are plotted against stimulus frequency, and the delays lie within the dotted lines. From Crow *et al.* (1978), Fig. 8.

source, but in *discriminating between* the directions of sound sources. The cyclic functions of Figs 6.12A and 7.10A, obtained when firing rates were measured for different interaural timing disparities, indicate how. Note that we can best discriminate *changes* in time disparity by looking, not at the peaks of the functions, but at the points of greatest slope. These generally occur for far smaller interaural disparities than the peaks, and will be in the range for real stimuli.

The role of binaural interaction in the brainstem in sound localization has been strongly supported by behavioural experiments. Moore *et al.* (1974) trained cats to discriminate the direction of sounds. The various tracts by which binaural interaction might occur were cut in different animals. Sound localization was affected only by cutting the crossing fibres in the trapezoid body. These are the fibres by which binaural interactions occur in the superior olivary complex. Transections of the fibres joining the inferior colliculi of both sides, or of the corpus callosum joining the two cerebral hemispheres, were without effect. The primacy of binaural interactions at the superior olive was further supported by cutting the output pathway of the superior olivary complex, the lateral lemniscus, on one side. Sound localization was rapidly relearned (Casseday and Neff, 1975). So if binaural interaction had already occurred, information travelling up only one side of the brainstem was able to subserve sound localization.

Brainstem mechanisms of sound localization are also dealt with in Chapter 6, Sections C, E and F. Cortical mechanisms are dealt with in Chapter 7, Sections A.3, B.2 and C.4.

G. Speech

The response of auditory nerve fibres to speech sounds can be predicted from the properties of their responses to tones, which were described in Chapter 4. When the sound intensity is so low as to stimulate only the sharply tuned tips of the tuning curves of auditory nerve fibres, the fibres will be responding to a limited spectral analysis of the sound. The fibres will only respond when the speech sound has significant energy in their frequency range. The firing rate will follow the temporal envelope of the frequency-filtered stimulus. Most of the energy of speech sounds is below 5 kHz, and in this frequency range the neural firings will be phase-locked to the individual cycles of the speech sound as it appears after filtering by the peripheral frequency analyser, although each fibre will of course not fire on every cycle of the stimulus. Dynamic factors will also affect the response; where there is a rapid change in stimulus intensity, the fibres will show peaks of activity analogous to their onset firing at the beginning of a tone burst.

At higher intensities the neural iso-intensity curves become broader (Fig.

4.7). Fibres of high characteristic frequency in particular, whose tuning curves have long tails stretching to low frequencies, will respond to all frequencies in the speech sound. In this case the only information transmitted during the steady portions of the speech sound will be temporal information. The firing will follow the temporal envelope of the speech waveform, and the firings, when they occur, will be phase-locked to the individual cycles of the stimulus. But even at high overall stimulus intensities, the quieter portions of the speech waveform may be within the dynamic ranges of the auditory nerve fibres, and in these regions mean firing rate information will continue to be useful.

Some of the changes in frequency analysis with intensity, and the following of the envelope of the sound stimulus, are shown in response to the sound 'shoo cat' in Fig. 9.15. At low intensities the firing only occurred during the 'a', when the stimulus had energy near the fibre's characteristic frequency. At higher intensities firing occurred during the whole stimulus, and followed its envelope.

Sachs and Young (1979) made the same point by sampling the responses of a very large number of auditory nerve fibres of different characteristic frequencies to a single vowel sound. The results give a picture of the activity evoked by the stimulus in the whole nerve fibre array. Below the intensities at which saturation of the firing occurred, peaks of activity occurred at the formants of the vowel (Fig. 9.12B). As the intensity was raised, the firing was driven into saturation, and the peaks disapeared.

Similarly an analysis of phase-locking to the stimulus showed peaks of phase-locking at the formant frequencies. The contrasts in the pattern of phase-locking did not deteriorate, and even improved, with intensity (Fig. 9.12C). This confirms what was shown previously, that when the firing of auditory nerve fibres is saturated, spectral information is preserved in the phase-locking but is not obvious in the mean firing rates. Whether or not this temporal information is actually *used* by the nervous system is another matter.

Although responses to vowel sounds of high intensity have not been measured in cells with strong inhibitory sidebands, we would expect spectral information to be preserved in the mean firing rate over the whole range of stimulus intensity. Recordings in the dorsal cochlear nucleus for instance suggest that the formants would be represented by separate peaks of activity, separated by bands of inhibition. We would expect this pattern to be preserved at many later stages of the auditory system. But even in the cochlear nucleus we expect other analyses, for instance the selective responses to frequency and intensity transitions, to be influencing the results. Other complexities, which are not fully understood, are also known. For instance, Moore and Cashin (1974) showed that energy in inhibitory sidebands could increase neurones' responses to the transients in speech sounds.

Even at this early stage, the neurones will therefore be responding to some of the higher level aspects of the stimulus. Such an analysis is continued to the cortex, where the responses of cells to speech sounds are complex and cannot be predicted from the responses to simple stimuli (Chapter 7).

In the cortex the region primarily involved in the analysis of speech seems

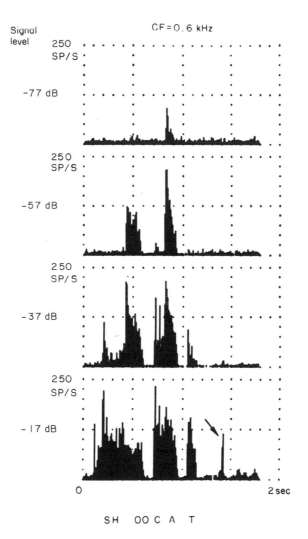

Fig. 9.15 The firing of an auditory nerve fibre in response to the sound 'shoo cat' is shown for different stimulus intensities. The stimulus was recorded on a tape loop and replayed repetitively, and a histogram of neuronal activity made with respect to the onset of the sound. The tape loop produced a stimulus artefact at the highest stimulus intensity (arrowed). From Kiang and Moxon (1972), Fig. 10.

to be Wernicke's area, part of the auditory association cortex on the posterior part of the temporal lobe on the dominant, generally left, hemisphere of the brain. The information originally came from the effects of localized brain lesions. Lesions here led to a disability known as sensory or Wernicke's aphasia, a disorder in the production of speech which was considered to have a perceptual basis because it was associated with disorders of comprehension and errors in word selection. Striking recent confirmation has come from studies in which the blood flow was measured by a radioactive tracer technique simultaneously in many regions of the brain while the subject was conscious (Lassen *et al.*, 1978). It seems that the local blood flow increases when neural activity is increased. When the subject passively listened to speech the greatest changes in blood flow were produced in Wernicke's area (Fig. 9.16). Activity in the primary auditory cortex was presumably underrepresented because in man the cortex lies in the lateral fissure. There was also a small activation of Broca's area, an area generally thought to be concerned with the *production* of speech and situated on the lower posterior part of the frontal lobe.

How are speech sounds analysed in the auditory cortex? Such electrophysiological studies as have been undertaken in animals suggest, as might be expected, that speech sounds undergo complex processing. But they have not indicated any special ways in which speech, as distinct from any other complex stimulus, is processed. We would not of course expect human speech to have any particular significance for nonhuman subjects, and some experimenters have tried to circumvent this by using the vocalizations of the

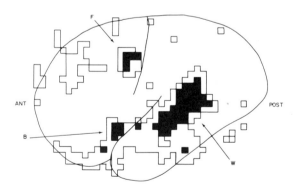

Fig. 9.16 When a conscious subject passively listens to speech, the greatest increases in blood flow are produced in Wernicke's area (W) in the dominant cerebral hemisphere. Increases were also produced in Broca's area (B) and the frontal eye fields (F).

Radioactive Xe[133] was dissoved in saline solution and injected into the arteries supplying the brain. The local concentration of the Xe[133] was measured by an array of scintillation counters placed over the skull. Areas of high relative blood flow are indicated by the contour lines. Adapted from Lassen *et al.* (1978).

species under investigation. However, these studies have not convincingly shown any special class of analysers that will respond specifically to speech-like sounds but not to other equally complex, non-speech, sounds. (e.g. Sovijärvi, 1975). In man, attempts have been made to use psychophysical evidence to show the ways in which speech sounds are processed differently from non-speech sounds. For instance Liberman *et al.* (1967) used psychoacoustic evidence to show that speech was processed in a special way, one that they called the 'speech mode'. As pointed out by Schouten (1980), many of the results on which they based their conclusions were determined by the basic psychoacoustic properties of the stimuli used. He suggested that their arguments could not be used to show that the processing of speech differs from that of other similarly complex non-speech sounds. At the moment it seems beyond our techniques to separate the processing of speech from that of all other complex stimuli. Nevertheless, there may be ways in which we can analyse the processing of certain of the attributes in which speech sounds are rich.

There is strong evidence that the processing of speech occurs in the dominant hemisphere, which in the great majority of subjects is on the left side of the brain. For instance, lesions of the auditory areas of the left cerebral hemisphere, but rarely of the right, affect the perception of speech. Each ear seems to project preferentially to the contralateral cerebral cortex, and the right ear, contralateral to the generally dominant cerebral hemisphere, has a small but significant advantage in the perception of speech. The advantage of the right ear is not confined to speech: some tasks involving the detection of temporal transitions also show a right ear advantage. For instance, Papçun *et al.* (1974) showed that trained Morse code operators, or naive subjects with small stimulus sequences, had a right ear advantage for the recognition of Morse code. They suggested that the dominant cerebral hemisphere was important for the analysis of stimuli into its sequential components. It may well be that the complexity of the temporal pattern in the stimulus determines the extent of the right ear advantage along a continuum. Halperin *et al.* (1973) asked subjects to repeat the order of stimuli which varied either in frequency, or in duration. Their result was that the more frequency or duration transitions the stimulus contained, the more the ear advantage shifted from left to right. This suggests that one of the special functions of the dominant cerebral hemisphere, and hence possibly of Wernicke's area, is the analysis of complex auditory stimuli in terms of sequential patterns, and that this is one of the reasons for its special role in speech. The implication of the time dimension in cortical function is reminiscent of some of the effects of cortical lesions in animals (Chapter 7).

Our understanding of the way in which the auditory system processes speech is in its infancy and unravelling the neuronal mechanisms involved is one of the supreme challenges of auditory physiology.

H. Summary

1. The behavioural absolute threshold lies just below the minimum thresholds of single auditory nerve fibres. Changes in mean discharge rate, rather than phase-locking, are probably the detection criterion used.

2. Frequency resolution describes the ability to filter out, on the basis of frequency, one stimulus component from another in a complex stimulus. The psychophysical resolving power of the auditory system seems to approximately match its neural resolving power. However on close analysis the agreement is seen not to be exact. Psychophysical resolution bandwidths, known as critical bandwidths, may well be larger than neural resolution bandwidths.

3. When critical bandwidths are measured psychophysically, a probe is usually presented simultaneously with a masker. But when nonsimultaneous masking techniques, such as forward masking, are used, the psychophysical frequency resolution bandwidths turn out to be rather narrower. They then match neural resolution bandwidths. The psychophysical filters determined with nonsimultaneous masking are often also surrounded by inhibitory sidebands. This suggests that nonsimultaneous masking techniques, rather than simultaneous masking techniques, provide an accurate picture of the neural representation of auditory stimuli. There are nevertheless some difficulties with this view, and the issue is still open.

4. In frequency discrimination, two tones are presented successively, and we have to tell whether there is a difference between them on the basis of frequency. This could be done by detecting a shift in the spatial pattern of excitation in the auditory system, or it could be done by detecting differences in the timing of nerve impulses. It is not possible to decide conclusively between these two theories. Many would support the view that temporal information is used at low frequencies, in the frequency range for neural phase-locking, and shifts in the spatial pattern of excitation are used at high frequencies.

5. The psychophysical frequency resolving power of the auditory system is maintained practically unchanged in the intensity range in which the firing of auditory nerve fibres is saturated. It is not known how their effective frequency resolving power is preserved in this intensity range. It is difficult to escape the conclusion that for a variety of causes the firing of all fibres is not quite saturated. It is also possible that phase-locking of neural firing, which does not deteriorate with intensity, is used.

6. The sensation of loudness seems to depend on the total quantity of activity in the auditory nerve.

7. Binaural influences on sound localization seem to depend primarily on binaural interactions in the superior olivary complex. In the owl, neurones in the homologue of the inferior colliculus form a spatial map of the environment. In mammals, many of the neurones investigated seem involved, not in representing the directions of sound sources, but in discriminating *between* the directions of sound sources.

8. Speech sounds are transmitted by the auditory nerve in a way that can be understood from its response to simpler stimuli. Depending on the position of the speech stimulus in the response area of the fibre, each fibre responds to a limited spectral analysis of the stimulus. The firings follow the temporal envelope of the stimulus, and are, at low frequencies, phase-locked to the individual cycles of the stimulus. In the higher centres of the auditory system, speech sounds undergo complex analyses, depending for instance on transitions of intensity and frequency. No single unit electrophysiological analysis has so far shown ways in which speech sounds are treated differently from complex non-speech sounds.

9. The cortical analysis of speech occurs primarily in Wernicke's area in the dominant cerebral hemisphere. The dominant cerebral hemisphere seems particularly important for analysing sounds in terms of their sequential patterns.

I. Further Reading

The psychophysics of hearing is dealt with by Tobias (1970, 1972), Plomp (1976), and Moore (1982).

Frequency discrimination and resolution, and their relation to physiology, are discussed by Evans (1978) and Moore (1982).

Brain stem mechanisms of sound localization are dealt with by Harrison (1978), and cortical mechanisms by Ravizza and Belmore (1978).

The representation of speech in the auditory nerve is discussed in articles in the *J. Acoustical Soc. Am.* (1980), **68**, between pp. 830 and 875. Articles by Kiang, Delgutte, Sachs and Young are recommended. Cortical mechanisms of speech are discussed by Ravizza and Belmore (1978), and Hecaen (1979). The volume containing Hecaen's article (*The Handbook of Behavioural Biology*, Vol. 2 (M. S. Gazzaniga, ed. Academic Press, New York) contains several other useful articles on brain mechanisms of speech.

X. Sensorineural Hearing Loss

Some forms of cochlear pathology can be induced experimentally, and changes found in the responses of auditory nerve fibres. The correlation of these changes with the changes that can be shown psychophysically will be described in this chapter. In addition, attempts to restore lost hearing by means of a cochlear prosthesis will be described. This chapter requires knowledge of Chapter 3 and the first part of Chapter 4 on the auditory nerve.

A. Types of Hearing Loss

Hearing loss arising in the auditory periphery is divided into two types, known as conductive and sensorineural loss.

Hearing loss due to an abnormality *before* the cochlea is known as conductive loss. It may arise because the impedance transformation in the middle ear is disrupted, because for instance the ossicles are immobilized, or because the differential transfer of pressure to the oval and round windows is otherwise impaired. Conductive loss produces a simple though frequency dependent attenuation of the stimulus, and can be compensated for by hearing aids. In many cases, the causes are amenable to treatment by antibiotics, and in severe cases the loss is amenable to surgical intervention, for instance by a prosthesis replacing an ossified stapes in the oval window.

Hearing loss arising in the cochlea or auditory nerve is known as sensorineural hearing loss. That arising in the nerve often results from a tumour. However the most common form of sensorineural impairment arises in the cochlea, when it is known by the rather cumbersome name of 'sensorineural hearing loss of cochlear origin'. In for instance middle and old age senile changes can produce a cochlear impairment known as presbycusis, that can be severe, progressive, and is completely without cure. Cochlear hearing loss can also be caused by noise trauma, drugs, infections, or may be congenital. In addition, many cases are encountered where no cause can be assigned. Particularly vulnerable sites are the sensitive transducer cells, namely the hair cells of the cochlea, and the stria vascularis. If the hair cells are destroyed they cannot be replaced. Because treatment is so often inadequate, because hearing aids prove to be of limited use, and because the condition is widespread, the importance of sensorineural deafness of cochlear origin cannot be overestimated. Physiological studies have recently revealed some of the physiological changes associated with cochlear damage, and it is these changes with which the present chapter will be mostly concerned, as well as some recent attempts to restore lost hearing by means of a cochlear prosthesis.

B. Sensorineural Hearing Loss of Cochlear Origin

1. Physiological Correlates

(a) Damage to outer hair cells

Nearly all nerve fibres synapse on inner hair cells rather than outer hair cells (p. 71), but it is likely that, in some way at present unknown, outer hair cells act to confer sensitivity on the inner hair cells.

In many of the forms of cochlear impairment that have been produced experimentally, the outer hair cells seem more vulnerable than the inner hair cells over the greater length of the cochlea. This is particularly true for the basal and middle turns. Ototoxic agents such as the aminoglycoside antibiotic kanamycin are often used experimentally to produce regulated cochlear damage. If the dosage is closely controlled, complete destruction of outer hair cells can be produced over large stretches of the cochlea without any obvious changes in inner hair cells. Figure 10.1A shows a common correlate in the tuning curves of auditory nerve fibres. The sensitive, sharply tuned, tip of the tuning curve is raised. Sensitivity is therefore lost, and frequency resolution decreases because the tip of the tuning curve becomes broader. We would expect this to have the psychophysical correlates of a severe loss in auditory sensitivity and a loss in frequency resolution for complex sounds. These are in fact observed.

The selective effect on the tip of the tuning curve is part of the evidence that outer hair cells somehow increase the sensitivity of inner hair cells, by a boost around the characteristic frequency.

Some researchers show a sharply tuned remnant of the tip on the high frequency slope of the tuning curve (Fig. 10.1B). This can be taken to mean that one component of the frequency selectivity of the organ of Corti is intact, but that the more broadly tuned increase in sensitivity provided by the outer hair cells is missing. The reason why the small sharp tip appears in some experiments and not others is not known — it may be the result of species differences. Nevertheless, we would expect both patterns to be associated with a loss in frequency resolution in most practical situations, because in most cases it is the broad bowl-shaped tail of the tuning curve that has the lowest threshold.

A third pattern of changes was noted by Liberman and Kiang (1978), who found that in some cases the low frequency tail of the tuning curve was *lowered* in threshold as well (Fig. 10.1C). The tuning curves therefore became W-shaped. This would again lead to a loss of resolution for some types of stimuli.

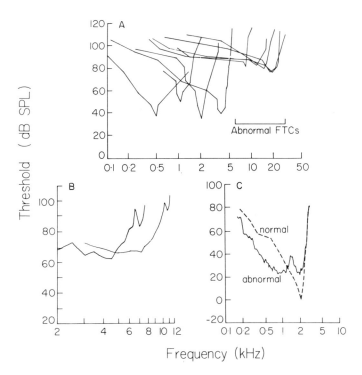

Fig. 10.1 The tuning curves of auditory nerve fibres can show a variety of patterns of abnormality after outer hair cell damage.

In A the sharply tuned tips are lost. In B the tip is still present but is shortened, and appears on the high frequency slope of the residual tuning curve. In C the sharply tuned tip is raised, and the broadly tuned tail is lowered in threshold.

A from Evans and Harrison (1975), Fig. 1, in the guinea-pig, B from Dallos *et al.* (1977), Fig 2, in the chinchilla, and C adapted from Liberman and Kiang (1978) in the cat.

Cochlear damage also reduces spontaneous activity in the auditory nerve. When the pathology is so severe as to reduce all the responses to sound, the spontaneous activity is abolished, or almost completely abolished (Kiang *et al*. 1970). In the few fibres that do fire spontaneously, the firing is sporadic, with a few spikes at short intervals, followed by long silent intervals (Liberman and Kiang, 1978).

The above changes have most usually been investigated with the aminoglycoside antibiotics. Anoxia, noise trauma, metabolic poisons such as cyanide, and ototoxic loop diuretics, produce broadly similar effects (e.g. Evans, 1976). Where different patterns of change have been produced, it is not known whether differences in the agent are responsible, or whether they are due to variation in species, in the degree of trauma produced, or in the extent to which other structures such as the inner hair cells or the stria vascularis are affected.

(b) Damage to inner hair cells

The majority of experimental manipulations affect outer hair cells rather than inner hair cells. In one study, however, careful histological examination of the cochlea showed regions where noise trauma had produced changes in inner hair cells and not outer hair cells (Liberman and Kiang, 1978). The changes in the inner hair cells were confined to the stereocilia, which had become clumped together. In these case, the neural tuning curves retained their normal V shape but were raised in threshold. The neural tuning was therefore unaffected, but the threshold was raised at all frequencies.

2. Psychophysical Correlates

(a) Sensitivity

The neural data should lead us to expect primarily a loss of sensitivity in sensorineural deafness of cochlear origin, and to the extent that the sharp tips of the neural tuning curves are widened, a loss in frequency resolution. These are observed.

The loss of sensitivity is of course an easily recognizable sign of deafness. High frequencies are generally affected first. The reasons are not known. In man there is in addition a puzzling phenomenon, seen particularly after noise trauma, of a selective hearing loss around 4 kHz. This produces what is known as the '4 kHz notch' in the audiogram. Again, the reasons are not known. It may correspond to a particular vulnerability of the cochlea in this frequency region. A 4 kHz notch is also seen in the behavioural audiograms of apparently normal cats (Fig. 4.4), and is also seen in the thresholds of auditory nerve fibres with characteristic frequencies in that region. These small losses in apparently normal animals seem to be pathological, because they are reduced in cats raised from birth in a soundproofed chamber.

(b) Frequency resolution

The change in neural frequency resolution similarly has a correlate in psychophysical data. Psychophysical tuning curves, which are thought to give a rough approximation to neural tuning curves (p. 254 and Fig. 9.2), are broadened (Fig. 10.2). The sharply tuned tip of the psychophysical tuning curve is reduced or abolished, and the low frequency slope in particular, becomes shallower (Leshowitz and Lindstrom, 1977). The changes are seen with both simultaneous and nonsimultaneous masking techniques (Nelson and Turner, 1980; Wightman *et al.*, 1977).

Critical bandwidths, being the bandwidths of the psychophysical filter (see p. 255), are also affected. For instance, estimates of the loudness of stimuli of different bandwidths can provide a measure of the critical bandwidth (Fig. 9.13). In patients with cochlear hearing loss such loudness measures show the ciritical band to be wider than normal (Bonding, 1979). In a different type of experiment, Pick *et al.* (1977) asked subjects to detect a probe tone in noise of rippled spectrum. They plotted the masked threshold as a function of the frequency spacing of the ripples, and used the results to calculate the shape of the psychophysical filter. With hearing losses of up to 40 dB, the main change was in the length of the sharply tuned tip segment of the psychophysical filter. For greater losses, the tip segment increased in bandwidth as well. These patterns have a parallel in the single unit data; for

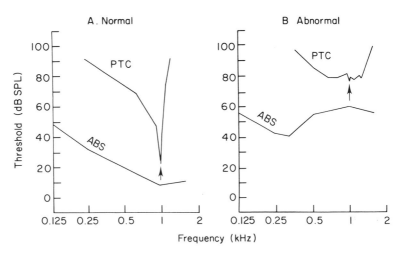

Fig. 10.2 Psychophysical tuning curves determined with forward masking in a normal subject (A), and in a subject with sensorineural hearing loss (B). ABS: absolute threshold (audiogram); Arrow: frequency and intensity of probe. From Nelson and Turner (1980), Figs 1 and 5.

small losses, the tips of the tuning curves are raised but do not become any broader; after a certain point, the tuning curves broaden substantially. There was also a large scatter in the psychophysical data, some patients with hearing losses of up to 70 dB showing normal frequency resolution bandwidths. Part of the scatter may arise because critical bandwidth tasks are comparatively difficult and complex anyway; but it may also be that the different patients were differently affected in the extent to which the sharply tuned tips of their tuning curves were affected. Some may have had tuning curves like those of Fig. 10.1A, with no sharply tuned tip segment, and others may have had ones like those of Fig. 10.1B and C, with a short remnant of the tip remaining.

The loss of frequency resolution may be one reason why speech perception is reduced in sensorineural hearing loss, and why even with amplification, speech perception cannot always be completely restored. Hearing aids may be able to restore *sensitivity*, and so the absolute threshold, but they cannot restore *resolution*.

(c) Loudness recruitment

Patients with sensorineural hearing loss show another characteristic feature, so specific that it can be used as a diagnostic tool — namely that of loudness recruitment. Loudness recruitment can also be explained in terms of the neural data. It can most readily be demonstrated if the hearing loss is unilateral, as can occur in Ménières's disease. The subject is asked to match the loudness of a stimulus in his abnormal ear with one in his normal ear. Near threshold, the stimuli are matched in loudness when the stimulus in the abnormal ear is raised by the amount of hearing loss (Fig. 10.3). But as the stimulus intensity is raised, the match occurs nearer and nearer normal levels, so that often by 80 dB SPL the match is made with the two stimuli at the same intensity. Loudness in the affected ear therefore grows abnormally quickly with intensity.

The neural explanation for loudness recruitment can be understood from the diagrams of Fig. 10.4. In part A, sample neural tuning curves from a normal cochlea are shown. It seems likely, as was explained in the last chapter (p. 275), that the loudness of a stimulus depends on the total amount of activity in the auditory nerve. As the stimulus intensity is raised, the number of fibres activated at first rises slowly, while only the tip segments of the curves are activated, and then more abruptly, when the tails of the tuning curves are encountered. In the pathological ear (part B), the tips of the tuning curves are missing, and as the stimulus intensity is raised the number of fibres activated increases rapidly, soon approaching normal levels.

A second factor also contributes to loudness recruitment. The rate-intensity functions of pathological fibres are steeper than normal, also leading to an abnormally fast increase of activity with intensity once threshold is reached.

(d) Tinnitus

One of the distressing accompaniments of sensorineural hearing loss is tinnitus, which can deprive the sufferer of even the dubious consolation of living in a silent world. Tinnitus is at the moment poorly controlled by drugs or surgery, and the only treatment of use is to mask it by external noise. This does not of course help if the patient is deaf anyway. Generally, sufferers just have to 'live with it'.

Until recently, it was thought useful to divide tinnitus into 'objective' and 'subjective' tinnitus. Objective tinnitus was thought to arise peripheral to the cochlea, in say the musculature of the middle ear, and could be recorded objectively with microphones or heard by other listeners. Subjective tinnitus arose in the receptors, or more centrally, and therefore could not be measured objectively outside the ear. The discovery of the evoked cochlear mechanical response by Kemp (1978) showed that objectively measurable sound could be produced by the cochlea itself, so that the division of tinnitus into the objective and subjective does not have the obvious anatomical correlate that it once did.

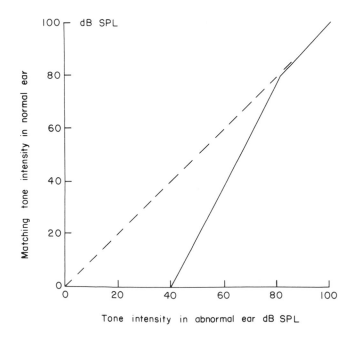

Fig. 10.3 Loudness recruitment with unilateral sensorineural hearing loss.

Figure 5.9 (p. 129) shows the recording of the sound pressure in one of these cases of externally recordable tinnitus of cochlear origin.

The origin of the evoked cochlear mechanical response is not certain, and some hypotheses were discussed in Chapter 5 (p. 128). It seems that when hair cells are activated some mechanical energy is fed back into the basilar membrane. The feedback could possibly arise from fluid flows across cell membranes associated with ion flows, or from active motility of the stereocilia on hair cells due to actin–myosin interactions in the stereocilia (Macartney *et al.*, 1980). If the frequency relations are right, mechanical energy may be reflected back and forth along the cochlea, further stimulating the hair cells, and leading to a self-sustaining oscillation, and so to tinnitus. Points in the cochlea at which its properties are changing abruptly seem particularly able to generate the oscillations, and it is possible that this type of tinnitus is associated with normal hair cells on the borders of regions of hearing loss.

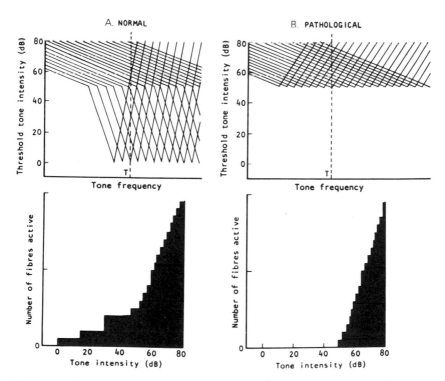

10.4 A neural explanation of loudness recruitment. Loudness in the abnormal ear grows abnormally quickly with intensity once threshold is reached, because the tips of the tuning curves are missing. From Evans (1975c), Fig. 8.

Although this is an intriguing explanation of one type of tinnitus, it is unlikely to explain the majority of cases encountered. We expect tinnitus associated with the evoked cochlear mechanical response to be continuous, and narrowband or tonal. Much tinnitus is discontinuous and atonal, like high pitched hissing or knocking noises. Moreover the evoked cochlear mechanical response disappears in experimental cochlear deafness, and tinnitus can be particularly strong in patients with severe hearing loss.

It is very likely that there will be many causes of other types of tinnitus and a single explanation may therefore not be adequate. In some cases, it is possible that tinnitus can arise from an increase in the spontaneous activity in the auditory nerve. High doses of salicylate (aspirin) can produce acute tinnitus in man, and Evans *et al.* (1981) showed in animal experiments that salicylate could temporarily increase the spontaneous activity of auditory nerve fibres. However it does seem that the tinnitus associated with some long term sensorineural hearing loss does not arise from an increase of activity in auditory nerve fibres, because the spontaneous activity of auditory nerve fibres is reduced rather than increased in some cases of experimental cochlear pathology (Kiang *et al.*, 1970). One explanation of tinnitus which might apply in these cases is that it arises centrally after a disappearance of an input from the cochlea. In an analogy that is sometimes given (e.g. Ballantyne, 1977), most normal subjects hear a 'noise in their heads' on entering a soundproofed room. It is suggested that normally this internal noise, possibly of central origin, is masked by external noise. When there is hearing loss, external noise does not mask the internal noise, and tinnitus is heard. Such an explanation does not by itself say why subjects with sensorineural impairment may hear their tinnitus as more disturbing than do normal subjects when deprived of sensory input in a soundproofed room. It is possible therefore that with continued deprivation, and perhaps a lack of spontaneous activity in the auditory nerve, a hypersensitivity akin to denervation hypersensitivity may occur in the central nervous system. There is further evidence that some tinnitus arises centrally, because cutting the auditory nerve is often an ineffective treatment. Moreover, where it is possible to reverse the deprivation, for instance by stimulating the cochlea electrically with a prosthesis, patients sometimes report an improvement in their tinnitus.

Gerken (1979) presented evidence that a denervation hypersensitivity did occur in the auditory system after cochlear damage. He implanted electrodes in a variety of auditory nuclei, and trained animals to respond behaviourally to electrical stimuli. Following cochlear damage, thresholds for the detection of electrical stimuli were lower in a wide range of auditory nuclei, including the first nucleus of the auditory pathway, the cochlear nucleus.

C. A Cochlear Prosthesis?

1. Introduction

When the hair cells of the cochlea are lost they cannot be replaced. Therefore hearing cannot be restored. Under these circumstances the best hope for restoring some auditory function seems to be to bypass the transducer mechanism, and to attempt to stimulate what remains of the auditory nerve directly, by electrical means. In recent years, groups in several laboratories have attempted to do this, by implanting electrodes in the cochlea or auditory nerve. It is hoped that by stimulating early in the auditory pathway, the complex and specialized signal processing capability of the auditory system will be utilized. Some of the results have been impressive; many of the others have not. The treatment is still in the experimental stage and it is not yet known whether it will be generally applicable.

The aims of electrical stimulation have ranged from the very conservative to the very advanced. At the most basic level, patients with implanted prostheses report that one of the benefits is just being in some sort of auditory contact with the environment. Being able to hear alarm signals and approaching traffic is obviously valuable. At a slightly more advanced level, even a few auditory cues can be of use in lip reading, particularly if they help distinguish differences which do not appear in the lips, such as the difference between voiced and unvoiced sounds. Furthermore, some feedback from the patient's own voice is invaluable in helping him control it. At a much more advanced level, some groups have the hope of eventually conveying speech completely through the prosthesis, with such preprocessing of the acoustic signal as may be necessary.

2. Physiological Background

(a) Condition of the nerve

One question is: are there any auditory nerve fibres left when all hearing has been lost through cochlear deafness? Kerr and Schuknecht (1968) counted cells of the spiral ganglion *post mortem* in 29 patients suffering from profound deafness. In 25% of the cases two-thirds or more of the spiral ganglion cells were present, and in 68% of cases less than one-third. The extent of the loss seemed to depend on the original cause of the deafness. There were large losses if the original deafness was due to bacterial labyrinthitis, but only small ones if due to ototoxic antibiotic administration. So it seems that there is a good survival in a quarter of patients which might justify an implant.

Before implanting a prosthesis, many laboratories test for the presence of auditory nerve fibres by stimulating the nerve extracochlearly and asking for patients' subjective reports or measuring brain stem evoked responses (e.g. Chouard, 1980). Such tests unfortunately only show if *some* fibres remain, and not how many.

A second problem is that insertion of the device into the cochlea may produce a further loss of nerve fibres. Schindler *et al.* (1977) showed that as long as there was no gross direct damage to the cochlear partitions when the device was inserted, the only degeneration was that of hair cells and not of nerve fibres. It further seemed that in cats with pre-existing cochlear pathology, insertion of the device and electrical stimulation caused no further neural degeneration.

(b) Responses of auditory nerve fibres to electrical stimulation

In normal subjects, useful information is transmitted by the auditory nerve as a result of, for instance, its frequency selectivity, and because the neural firings follow the stimulus waveform. It is worth therefore considering the extent to which the different aspects of normal processing can be reproduced by electrical stimulation.

Kiang and Moxon (1972) recorded the responses of cat auditory nerve fibres to electrical stimuli applied to the round window. The responses showed that auditory nerve fibres were not selectively tuned to electrical stimuli at all (Fig. 10.5). Therefore if frequency information is to be transmitted as place information in the auditory nerve, ways must be found of restricting the stimulus to local regions of the cochlea. Such localized stimulation seems rather difficult. Bipolar electrode arrays show that the sharpest tuning curves that could be produced have slopes equivalent to 20 dB/octave, about a tenth of those occurring naturally. Temporal information is on the other hand preserved. Phase-locking is maintained, and the neural

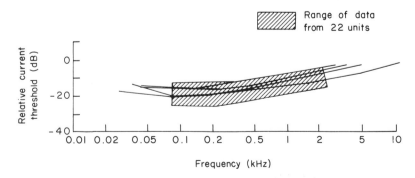

Fig. 10.5 Auditory nerve fibres show negligible tuning to electrical stimuli applied across the cochlea. These broad 'tuning curves' should be compared with the sharp tuning curves to acoustic stimuli in the normal cochlea, shown in Fig. 4.3. From Kiang and Moxon (1972), Fig. 1.

firings can sometimes be restricted more closely to one point on the stimulating waveform.

Kiang and Moxon (1972) also showed that rate-intensity functions to electrical stimuli were very steep, with a dynamic range of less than 10 dB (Fig. 10.6). This means that very reliable amplitude compression of the stimulus is necessary.

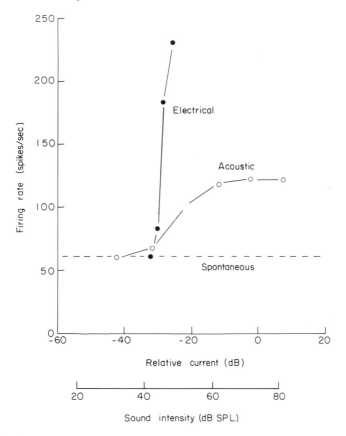

Fig. 10.6 The steep rate-intensity function seen with electrical stimuli, compared with the function found with acoustic stimuli. From Kiang and Moxon (1972), Fig. 3.

3. Results

(a) Intensity coding

As expected from the physiological experiments, the dynamic range, being the range between threshold and discomfort, is small, never more than 20 dB and often less than 10 dB (e.g. Fourcin *et al.*, 1979; Walsh *et al.*, 1980). It might be thought that if the stimulus were localized in the cochlea, increased current spread with intensity might increase the dynamic range. However, groups using bipolar stimulation and so a localized stimulus do not report wider dynamic ranges than those who do not.

The narrow dynamic range, presumably associated with a steep dependence of loudness on stimulus intensity, does not seem to have a correlate of particularly small difference limens for intensity. Differential intensity limens are about 1 dB, similar to those found with acoustic stimuli (e.g. Dillier *et al.*, 1980). Over the whole dynamic range, therefore, there may only be about 20 just noticeable differences for intensity, as compared with over 300 for acoustic stimuli in normal hearing.

(b) Frequency, pitch, and stimulus quality

If we believe the extreme position that at low frequency, information is carried purely by the temporal pattern of nerve impulses, then periodic electrical stimulation should produce faithful auditory sensations and good discrimination of frequencies.

The results of electrical stimulation have on the whole been disappointing for such a prediction. In only a few cases do electrical stimuli seem to produce clear tonal sensations. A typical report is that tones sound like 'comb and paper' or 'scratchy' (e.g. Fourcin *et al.*, 1979). Two possible reasons for this poor quality of sensation were discussed in Chapter 9 (p. 267). To summarize, they were, firstly, that the frequency limit of phase-locking to electrical stimuli, set by the refractory period of the axonal membrane, is well below that normally found for acoustic stimuli. Secondly, the electrical stimuli were applied to the basal, high frequency, end of the cochlea, and it is known that high frequency fibres are particularly poor at generating low pitch sensations.

Even when electrical stimuli of different frequencies can be discriminated or ranked, frequency discrimination limens are no better than 5%, an order of magnitude poorer than for acoustic stimuli. But in many cases this level of performance cannot be attained, and it is one of the surprising findings that although many patients can ascribe a high or low pitch to an electrical stimulus, they are remarkably bad at telling the difference between stimuli or at ranking them. In a similar way, complex stimuli such as speech seem very distorted, and are very poorly discriminated.

When frequencies could be ranked or matched, the frequency associated with the perceived pitch did not necessarily increase in proportion to the stimulus frequency. In a typical report, Simmons *et al.* (1979) found that pitch increased linearly with stimulus frequency up to 150–200 Hz, and then at an increasingly accelerating rate up to a stimulus frequency of 400 Hz, after which no further pitch changes were produced.

The discussion so far has been concerned with the subjective correlate of the periodicity of the stimulus. But the place of stimulation in the cochlea seems to have a subjective frequency correlate as well. In general, and as might be expected from the physiology, stimulation near the base gave rise to a sharp timbre, and that nearer the apex to a dull timbre. One patient for instance described the basal stimulus as producing a 'zing' and the more apical one a 'flug' (Dillier *et al.*, 1980). A patient of Eddington *et al.* (1978) similarly ascribed high pitches to basal electrodes and low pitches to apical ones, in a way that changed monotonically along the cochlea. There seemed to be a periodicity component as well, because increasing the stimulus frequency at any electrode increased the pitch sensation produced.

(c) Speech

The main goal in research on the auditory prosthesis has been to convey speech. As might already have been suspected from the quality of the sensations produced, electrical stimulation has not permitted the unaided perception of speech. Any good perception of words has been possible only with restricted word lists and long periods of training (Chouard, 1980).

The more realizable goal seems to be that of assisting lip reading. Many groups report improvements in lip reading, some dramatic, other less so (e.g. Chouard, 1980; cf. Bilger *et al.*, 1977). Even when the improvement in lip reading has not been dramatic, patients report at being delighted by the extra cues available (Fourcin *et al.*, 1979).

Such assistance also has the benefit of reducing the considerable strain associated with lip reading, and also produces a rewarding sense of emotional contact with the speaker.

(d) Conclusions

Work so far with the auditory prosthesis indicates that it is still in the experimental stage, and is not yet ready for large scale implantation.

It does not yet seem adequate for speech discrimination. Exploitation of many channels of stimulation seems one hopeful way of improving the performance of the device. Eddington (1980) for instance reported that four channels, with frequency specific signals fed to each channel, produced better speech discrimination than one channel alone. Multichannel prostheses bring their own disadvantages of a greater necessary intrusion into the cochlea, and a concomitantly greater danger of damage to the remaining neural elements, together with a larger tissue reaction, as well as requiring a larger surviving neural population. The latter requirement means that it is only applicable to a more restricted set of patients.

Preprocessing of the signal, to take into account the peculiar transformation of stimuli through the device, may also help intelligibility.

Although hopes for improvement direct our attention to more sophistication in the auditory prosthesis, we should not lose sight of the benefits to be gained from simpler versions, including the detection of environmental warning signals, assistance with lip reading, and the sense of emotional contact. In view of the simpler surgery needed for the more basic devices, the relative payoff may turn out to be greater.

D. Summary

1.   Hearing loss arises either in the conductive apparatus before the oval window, where it is known as conductive loss, or in the cochlea, or more centrally. If it arises in the cochlea, it is known as sensorineural hearing loss of cochlear origin.

2.   In experimental sensorineural hearing loss of cochlear origin, the tips of the tuning curves of auditory nerve fibres are primarily affected. Sometimes the tips are lost completely, so that in addition to a severe loss in neural threshold, there is a loss of frequency resolution. Sometimes a short, sharp, remnant of the tip remains. Sometimes the tail of the tuning curve is lowered in threshold as well.

3.   Psychophysically, a loss in frequency resolution is often seen in addition to the loss in sensitivity. The loss in frequency resolution can be seen in widened psychophysical tuning curves and in widened critical bandwidths.

4.   Loudness recruitment, also seen in sensorineural hearing loss of cochlear origin, can similarly be explained in terms of the abnormal neuronal responses. In normal ears, as the intensity of a tone is raised from low levels, at first only a few fibres are activated while the low level tips of the tuning curves are stimulated, and then a much larger number as the high threshold tails are encountered. Where the tips are missing, a large number of tails of tuning curves are encountered as soon as threshold is reached, and so loudness grows abnormally quickly. Rate-intensity functions for individual nerve fibres are also steeper when the tip of the tuning curve is missing.

5.   Some forms of tinnitus arising in the cochlea may give rise to objectively measurable sound emissions in the ear canal, as a result of the evoked cochlear mechanical response. However, in many cases of sensorineural

loss, it seems that evoked and spontaneous activity in the auditory nerve both decrease. The tinnitus therefore probably arises centrally, perhaps as a result of the hypersensitivity of a system deprived of its normal input. There is some evidence that denervation hypersensitivity occurs in the central auditory nervous system.

6. Attempts have been made to restore hearing in cases of profound hearing loss by means of an auditory prosthesis, with electrical stimulation of the cochlea or auditory nerve. It has not so far been possible to convey speech entirely through the prosthesis. The dynamic range of stimulus intensity, the frequency range, and the tonal quality seem poor. However, there is hope that simple stimuli may be conveyed usefully by the device.

E. Further Reading

For an introduction to deafness and audiometry, see a standard introductory textbook such as *Deafness*, by J. Ballantyne (1977) (Edinburgh, Churchill-Livingstone). *The Nervous System*, Vol. 3 (1975) (ed. in chief, D. B. Tower; volume ed. E. L. Eagles), New York, Raven Press, has many useful chapters. See also Dirks (1978).

Evans (1975b, 1976) discusses correlates of sensorineural deafness in the responses of auditory nerve fibres.

Progress on the cochlear prosthesis is reviewed in several articles in *Audiology* **19** (1980), part 2, pp. 105–187. Ballantyne *et al.* (1978) review work from a variety of laboratories.

Mechanisms of ototoxicity are discussed by Brown and Feldman (1978). The morphological changes associated with noise damage to the cochlea are discussed by Bohne (1976).

Appendix

Relation Between the Resistance and Depolarization of Hair Cells on Davis's Model.

The variable resistance at the apex of the hair cell, R_a, and the resistance at the base, R_b, form a voltage divider swinging the intracellular voltage V_i between the endocochlear potential V_o and the voltage defined by the equilibrium potentials of ions crossing the resistance of the basal membrane of the hair cell. Let all voltages be measured with respect to this latter voltage.

From the voltage divider:

$$V_i/V_o = R_b/(R_a + R_b)$$

If the total resistance of the cell as measured by an intracellular electrode is R, $1/R = 1/R_a + 1/R_b$ because it is connected to ground through the basal and apical resistances in parallel.

Solving for the variable resistance R_a:

$$R_a = R.R_b/(R_b - R)$$

Substituting in the expression for the voltage:

$$V_i/V_o = 1 - (R/R_b)$$

This relation shows that the intracellular voltage *increases* linearly as the total cell membrane resistance *decreases*. The linear relation requires that R_b, the resistance of the basal membrane of the hair cell, stays constant.

References

Abeles, M. and Goldstein, M. H. (1970). Functional architecture in cat primary auditory cortex: columnar organization and organization according to depth. *J. Neurophysiol.* **33**, 172–187.

Abeles, M. and Goldstein, M. H. (1972). Responses of single units in the primary auditory cortex of the cat to tones and to tone pairs. *Brain Res.* **42**, 337–352.

Adams, J. C. (1979). Ascending projections to the inferior colliculus. *J. Comp. Neurol.* **183**, 519–538.

Adams, J. C. and Warr, W. B. (1976). Origins of axons in the cat's acoustic striae determined by injection of horseradish peroxidase into severed tracts. *J. Comp. Neurol.* **170**, 107–122.

Ades, H. W. and Engström, H. (1974). Anatomy of the inner ear. In *Handbook of Sensory Physiology* Vol. 5/1 (eds W. D. Keidel and W. D. Neff), pp. 125–158. Springer, Berlin.

Adrian, E. D. (1931). The microphonic action of the cochlea: an interpretation of Wever and Bray's experiments. *J. Physiol. (Lond.)* **71**, xxviii–xxix.

Adrian, E. D., Bronk, D. W. and Phillips, G. (1931). The nervous origin of the Wever and Bray effect. *J. Physiol. (Lond.)* **73**. 2–3P.

Aitkin, L. M. (1973). Medial geniculate body of the cat: responses to tonal stimuli of neurons in medial division. *J. Neurophysiol.* **36**, 275–283.

Aitkin, L. M. and Prain, S. M. (1974). Medial geniculate body: unit responses in the awake cat. *J. Neurophysiol.* **37**, 512–521.

Aitkin, L. M. and Webster, W. R. (1972). Medial geniculate body of the cat: organization and responses to tonal stimuli of neurons in ventral division. *J. Neurophysiol.* **35**, 365–380.

Aitkin, L. M., Anderson, D. J. and Brugge, J. F. (1970). Tonotopic organization and discharge characteristics of single neurons in nuclei of the lateral lemniscus of the cat. *J. Neurophysiol.* **33**, 421–440.

Aitkin, L. M., Webster, W. R., Veale, J. C. and Crosby, D. C. (1975). Inferior colliculus — I. Comparison of response properties of neurons in central, pericentral and external nuclei of adult cat. *J. Neurophysiol.* **38**, 1196–1207.

Aitkin, L. M., Dickhaus, H., Schult, W. and Zimmerman, M. (1978). External nucleus of inferior colliculus: auditory and spinal somatosensory afferents and their interactions. *J. Neurophysiol.* **41**, 837–847.

Allen, J. B. (1980). Cochlear micromechanics — a physical model of transduction. *J. Acoust. Soc. Am.* **68**, 1660–1670.

Allen, W. F. (1945). Effect of destroying three localized cerebral cortical areas for sound on correct conditioned differential responses of the dog's foreleg. *Amer. J. Physiol.* **144**, 415–428.

Altman, J. A., Syka, J. and Shmigidina, G. N. (1970). Neuronal activity in the medial geniculate body of the cat during monaural and binaural stimulation. *Exp. Brain Res.* **10**, 81–93.

Andersen, P., Junge, K. and Sveen, O. (1972). Cortico-fugal facilitation of thalamic transmission. *Brain Behav. Evol.* **6**, 170–184.

Anderson. S. D. (1980). Some ECMR properties in relation to other signals from the auditory periphery. *Hearing Res.* **2**, 273–296.

Antoli-Candela, F. Jr. and Kiang, N. Y.-S. (1978). Unit activity underlying the N_1 potential of the cochlea. In *Evoked Electrical Activity in the Auditory Nervous System* (eds R. F. Naunton and C. Fernandez), pp. 165–189. Academic Press, New York and London.

Arthur, R. M., Pfeiffer, R. R. and Suga, N. (1971). Properties of 'two-tone inhibition" in primary auditory neurones. *J. Physiol. (Lond.)* **212**, 593–609.

Ballantyne, J. (1977). *Deafness*. Churchill-Livingstone, Edinburgh.

Ballantyne, J. C., Evans, E. F. and Morrison, A. W. (1978). Electrical auditory stimulation in the management of profound hearing loss. *J. Laryngol. Otol.* **92**, Suppl. 1, 1–117.

Banks, W. F., Saunders, J. C. and Lowry, L. D. (1979). Olivocochlear bundle activity recorded in awake cats. *Otolaryngol. Head Neck Surg.* **87**, 463–471.

Baru, A. V. and Karaseva, T. A. (1972). *The Brain and Hearing*. Consultants Bureau, New York.

Beaton, R. and Miller, J. M. (1975). Single cell activity in the auditory cortex of the unanesthetised, behaving, monkey: correlation with stimulus controlled behavior. *Brain Res.* **100**, 543–562.

von Békésy, G. (1952). DC resting potentials inside the cochlear partition. *J. Acoust. Soc. Am.* **24**, 72–76.

von Békésy, G. (1960). *Experiments in Hearing*. Wiley, New York.

Bennett, M. V. L. (1967). Mechanisms of electroreception. In *Lateral Line Detectors* (ed. P. Cahn), pp. 313–393. Indiana University Press, Bloomington.

Benson, D. A. and Heinz, R. D. (1978). Single unit activity in the auditory cortex of monkeys selectively attending left vs. right ear stimuli. *Brain Res.* **159**, 307–320.

Benson, D. A. and Teas, D. C. (1976). Single unit study of binaural interaction in the auditory cortex of the chinchilla. *Brain Res.* 103, 313–338.

Berlin, C. I. and McNeil, M. R. (1976). Dichotic listening. In *Contemporary Issues in Experimental Phonetics* (ed. N. J. Lass), pp. 327–388. Academic Press, New York and London.

Bilger, R. C., Black, F. O. and Hopkinson, N. T. (1977). Evaluation of subjects presently fitted with implanted auditory prostheses. *Ann. Otol. Rhinol. Laryngol.* **86**, Suppl. 38.

Birt, D., Nienhuis, R. and Olds, M. (1979). Separation of associative from non-associative short latency changes in medial geniculate and inferior colliculus during differential conditioning and reversal in rats. *Brain Res.* **167**, 129–138.

Bock, G. R. and Webster, W. R. (1974). Coding of spatial location by single units in the inferior colliculus of the alert cat. *Exp. Brain Res.* **21**, 387–398.

Bock, G. R., Webster, W. R. and Aitkin, L. M. (1972). Discharge patterns of single units in inferior colliculus of the alert cat. *J. Neurophysiol.* **35**, 265–277.

de Boer, E. (1969). Reverse correlation. II. Initiation of nerve impulses in the inner ear. *Proc. Kon. Nederl. Adad. Wet.* **72**, 129–151.

Bogert, B. P. (1951). Determination of the effects of dissipation in the cochlear partition by means of a network representing the basilar membrane. *J. Acoust. Soc. Am.* **23**, 151–154.

Bohne, B. (1976). Mechanisms of noise damage in the inner ear. In *Effects of Noise on Hearing* (eds D. Henderson, R. P. Hamernik, D. S. Dosanjh and J. H. Mills), pp. 41–67. Raven Press, New York.

Bonding, P. (1979). Critical bandwidth in patients with a hearing loss induced by salicylates. *Audiology* **18**, 133–144.

Borg, E. (1971). Efferent inhibition of afferent acoustic activity in the unanaesthetised rabbit. *Exp. Neurol.* **31**, 301–312.

Borg, E. (1973). On the neuronal organization of the acoustic middle ear reflex. A physiological and anatomical study. *Brain Res.* **49**, 101–123.

Bosher, S. K. and Warren, R. L. (1968). Observations on the electrochemistry of the cochlear endolymph of the rat. *Proc. Roy. Soc. (Lond.)* B, **171**, 227–247.

Brawer, J. R., Morest, D. K. and Kane, E. C. (1974). The neuronal architecture of the cochlear nucleus of the cat. *J. Comp. Neurol.* **155**, 251–299.

Britt, R. and Starr, A. (1976a). Synaptic events and discharge patterns of cochlear nucleus cells. I. Steady-frequency tone bursts. *J. Neurophysiol.* **39**. 162–178.

Britt, R. and Starr, A. (1976b). Synaptic events and discharge patterns of cochlear nucleus cells. II. Frequency-modulated tones. *J. Neurophysiol.* **39**, 179–194.

Broadbent, D. E. (1958). *Perception and Communication.* Pergamon, London.

Brown, R. D. and Feldman, A. M. (1978). Pharmacology of hearing and ototoxicity. *Ann. Rev. Pharmacol. Toxicol.* **18**, 233–252.

Brownell, W. E., Manis, P. B. and Ritz, L. A. (1979). Ipsilateral inhibitory responses in the cat lateral superior olive. *Brain Res.* **177**, 189–193.

Brugge, J. F. and Geisler, C. D. (1978). Auditory mechanisms of the lower brainstem. *Ann. Rev. Neurosci.* **1**, 363–394.

Brugge, J. F. and Merzenich, M. M. (1973). Responses of neurons in auditory cortex of the macaque monkey to monaural and binaural stimulation. *J. Neurophysiol.* **36**, 1138–1158.

Brugge, J. F., Dubrovsky, N. A., Aitkin, L. M. and Anderson, D. J. (1969). Sensitivity of single neurons in auditory cortex of cat to binaural tone stimulation; effects of varying interaural time and intensity. *J. Neurophysiol.* **32**, 1005–1024.

Buño, W. (1978). Auditory nerve fiber activity influenced by contralateral ear sound stimulation. *Exp. Neurol.* **59**, 62–74.

Buño, W., Velluti, R., Handler, P. and Garcia-Austt, E. (1966). Neural control of the cochlear input in the wakeful free guinea pig. *Physiol. Behav.* **1**, 23–35.

Burian, K., Hochmair, E., Hochmair-Desoyer, I. and Lessel, M. R. (1980). Electrical stimulation with multichannel electrodes in deaf patients. *Audiology* **19**, 128–136.

Butler, R. A., Diamond, I. T. and Neff, W. D. (1957). Role of auditory cortex in discrimination of changes in frequency. *J. Neurophysiol.* **20**, 108–120.

Cajal, S. R. Y. (1909). *Histologie du Système Nerveux de l'Homme et des Vertébrés,* Vol. 1. Maloine, Paris.

Cant, N. B. and Morest, D. K. (1978). Axons from non-cochlear sources in the anteroventral cochlear nucleus of the cat. A study with the rapid Golgi method. *Neuroscience* **3**, 1003–1029.

Capps, M. J. and Ades, H. W. (1968). Auditory frequency discrimination after transection of the olivocochlear bundle in squirrel monkeys. *Exp. Neurol.* **21**, 147–158.

Carmel, P. W. and Starr, A. (1963). Acoustic and non-acoustic factors modifying middle-ear muscle activity in waking cats. *J. Neurophysiol.* **26**, 598–616.

Casseday, J. H. and Neff, W. D. (1975). Auditory localization: role of auditory pathways in brainstem of the cat. *J. Neurophysiol.* **38**, 842–858.

Cherry, E. C. (1953). Some experiments on the recognition of speech, with one and with two ears. *J. Acoust. Soc. Am.* **25**, 975–979.

Chorazyna, H. and Stepien, L. (1963). Effect of bilateral Sylvian gyrus ablations on auditory conditioning in dogs. *Bull. Acad. Polon. Sci. Ser. Sci. Biol.* **11**, 43–45.

Chouard, C. H. (1980). The surgical rehabilitation of total deafness with the multi-channel cochlear implant. *Audiology* **19**, 137–145.

Christiansen, J. A., Jensen, C. E. and Vilstrup, Th. (1961). Displacement potentials and bending of rod-like polyelectrolytes. *Nature* **191**, 484–485.

Citron, L., Dix, M. R., Hallpike, C. S. and Hood, J. D. (1963). A recent clinico-pathological study of cochlear nerve degeneration resulting from tumor pressure and disseminated sclerosis, with particular reference to the finding of normal threshold sensitivity for pure tones. *Acta Otolar.* **56**, 330–337.

Colativa, F. B. (1972). Auditory cortical lesions and visual pattern discrimination in cat. *Brain Res.* **39**, 437–447.

Colativa, F. B. (1974). Insular-temporal lesions and vibrotactile temporal pattern discrimination in cats. *Psychol. Behav.* **12**, 215–218.

Colativa, F. B., Szeligo, F. V. and Zimmer, S. D. (1974). Temporal pattern discrimination in cats with insular-temporal lesions. *Brain Res.* **79**, 153–156.

Comis, S. D. (1970). Centrifugal inhibitory processes affecting neurones in the cat cochlear nucleus. *J. Physiol. (Lond.)* **210**, 751–760.

Comis, S. D. and Daves, W. E. (1969). Acetylcholine as a transmitter in the cat auditory system. *J. Neurochem.* **16**, 423–429.

Comis, S. D. and Whitfield, I. C. (1968). Influence of centrifugal pathways on unit activity in the cochlear nucleus. *J. Neurophysiol.* **31**, 62–68.

Corey, D. P. and Hudspeth, A. J. (1979a). Ionic basis of the receptor potential in a vertebrate hair cell. *Nature* **281**, 675–677.

Corey, D. P. and Hudspeth, A. J. (1979b). Response latency of vertebrate hair cells. *Biophys. J.* **26**, 499–506.

Cornwell, P. (1967). Loss of auditory pattern discrimination following insular-temporal lesions in cats. *J. Comp. Physiol. Psychol.* **63**, 165–168.

Cowey, A. and Weiskrantz, L. (1976). Auditory sequence discrimination in *Macaca Mulatta*: the role of the superior temporal cortex. *Neuropsychologia* **14**, 1–10.

Cranford, J. L. (1975). Role of neocortex in binaural hearing in the cat. I. Contra-lateral masking. *Brain Res.* **100**, 395–406.

Cranford, J. L. (1979a). Auditory cortex lesions and interaural intensity and phase-angle discrimination in cats. *J. Neurophysiol.* **42**, 1518–1526.

Cranford, J. L. (1979b). Detection versus discrimination of brief tones by cats with auditory cortex lesions. *J. Acoust. Soc. Am.* **65**, 1573–1575.

Cranford, J. L., Igarashi, M. and Stramler, J. H. (1976a). Effect of auditory neo-cortical ablation on pitch perception in the cat. *J. Neurophysiol.* **39**, 143–152.

Cranford, J. L., Igarashi, M. and Stramler, J. H. (1976b). Effect of auditory neo-cortex ablation on identification of click rates in cats. *Brain Res.* **116**, 69–81.

Crawford, A. C. and Fettiplace, R. (1979). Reversal of hair cell responses by current. *J. Physiol. (Lond.)* **295**, 66P.

Crawford, A. C. and Fettiplace, R. (1980) The frequency selectivity of auditory nerve fibres and hair cells in the cochlea of the turtle. *J. Physiol. (Lond.)* **306**, 79–125.

Crawford, A. C. and Fettiplace, R. (1981a). An electrical tuning mechanism in turtle cochlear hair cells. *J. Physiol. (Lond.)* **312**, 377–422.

Crawford, A. C. and Fettiplace, R. (1981b) Non-linearities in the responses of turtle hair cells. *J. Physiol. (Lond.)* **315**, 317–338.

Crow, G., Rupert, A. L. and Moushegian, G. (1978). Phase-locking in monaural and binaural medullary neurons: implications for binaural phenomena. *J. Acoust. Soc. Am.* **64**, 493–501.

Dallos, P. (1973a). *The Auditory Periphery*. Academic Press, New York and London.

Dallos, P. (1973b). Cochlear potentials and cochlear mechanics. In *Basic Mechanisms in Hearing* (ed. A. Møller), pp. 335–372. Academic Press, New York and London.

Dallos, P. (1975). Cochlear potentials. In *The Nervous System*, Vol. 3 (ed. D. B. Tower), pp. 69–80. Raven Press, New York.

Dallos, P. (1978). Biophysics of the cochlea. In *Handbook of Perception*, Vol. 4 (eds E. C. Carterette and M. P. Friedman), pp. 125–162. Academic Press, New York and London.

Dallos, P. (1981). Cochlear physiology. *Ann. Rev. Psychol.* **32**, 153–190.

Dallos, P. and Harris, D. (1978). Properties of auditory nerve responses in absence of outer hair cells. *J. Neurophysiol.* **41**, 365–383.

Dallos, P. and Wang, C.-Y. (1974). Bioelectric correlates of kanamycin intoxication. *Audiology* **13**, 277–289.

Dallos, P., Schoeny, Z. G. and Cheatham, M. A. (1972). Cochlear summating potentials: descriptive aspects. *Acta Otolar.* Suppl **302**, 1–46.

Dallos, P., Ryan, A., Harris, D., McGee, T. and Ödzamar, Ö. (1977). Cochlear frequency selectivity in the presence of hair cell damage. In *Psychophysics and Physiology of Hearing* (eds E. F. Evans and J. P. Wilson), pp. 249–258. Academic Press, London and New York.

Dallos, P., Harris, D. M., Relkin, E. and Cheatham, M. A. (1980). Two-tone suppression and intermodulation distortion in the cochlea: effect of outer hair cell lesions. In *Psychophysical, Physiological, and Behavioural Studies in Hearing* (eds G. van den Brink and F. A. Bilsen), pp. 242–249. Delft University Press, Delft.

David, E., Keidel, W. D., Kallert, S., Bechtereva, N. P. and Bundzen, P. V. (1977). Decoding processes in the auditory system and human speech analysis. In *Psychophysics and Physiology of Hearing* (eds E. F. Evans and J. P. Wilson), pp. 509–516. Academic Press, London and New York.

Davis, H. (1958). Transmission and transduction in the cochlea. *Laryngoscope* **68**, 359–382.

Davis, H. (1965). A model for transducer action in the cochlea. *Cold Spring Harbor Symp. Quant. Biol.* **30**, 181–189.

Davis, H. (1968). Mechanisms of the inner ear. *Ann. Otol. Rhinol. Laryngol.* **77**, 644–655.

Delgutte, B. (1980). Representation of speech-like sounds in the discharge patterns of auditory-nerve fibers. *J. Acoust. Soc. Am.* **68**, 843–857.

Densert, O. and Flock, A. (1974). An electron-microscopic study of adrenergic innervation in the cochlea. *Acta Otolar.* **77**, 185–197.

DeRosier, D. J., Tilney, L. G. and Egelman, E. (1980). Actin in the inner ear: the remarkable structure of the stereocilium. *Nature* **287**, 291–296.

Desmedt, J. E. (1975). Physiological studies of the efferent recurrent auditory system. In *Handbook of Sensory Physiology* Vol. 5/2 (eds W. D. Keidel and W. D. Neff), pp. 219–246. Springer, Berlin.

Desmedt, J. E. and Mechelse, K. (1958). Suppression of acoustic input by thalamic stimulation. *Proc. Soc. Exp. Biol. N.Y.* **99**, 772–775.

Desmedt, J. E. and Robertson, D. (1975). Ionic mechanism of the efferent olivocochlear inhibition studied by cochlear perfusion in the cat. *J. Physiol. (Lond.)* **247**, 407–428.

Dewson, J. H. (1964). Speech sound discrimination by cats. *Science* **144**, 555–556.

Dewson, J. H. (1968). Efferent olivocochlear bundle: some relationships to stimulus discrimination in noise. *J. Neurophysiol.* **31**, 122–130.

Dewson, J. H., Nobel, K. W. and Pribram, K. H. (1966). Corticofugal influence at cochlear nucleus of the cat: some effects of ablation of insular-temporal cortex. *Brain Res.* **2**, 151–159.

Dewson, J. H., Pribram, K. H. and Lynch, J. C. (1969). Effects of ablations of temporal cortex upon speech sound discrimination in the monkey. *Exp. Neurol.* **24**, 579–591.

Dewson, J. H., Cowey, A. and Weiskrantz, L. (1970). Disruptions of auditory sequence discrimination by unilateral and bilateral cortical ablations of superior temporal gyrus in the monkey. *Exp. Neurol.* **28**, 529–548.

Diamond, I. T. and Neff, W. D. (1957). Ablation of temporal cortex and discrimination of auditory patterns. *J. Neurophysiol.* **20**, 300–315.

Diamond, I. T., Jones, E. G. and Powell, T. P. S. (1969). The projection of the auditory cortex upon the diencephalon and the brain stem of the cat. *Brain Res.* **15**, 305–340.

Dillier, N., Spillmann, T., Fisch, U. P. and Leifer, L. J. (1980). Encoding and decoding of auditory signals in relation to human speech and its application to human cochlear implants. *Audiology* **19**, 146–163.

Dirks, D. D. (1978). Effects of hearing impairment on the auditory system. In *Handbook of Perception*, Vol 4 (eds E. C. Carterette and M. P. Friedman), pp. 567–608. Academic Press, New York and London.

Dohlman, G. F. (1960). Histochemical studies of vestibular mechanisms. In *Neural Mechanisms of the Auditory and Vestibular Systems* (eds G. L. Rasmussen and W. F. Windle), pp. 258–275. Thomas, Springfield.

Duifhuis, H. (1976). Cochlear nonlinearity and second filter: possible mechanisms and implications. *J. Acoust. Soc. Am.* **59**, 408–423.

Economo, C. von and Horn, L. (1930). Über Windungsrelief, Masse und Rindenarchitektonik der Supratemporalfläche, ihre individuellen und ihre Seitenunterschiede. *Z. Ges. Neurol. Psychiat.* **130**, 678–757.

Eddington, D. K. (1980). Speech discrimination in deaf subjects with cochlear implants. *J. Acoust. Soc. Am.* **68**, 885–891.

Eddington, D. K., Dobelle, W. H., Brackman, D. E., Mladejovsky, M. G. and Parkin, J. L. (1978). Auditory prostheses research with multiple channel intracochlear stimulation in man. *Ann. Otol. Rhinol. Laryngol.* **87**, Suppl. **53**, 1–39.

Egan, J. P. and Hake, H. W. (1950). On the masking pattern of a simple auditory stimulus. *J. Acoust. Soc. Am.* **22**, 622–630.

Eisenman, L. M. (1974). Neural encoding of sound location: an electrophysiological study in auditory cortex (AI) of the cat using free field stimuli. *Brain Res.* **75**, 203–214.

Eldredge, D. H. (1974). Inner ear — cochlear mechanics and cochlear potentials. In *Handbook of Sensory Physiology* Vol. 5/1 (eds W. D. Keidel and W. D. Neff), pp. 549–584. Springer, Berlin.

Elliott, D. N. and Trahiotis, C. (1970). Cortical lesions and auditory discrimination. *Psychol. Bull.* **77**, 198–222.

Elliott, D. N., Stein, L. and Harrison, M. J. (1960). Discrimination of absolute-intensity thresholds and frequency-difference thresholds in cats. *J. Acoust. Soc. Am.* **32**, 380–384.

Elverland, H. H. (1977). Descending connections between the superior olivary and cochlear nucleus complexes in the cat studied by autoradiographic and horseradish peroxidase methods. *Exp. Brain Res.* **27**, 397–412.

Elverland, H. H. (1978). Ascending and intrinsic projections of the superior olivary complex in the cat. *Exp. Brain Res.* **32**, 117–134.

Engerbretson, A. M. and Eldredge, D. H. (1968). Model for the nonlinear characteristics of cochlear potentials. *J. Acoust. Soc. Am.* **44**, 548–554.

Engström, H. (1960). The cortilymph, the third lymph of the inner ear. *Acta Morphol. Neer. Scand.* **3**, 195–204.

Engström, H. and Engström, B. (1978). Structure of hairs on cochlear sensory cells. *Hearing Res.* **1**, 49–66.

Engström, H., Ades, H. W. and Hawkins, J. E. (1965). Cellular pattern, nerve structures and fluid spaces of the organ of Corti. In *Contributions to Sensory Physiology*, Vol 1. (ed. W. D. Neff), pp. 1–37. Academic Press, New York.

Erulkar, S. D. (1959). The responses of single units of the inferior colliculus of the cat to acoustic stimulation. *Proc. Roy. Soc. (Lond)* B, **150**, 336–355.

Erulkar, S. D. (1975). Physiological studies of the inferior colliculus and medial geniculate complex. In *Handbook of Sensory Physiology* Vol. 5/2 (eds W. D. Keidel and W. D. Neff), pp. 145–198. Springer, Berlin.

Erulkar, S. D., Rose, J. E. and Davies, P. W. (1956). Single unit activity in the auditory cortex of the cat. *Bull. Johns Hopkins Hosp.* **99**, 55–86.

Evans, E. F. (1968). Cortical representation. In *Hearing Mechanisms in Vertebrates* (eds A. V. S. de Reuck and J. Knight), pp. 272–287. Churchill, London.

Evans, E. F. (1972). The frequency response and other properties of single fibres of the guinea-pig cochlear nerve. *J. Physiol. (Lond.)* **226**, 263–287.

Evans, E. F. (1975a). Cochlear nerve and cochlear nucleus. In *Handbook of Sensory Physiology* Vol. 5/2 (eds W. D. Keidel and W. D. Neff), pp. 1–108. Springer, Berlin.

Evans, E. F. (1975b). Normal and abnormal functioning of the cochlear nerve. *Symp. Zool. Soc. Lond.* **37**, 133–165.

Evans, E. F. (1975c). The sharpening of cochlear frequency selectivity in the normal and abnormal cochlea. *Audiology* **14**, 419–442.

Evans, E. F. (1976). Temporary sensorineural hearing losses and 8th nerve changes. In *Effects of Noise on Hearing* (eds D. Henderson, R. P. Hamernik, D. S. Dosanjh and J. H. Mills), pp. 199–221. Raven Press, New York.

Evans, E. F. (1977). Frequency selectivity at high signal levels of single units in cochlear nerve and nucleus. In *Psychophysics and Physiology of Hearing* (eds E. F. Evans and J. P. Wilson), pp. 185–192. Academic Press, New York and London.

Evans, E. F. (1978). Place and time coding of frequency in the peripheral auditory system: some physiological pros and cons. *Audiology* **17**, 369–420.

Evans, E. F. and Harrison, R. V. (1975). Correlation between outer hair cell damage and deterioration of cochlear nerve tuning properties in the guinea pig. *J. Physiol. (Lond.)* **256**, 43–44P.

Evans, E. F. and Nelson, P. G. (1973a). The responses of single neurones in the cochlear nucleus of the cat as a function of their location and anaesthetic state. *Exp. Brain Res.* **17**, 402–427.

Evans, E. F. and Nelson, P. G. (1973b). On the functional relationship between the dorsal and ventral divisions of the cochlear nucleus of the cat. *Exp. Brain Res.* **17**, 428–442.

Evans, E. F. and Palmer, A. R. (1975). Responses of single units in the cochlear nerve and nucleus of the cat to signals in the presence of bandstop noise. *J. Physiol. (Lond.)* **252**, 60–62P.

Evans, E. F. and Whitfield, I. C. (1964). Classification of unit responses in the auditory cortex of the unanaesthetised cat. *J. Physiol.* (Lond.) **171**, 476–493.

Evans, E. F. and Wilson, J. P. (1975). Cochlear tuning properties: concurrent basilar membrane and single nerve fiber measurements. *Science* **190**, 1218–1221.

Evans, E. F. and Wilson, J. P. (1977). *Psychophysics and Physiology of Hearing.* Academic Press, London and New York.

Evans, E. F., Ross, H. F. and Whitfield, I. C. (1965). The spatial distribution of unit characteristic frequency in the primary auditory cortex of the cat. *J. Physiol. (Lond.)* **179**, 238–247.

Evans, E. F., Wilson, J. P. and Borerwe, T. A. (1981). Animal models of tinnitus. In *Tinnitus* (eds D. Evered and G. Lawrenson), pp. 108–129. *CIBA Symposium* **85**, Pitman Medical, London.

Fernandez, C. (1951). The innervation of the cochlea (guinea pig). *Laryngoscope* **61**, 1152–1172.

Fettiplace, R. and Crawford, A. C. (1980). The origin of tuning in turtle cochlear hair cells. *Hearing Res.* **2**, 447–454.

Fex, J. (1959). Augmentation of the cochlear microphonics by stimulation of efferent fibres to cochlea. *Acta Otolar.* **50**, 540–541.

Fex, J. (1962). Auditory activity in centrifugal and centripetal cochlear fibres in cat. *Acta Physiol. Scand.* **55**, Suppl. **189**. 5–68.

Fex, J. (1967). Efferent inhibition in the cochlea related to hair-cell dc activity: study of postsynaptic activity of the crossed olivocochlear fibres in the cat. *J. Acoust. Soc. Am.* **41**, 666–675.

Fex, J. (1973). Neuropharmacology and potentials of the inner ear. In *Basic Mechanisms in Hearing* (ed. A. Møller), pp. 377–420. Academic Press, New York and London.

Fex, J. (1974). Neural excitatory processes of the inner ear. In *Handbook of Sensory Physiology* Vol. 5/1 (eds W. D. Keidel and W. D. Neff), pp. 585–646. Springer, Berlin.

Finlayson, L. H. and Osborne, M. P. (1975). Secretory activity of neurons and related electrical activity. *Adv. Comp. Physiol. and Biochem.* **6**, 165–258.

Fletcher, H. (1940). Auditory patterns. *Revs Modern Phys.* **12**, 47–65.

Flock, A. (1971). Sensory transduction in hair cells. In *Handbook of Sensory Physiology*, Vol. 1 (ed. W. R. Loewenstein), pp. 396–441. Springer, Berlin.

Flock, A. (1977). Physiological properties of sensory hairs in the ear. In *Psychophysics and Physiology of Hearing* (eds E. F. Evans and J. P. Wilson), pp. 15–25. Academic Press, London and New York.

Fourcin, A. J., Rosen, S. M., Moore, B. C. J., Douek, E. E., Clarke, G. P., Dodson, H. and Bannister, L. H. (1979). External electrical stimulation of the cochlea: clinical, psychophysical, speech-perceptual and histological findings. *Brit. J. Audiol.* **13**, 85–107.

Fox, J. E. (1979). Habituation and prestimulus inhibition of the auditory startle reflex in decerebrate rats. *Physiol. Beh.* **23**, 291–297.

Fujita, S. and Elliott, D. N. (1965). Thesholds of audition for three species of monkey. *J. Acoust. Soc. Am.* **37**, 139–144.

Funkenstein, H. H. and Winter, P. (1973). Responses to acoustic stimuli of units in the auditory cortex of awake squirrel monkeys. *Exp. Brain Res.* **18**, 464–488.

Furukawa, T. and Ishii, Y. (1967). Neurophysiological studies of hearing in goldfish. *J. Neurophysiol.* **30**, 1377–1403.

Galambos, R. (1956). Suppression of auditory nerve activity by stimulation of efferent fibers to cochlea. *J. Neurophysiol.* **19**, 424–437.

Galambos, R. (1960). Studies of the auditory system with implanted electrodes. In *Neural Mechanisms of the Auditory and Vestibular Systems* (eds G. L. Rasmussen and W. F. Windle), pp. 137–151. Thomas, Springfield.

Gässler, G. (1954). Uber die Hörshwelle für Schallereignisse mit verschieden breitem Frequenzspectrum. *Acustica* 4, 408–414.

Gazzaniga, M. S. and Sperry, R. W. (1967). Language after section of the cerebral commissures. *Brain* 90, 131–148.

Geisler, C. D. (1976). Mathematical models of the mechanics of the inner ear. In *Handbook of Sensory Physiology* Vol. 5/3 (eds W. D. Keidel and W. D. Neff), pp. 391–415. Springer, Berlin.

Geisler, C. D., Rhode, W. S. and Kennedy, D. T. (1974). Responses to tonal stimuli of single auditory nerve fibers and their relation to basilar membrane motion in the squirrel monkey. *J. Neurophysiol.* 37, 1156–1172.

Geisler, C. D., Mountain, D. C., Hubbard, A. E., Adrian, H. O. and Ravindran, A. (1977). Alternating electrical-resistance changes in the guinea-pig cochlea caused by acoustic stimuli. *J. Acoust. Soc. Am.* 61, 1557–1566.

Geisler, C. D., Mountain, D. C. and Hubbard, A. E. (1980). Sound-induced resistance changes in the inner ear. *J. Acoust. Soc. Am.* 67, 1729–1735.

Geniec, P. and Morest, D. K. (1971). The neuronal architecture of the human posterior colliculus: a study with the Golgi method. *Acta Otolar.* Suppl. 295, 1–35.

Gerken, G. M. (1979). Central denervation hypersensitivity in the auditory system of the cat. *J. Acoust. Soc. Am.* 66, 721–727.

Gershuni, G. V., Baru, A. V. and Karaseva, T. A. (1967). Role of auditory cortex in discrimination of acoustic stimuli. *Neural Sciences Trans.* 1, 370–382.

Gilbert, A. G. and Pickles, J. O. (1980). Responses of auditory nerve fibres to noise bands of different widths. *Hearing Res.* 2, 327–333.

Glaser, E. M., van der Loos, H. and Gissler, M. (1979). Tangential orientation and spatial order in dendrites of cat auditory cortex: a computer microscope study of Golgi-impregnated material. *Exp. Brain Res.* 36, 411–431.

Goblick, T. and Pfeiffer, R. R. (1969). Time domain measurements of cochlear nonlinearities using combination click stimuli. *J. Acoust. Soc. Am.* 46, 924–938.

Godfrey, D. A., Kiang, N. Y.-S. and Norris, B. E. (1975a). Single unit activity in the posteroventral cochlear nucleus of the cat. *J. Comp. Neurol.* 162, 247–268.

Godfrey, D. A., Kiang, N. Y.-S. and Norris, B. E. (1975b). Single unit activity in the dorsal cochlear nucleus of the cat. *J. Comp. Neurol.* 162, 269–284.

Godfrey, D. A., Carter, J. A., Berger, S. J., Lowry, O. H. and Matchinsky, F. M. (1977). Quantitative histochemical mapping of candidate transmitter amino acids in cat cochlear nucleus. *J. Histochem. Cytochem.* 25, 417–431.

Goldberg, J. M. (1975). Physiological studies of auditory nuclei of the pons. In *Handbook of Sensory Physiology* Vol. 5/2 (eds W. D. Keidel and W. D. Neff), pp. 109–144. Springer, Berlin.

Goldberg, J. M. and Brown, P. B. (1968) Functional organization of the dog superior olivary complex: an anatomical and electrophysiological study. *J. Neurophysiol.* 31, 639–656.

Goldberg, J. M. and Brown, P. B. (1969). Response of binaural neurons of dog superior olivary complex to dichotic tonal stimuli: some physiological mechanisms of sound localization. *J. Neurophysiol.* 32, 613–636.

Goldberg, J. M. and Brownell, W. E. (1973). Response characteristics of neurons in anteroventral and dorsal cochlear nuclei of cat. *Brain Res.* 64, 35–54.

Goldberg, J. M., Diamond, I. T. and Neff, W. D. (1957). Auditory discrimination after ablation of temporal and insular cortex in cat. *Fed. Proc.* 16, 204.

Goldberg, J. M., Adrian, H. O. and Smith, F. D. (1964). Response of neurons of the superior olivary complex of the cat to acoustic stimuli of long duration. *J. Neurophysiol.* **27**, 706–749.

Goldstein, J. L. (1967). Auditory nonlinearity. *J. Acoust. Soc. Am.* **41**, 676–689.

Goldstein, J. L. and Kiang, N. Y.-S. (1968). Neural correlates of the aural combination tone $2f_1 - f_2$. *Proc. I.E.E.E.* **56**, 981–992.

Goldstein, M. H. and Abeles, M. (1975). Single unit activity of the auditory cortex. In *Handbook of Sensory Physiology*, Vol. 5/2 (eds W. D. Keidel and W. D. Neff), pp. 199–218. Springer, Berlin.

Goldstein, M. H., Hall, J. L. and Butterfield, B. O. (1968). Single-unit activity in the primary auditory cortex of unanesthetised cats. *J. Acoust. Soc. Am.* **43**, 444–455.

Green, D. M. (1976). *An Introduction to Hearing.* Wiley, New York.

Greenwood, D. D. (1977). Comment on the above paper. In *Psychophysics and Physiology of Hearing* (eds E. F. Evans and J. P. Wilson), p. 40. Academic Press, London and New York.

Greenwood, D. D. and Goldberg, J. M. (1970). Response of neurons in the cochlear nuclei to variations in noise bandwidths and to tone-noise combinations. *J. Acoust. Soc. Am.* **47**, 1022–1040.

Griffin, D. R., Dunning, D. C., Cahlander, D. A. and Webster, F. A. (1962). Correlated orientation sounds and ear movements of horseshoe bats. *Nature* **196**, 1185–1186.

Groen, J. J. (1964). Super- and subliminal binaural beats. *Acta Otolar.* **57**, 224–230.

Guild, S. R. (1932). Correlations of histologic observations and the acuity of hearing. *Acta Otolar.* **17**, 207–249.

Guinan, J. J. and Peake, W. T. (1967). Middle ear characteristics of anesthetised cats. *J. Acoust. Soc. Am.* **41**, 1237–1261.

Guinan, J. J., Guinan, S. S. and Norris, B. E. (1972). Single auditory units in the superior olivary complex. I. Responses to sounds and classification based on physiological properties. *Int. J. Neurosci.* **4**, 101–120.

Hall, J. L. (1972). Auditory distortion products $f_2 - f_1$ and $2f_1 - f_2$. *J. Acoust. Soc. Am.* **51**, 1863–1871.

Hall, J. L. (1980). Cochlear models: two-tone suppression and the second filter. *J. Acoust. Soc. Am.* **67**, 1722–1728.

Halperin, Y., Nachson, I. and Carmon, A. (1973). Shift of ear superiority in dichotic listening to temporally-patterned nonverbal stimuli. *J. Acoust. Soc. Am.* **53**, 46–50.

Harris, D. M. (1979). Action potential suppression, tuning curves and thresholds: comparison with single fiber data. *Hearing Res.* **1**, 133–154.

Harris, D. M. and Dallos, R. D. (1979). Forward masking of auditory nerve fiber responses. *J. Neurophysiol.* **42**, 1083–1107.

Harrison, J. M. (1978). Functional properties of the auditory system of the brain stem. In *Handbook of Behavioural Neurobiology* Vol. 1 (ed. R. B. Masterton), pp. 409–458. Plenum Press, New York.

Harrison, J. M. and Howe, M. E. (1974a). Anatomy of the afferent auditory nervous system of mammals. In *Handbook of Sensory Physiology* Vol. 5/1 (eds W. D. Keidel and W. D. Neff), pp. 283–336. Springer, Berlin.

Harrison, J. M. and Howe, M. E. (1974b). Anatomy of the descending auditory system (mammalian), In *Handbook of Sensory Physiology* Vol. 5/1 (eds W. D. Keidel and W. D. Neff), pp. 363–388. Springer, Berlin.

Hebrank, J. and Wright, D. (1974). Spectral cues used in the localization of sound sources in the median plane. *J. Acoust. Soc. Am.* **56**, 1829–1834.

Hecaen, H. (1979). Aphasias. In *Handbook of Behavioural Neurobiology*, Vol. 2 (ed. M. S. Gazzaniga), pp. 239–292. Academic Press, New York and London.
Heffner, H. (1978). Effect of auditory cortex ablation on localization and discrimination of brief sounds. *J. Neurophysiol.* **41**, 963–976.
Heffner, H. and Masterton, R. B. (1975). Contribution of auditory cortex to sound localization in the monkey (*Macaca mulatta*). *J. Neurophysiol.* **38**, 1340–1358.
Heffner, R., Heffner, H. and Masterton, B. (1971). Behavioral measurements of absolute and frequency difference thresholds in guinea-pig. *J. Acoust. Soc. Am.* **49**, 1888–1895.
Held, G. (1893). Die centrale Gehörleitung. *Arch. Anat. Physiol. Anat. Abt.* (**1893**) 201–248.
Helmholtz, H. L. F. (1863). *Die Lehre von den Tonempfindungen als Physiologische Grundlage für die Theorie der Musik.* Eng. Trans. of 3rd. ed. by A. J. Ellis, *On the Sensations of Tone*, 1875. Longmans, Green, London.
Hendry, B. M., Urban, B. W. and Haydon, D. A. (1978). The blockage of the electrical conductance in a pore-containing membrane by the n-alkanes. *Biochim. Biophys. Acta.* 513, 106–116.
Hernandez-Peon, R., Scherrer, H. and Jouvet, M. (1956). Modification of electric activity in cochlear nucleus during "attention" in unanesthetised cats. *Science*, **123**, 331–332.
Hodgkin, A. L. and Huxley, A. F. (1952). A quantitative description of membrane current and its application to conduction and excitation in nerve. *J. Physiol. (Lond.)* **117**, 500–544.
Honrubia, V. and Ward, P. H. (1968). Longitudinal distribution of the cochlear microphonics inside the cochlear duct (guinea pig). *J. Acoust. Soc. Am.* **44**, 951–958.
Honrubia, V. and Ward, P. H. (1969). Properties of the summating potential of the guinea pig's cochlea. *J. Acoust. Soc. Am.* **45**, 1443–1450.
Honrubia, V., Strelioff, D. and Sitko, S. T. (1976). Physiological basis of cochlear transduction and sensitivity. *Ann. Otol. Rhinol. Laryngol.* **85**, 697–710.
Hopkins, C. D. (1976). Stimulus filtering and electroreception: tuberous electroreceptors in three species of gymnotoid fish. *J. Comp. Physiol.* **111**, 171–207.
Houtgast,T. (1972). Psychophysical evidence for lateral inhibition in hearing. *J. Acoust. Soc. Am.* **51**, 1885–1894.
Houtgast, T. (1973). Psychophysical experiments on 'tuning curves' and 'two-tone inhibition'. *Acustica* **29**, 168–179.
Houtgast, T. (1974). *Lateral Suppression in Hearing.* Inst TNO, Soesterberg.
Houtgast, T. (1977). Auditory-filter characteristics derived from direct-masking data and pulsation-threshold data with a rippled-noise masker. *J. Acoust. Soc. Am.* **62**, 409–415.
Hubbard, A. E., Geisler, C. D. and Mountain, D. C. (1979). Comparison of the spectra of the cochlear microphonic and of the sound-elicited electrical impedance changes measured in scala media of the guinea pig. *J. Acoust. Soc. Am.* **66**, 431–445.
Hubel, D. H. and Wiesel, T. N. (1962). Receptive fields, binocular interaction and functional architecture in the cat's visual cortex. *J. Physiol. (Lond.)* **160**, 106–154.
Hubel, D. H. and Wiesel, T. N. (1963). Shape and arrangement of columns in cat's striate cortex. *J. Physiol. (Lond.)* **165**, 559–568.
Hubel, D. H., Henson, C. O., Rupert, A. and Galambos, R. (1959). "Attention" units in the auditory cortex. *Science* **129**, 1279–1280.
Hudspeth, A. J. and Corey, D. P. (1977). Sensitivity, polarity, and conductance

314   *An Introduction to the Physiology of Hearing*

change in the response of vertebrate hair cells to controlled mechanical stimuli. *Proc. Natl. Acad. Sci. USA.* **74**, 2407–2411.

Hudspeth, A. J. and Jacobs, R. (1979). Stereocilia mediate transduction in vertebrate hair cells. *Proc. Natl. Acad. Sci. USA.* **76**, 1506–1509.

Ilberg, Ch. v. and Vosteen, K. H. (1969). Permeability of the inner-ear membranes. *Acta Otolar.* **67**, 165–170.

Imig, T. J. and Adrian, H. O. (1977). Binaural columns in the primary field (AI) of cat auditory cortex. *Brain Res.* **138**, 241–257.

Imig, T. J., Ruggero, M. A., Kitzes, L. M., Javel, E. and Brugge, J. F. (1977). Organization of auditory cortex in the owl monkey (*Aotus trivirgatus*). *J. Comp. Neurol.* **171**, 111–128.

Jane, J. A., Masterton, R. B. and Diamond, I. T. (1965). The function of the tectum for attention to auditory stimuli in the cat. *J. Comp. Neurol.* **125**, 165–192.

Javel, E. (1981). Suppression of auditory nerve responses. I. Temporal analysis, intensity effects and suppression contours. *J. Acoust. Soc. Am.* **69**, 1735–1745.

Jerger, J., Weikers, N. J., Sharbrough, F. W. and Jerger, S. (1969). Bilateral lesions of the temporal lobe. *Acta Otolar.* Suppl. **258**, 1–51.

Johnstone, B. M. and Boyle, A. J. F. (1967). Basilar membrane vibration examined with the Mössbauer technique. *Science* **158**, 389–390.

Johnstone, B. M. and Sellick, P. M. (1972). The peripheral auditory apparatus. *Quart. Revs. Biophys.* **5**, 1–57.

Johnstone, B. M., Johnstone, J. R. and Pugsley, I. D. (1966). Membrane resistance in endolymphatic walls of the first turn of the guinea pig cochlea. *J. Acoust. Soc. Am.* **40**, 1398–1404.

Johnstone, B. M., Taylor, K. J. and Boyle, A. J. (1970). Mechanics of the guinea pig cochlea. *J. Acoust. Soc. Am.* **47**, 504–509.

Johnstone, J. R. and Johnstone, B. M. (1966). Origin of summating potential. *J. Acoust. Soc. Am.* **40**, 1405–1413.

Kaas, J., Axelrod, S. and Diamond, I. T. (1967). An ablation study of the auditory cortex in the cat using binaural tonal patterns. *J. Neurophysiol.* **30**, 710–724.

Kane, E. C. (1973). Octopus cells in the cochlear nucleus of the cat: heterotypic synapses on homeotypic neurons. *Intern. J. Neurosci.* **5**, 251–279.

Karaseva, T. A. (1972). The role of the temporal lobe in human auditory perception. *Neuropsychology* **10**, 277–231.

Katsuki, Y., Sumi, T., Uchiyama, H. and Watanabe, T. (1958). Electrical responses of auditory neurons in cat to sound stimulation. *J. Neurophysiol.* **21**, 569–588.

Katsuki, Y., Watanabe, T. and Maruyama, N. (1959). Activity of auditory neurons in upper levels of brain of cat. *J. Neurophysiol.* **22**, 343–359.

Katsuki, Y., Suga, N. and Kanno, Y. (1962). Neural mechanism of the peripheral and central auditory system in monkeys. *J. Acoust. Soc. Am.* **34**, 1396–1410.

Keidel, W. D. (1974). Information processing in the higher parts of the auditory pathway. In *Facts and Models in Hearing* (eds E. Zwicker and E. Terhardt), pp. 216–226. Springer, Berlin.

Kelly, J. B. and Whitfield, I. C. (1971). Effects of auditory cortical lesions on discriminations of rising and falling frequency-modulated tones. *J. Neurophysiol.* **34**, 802–816.

Kemp, D. T. (1978). Stimulated acoustic emissions from within the human auditory system. *J. Acoust. Soc. Am.* **64**, 1386–1391.

Kemp, D. T. and Chum, R. (1980). Properties of the generator of stimulated acoustic emissions. *Hearing Res.* **2**, 213–232.

Kerr, A. and Schuknecht, H. F. (1968). The spiral ganglion in profound deafness. *Acta Ololar.* **65**, 586–598.

Kesner, R. P. (1966). Subcortical mechanisms of audiogenic seizure. *Exp. Neurol.* **15**, 192–205.

Kessel, R. G. and Kardon, R. H. (1979). *Tissues and Organs.* W. H. Freeman and Company, San Fransisco.

Khanna, S. M. and Tonndorf, J. (1971). The vibratory pattern of the round window in cats. *J. Acoust. Soc. Am.* **50**, 1475–1483.

Khanna, S. M. and Tonndorf, J. (1972). Tympanic membrane vibration in cats studied by time-averaged holography. *J. Acoust. Soc. Am.* **51**, 1904–1920.

Kiang, N. Y.-S. (1965). Stimulus coding in the auditory nerve and cochlear nucleus. *Acta Otolar.* **59**, 186–200.

Kiang, N. Y.-S. (1968). A survey of recent developments in the study of auditory physiology. *Ann. Otol. Rhinol. Laryngol.* **77**, 656–675.

Kiang, N. Y.-S. (1975). Stimulus representation in the discharge patterns of auditory neurons. In *The Nervous System*, Vol. 3 (ed. D. B. Tower), pp. 81–96. Raven Press, New York.

Kiang, N. Y.-S. (1980). Processing of speech by the auditory nervous system. *J. Acoust. Soc. Am.* **68**, 830–835.

Kiang, N. Y.-S. and Moxon, E. C. (1972). Physiological considerations in artificial stimulation of the inner ear. *Ann. Otol. Rhinol. Laryngol.* **81**, 714–730.

Kiang, N. Y.-S., Watanabe, T., Thomas, E. C. and Clark, L. F. (1965). Discharge Patterns of Single Fibers in the Cat's Auditory Nerve (*Res. Monogr.* no. **35**) M.I.T. Press, Cambridge.

Kiang, N. Y.-S., Sachs, M. B. and Peake, W. T. (1967). Shapes of tuning curves for single auditory-nerve fibers. *J. Acoust. Soc. Am.* **42**, 1341–1342.

Kiang, N. Y.-S., Moxon, E. C. and Levine, R. A. (1970). Auditory-nerve activity in cats with normal and abnormal cochleas. In *Sensorineural Hearing Loss* (eds G. E. W. Wolstenholme and J. Knight), pp. 241–268. CIBA Foundation Symposium. Churchill, London.

Kim, D. O. and Molnar, C. E. (1975). Cochlear mechanics: measurements and models. In *The Nervous System*, Vol. 3 (ed. D. B. Tower), pp. 57–68. Raven Press, New York.

Kim, D. O., Molnar, C. E. and Pfeiffer, R. R. (1973). A system of nonlinear differential equations modeling basilar-membrane motion. *J. Acoust. Soc. Am.* **54**, 1517–1529.

Kim, D. O., Siegel, J. H. and Molnar, C. E. (1979). Cochlear nonlinear phenomena in two-tone responses. *Scand. Audiol.* Suppl **9**, 63–81.

Kim, D. O., Molnar, C. E. and Matthews, J. W. (1980). Cochlear mechanics: nonlinear behavior in two-tone responses as reflected in cochlear-nerve-fiber responses and in ear-canal sound pressure. *J. Acoust. Soc. Am.* **67**, 1704–1721.

Klinke, R. and Galley, N. (1974). Efferent innervation of vestibular and auditory receptors. *Physiol. Revs.* **54**, 316–357.

Klinke, R., Boerger, G. and Gruber, J. (1969). Studies on the functional significance of efferent innervation in the auditory system: afferent neuronal activity as influenced by contralaterally-applied sound. *Pflüger's Arch. Ges. Physiol.* **306**, 165–175.

Knight, P. L. (1977). Representation of the cochlea within the anterior field (AAF) of the cat. *Brain Res.* **130**, 447–467.

Knudsen, E. I. and Konishi, M. (1978). A neural map of auditory space in the owl. *Science* **200**, 795–797.

Koenig, E. (1957). The effects of auditory pathway interruption on the incidence of sound-induced seizures in rats. *J. Comp. Neurol.* **108**, 383–392.

Kohllöffel, L. U. E. (1972a). A study of basilar membrane vibrations. II. The vibratory amplitude and phase pattern along the basilar membrane (post mortem). *Acustica* **27**, 66–81.

Kohllöffel, L. U. E. (1972b). A study of basilar membrane vibrations. III. The basilar membrane frequency response curve in the living guinea pig. *Acustica* **27**, 82–89.

Konishi, T. and Yasuno, T. (1963). Summating potential of the cochlea in the guinea pig. *J. Acoust. Soc. Am.* **35**, 1448–1452.

Kronester-Frei, A. (1979). Localization of the marginal zone of the tectorial membrane *in situ*, unfixed and *in vivo*-like ionic milieu. *Arch. Oto-rhino-laryngol.* **224**, 3–9.

Kryter, K. D. and Ades, H. W. (1943). Studies on the function of the higher acoustic centers in the cat. *Am. J. Psychol.* **56**, 501–536.

Kuijpers, W. and Bonting, S. L. (1969). Studies on the (Na^+-K^+)-activated ATPase. XXIV. Localization and properties of ATPase in the inner ear of the guinea pig. *Biochim. Biophys. Acta.* **173**, 477–485.

Kuijpers, W. and Bonting, S. L. (1970). The cochlear potentials. I. The effect of ouabain on the cochlear potentials of the guinea pig. *Pflügers Arch. Ges. Physiol.* **320**, 348–358.

Kuwada, S., Yin, T. C. T., Haberly, L. B. and Wickesberg, R. E. (1980). Binaural interaction in the cat inferior colliculus: physiology and anatomy. In *Psychophysical, Physiological and Behavioural Studies in Hearing*. (eds G. van den Brink and F. A. Bilsen), pp. 401–408. Delft University Press, Delft.

Lassen, N. A., Ingvar, D. H. and Skinhøj, E. (1978). Brain function and blood flow. *Scientific Am.* **239**, (4) 50–59.

Lepage, E. and Johnstone, B. M. (1980). Nonlinear mechanical behaviour of the basilar membrane in the basal turn of the guinea pig. *Hearing Res.* **2**, 183–189.

Leshowitz, B. and Lindström, R. (1977). Measurement of nonlinearities in listeners with sensorineural hearing loss. In *Psychophysics and Physiology of Hearing* (eds E. F. Evans and J. P. Wilson), pp. 283–292. Academic Press, London and New York.

Liberman, A. M., Cooper, F. S., Shankweiler, D. P. and Studdert-Kennedy, M. (1967). Perception of the speech code. *Psychol. Rev.* **74**, 431–461.

Liberman, M. C. (1978). Auditory-nerve responses from cats raised in a low-noise chamber. *J. Acoust. Soc. Am.* **63**, 442–455.

Liberman, M. C. and Kiang, N. Y.-S. (1978). Acoustic trauma in cats. *Acta Otolar.* Suppl. **358**, 1–63.

Lim, D. J. (1980). Cochlear anatomy related to cochlear micromechanics. A review. *J. Acoust. Soc. Am.* **67**, 1686–1695.

Llinas, R. (1979). The role of calcium in neuronal function. In *The Neurosciences: Fourth Study Program* (eds F. O. Schmitt and F. G. Worden), pp. 555–571. M.I.T. Press, Cambridge.

Lovick, T. A. and Zbrozyna, A. W. (1975). Classical conditioning of the corneal reflex in the chronic decerebrate rat. *Brain Res.* **89**, 337–340.

Lowenstein, O. and Sand, A. (1940). The mechanism of the semicircular canal. A study of the responses of single-fibre preparations to angular accelerations and rotation at constant speed. *Proc. Roy. Soc. (Lond.)* B **129**, 256–275.

Lowenstein, O. and Wersäll, J. (1959). A functional interpretation of the electron-microscopic structure of sensory hairs in the cristae of the elasmobranch *Raja Clavata* in terms of directional sensitivity. *Nature* **184**, 1807–1808.

Macartney, J. C., Comis, S. D. and Pickles, J. O. (1980). Is myosin in the cochlea a basis for active motility? *Nature* **288**, 491–492.

Majorossy, K. and Kiss, A. (1976). Specific patterns of neuron arrangement and of synaptic articulation in the medial geniculate body. *Exp. Brain Res.* **26**, 1–17.

Manley, J. A. and Müller-Preuss, P. (1978). Response variability of auditory cortex cells in the squirrel monkey to constant acoustic stimuli. *Exp. Brain Res.* **32**, 171–180.

Marin, O. S., Schwartz, M. F. and Saffran, E. M. (1979). Origins and distribution of language. In *Handbook of Behavioral Neurobiology*, Vol. 2, (ed. M. S. Gazzaniga), pp. 179–213. Academic Press, New York and London.

Massopust, L. C. and Ordy, J. M. (1962). Auditory organization of the inferior colliculi in the cat. *Exp. Neurol.* **6**, 465–477.

Mast, T. E. (1970). Binaural interaction and contralateral inhibition in dorsal cochlear nucleus of the chinchilla. *J. Neurophysiol.* **33**, 108–115.

Mast, T. E. (1973). Dorsal cochlear nucleus of the chinchilla: excitation by contralateral sound. *Brain Res.* **62**, 61–70.

Masterton, R. B. and Diamond, I. T. (1964). Effects of auditory cortex ablation on discrimination of small binaural time differences. *J. Neurophysiol.* **27**, 15–36.

Masterton, B. and Diamond, I. T. (1967). The medial superior olive and sound localization. *Science* **155**, 1696–1697.

Merzenich, M. M. and Brugge, J. F. (1973). Representation of the cochlear partition on the superior temporal plane of the macaque monkey. *Brain Res.* **50**, 275–296.

Merzenich, M. M., Knight, P. L. and Roth, G. L. (1975). Representation of cochlea within primary auditory cortex in the cat. *J. Neurophysiol.* **38**, 231–249.

Merzenich, M. M., Roth, G. L., Andersen, R. A., Knight, P. L. and Colwell, S. A. (1977). Some basic features of organization of the central auditory nervous system. In *Psychophysics and Physiology of Hearing* (eds E. F. Evans and J. P. Wilson), pp. 485–497. Academic Press, London and New York.

Meyer, D. R. and Woosey, C. N. (1952). Effects of localized cortical destruction on auditory discriminative conditioning in cat. *J. Neurophysiol.* **15**, 149–162.

Middlebrooks, J. C., Dykes, R. W. and Merzenich, M. M. (1980). Binaural response-specific bands in primary auditory cortex (AI) of the cat: topographical organization orthogonal to isofrequency contours. *Brain Res.* **181**, 31–48.

Milner, B. (1962). Laterality effects in audition. In *Interhemispheric Relations and Cerebral Dominance* (ed. V. B. Mountcastle), pp. 177–195. Johns Hopkins Press, Baltimore.

Møller, A. R. (1965). An experimental study of the acoustic impedance of the middle ear and its transmission properties. *Acta Otolar.* **60**, 129–149.

Møller, A. R. (1969). Unit responses in the rat cochlear nucleus to repetitive, transient, sounds. *Acta Physiol. Scand.* **75**, 542–551.

Møller, A. R. (1974). Function of the middle ear. In *Handbook of Sensory Physiology* Vol. 5/1 (eds W. D. Keidel and W. D. Neff), pp. 491–517. Springer, Berlin.

Møller, A. R. (1976). Dynamic properties of the responses of single neurones in the cochlear nucleus of the rat. *J. Physiol. (Lond.)* **259**, 63–82.

Møller, A. R. (1977). Frequency selectivity of single auditory nerve fibers in response to broadband noise stimuli. *J. Acoust. Soc. Am.* **62**, 135–142.

Møller, A. R. (1978). Coding of time-varying sounds in the cochlear nucleus. *Audiology* **17**, 446–468.

Moore, B. C. J. (1973). Frequency difference limens for short-duration tones. *J. Acoust. Soc. Am.* **54**, 610–619.

Moore, B. C. J. (1975). Mechanisms of masking. *J. Acoust. Soc. Am.* **57**, 391–399.

Moore, B. C. J. (1980). Detection cues in forward masking. In *Psychophysical, Physiological and Behavioural Studies in Hearing* (eds G. van den Brink and F. A. Bilsen), pp. 222–229. Delft University Press, Delft.

Moore, B. C. J. (1982). *An Introduction to the Psychology of Hearing.* Academic Press, London and New York.

Moore, T. J. and Cashin, J. L. (1974). Response patterns of cochlear nucleus neurons to excerpts from sustained vowels. *J. Acoust. Soc. Am.* **56**, 1565–1576.

Moore, C. N., Casseday, J. H. and Neff, W. D. (1974). Sound localization: the role of the commissural pathways of the auditory system of the cat. *Brain Res.* **82**, 13–26.

Morest, D. K. (1964). The neuronal architecture of the medial geniculate body of the cat. *J. Anat.* **98**, 611–630.

Morest, D. K. (1965). The laminar structure of the medial geniculate body of the cat. *J. Anat. (Lond.)* **99**, 143–160.

Morest, D. K. (1975). Synaptic relationships of Golgi type II cells in the medial geniculate body of the cat. *J. Comp. Neurol.* **162**, 157–194.

Morest, D. K., Kiang, N. Y.-S., Kane, E. C., Guinan, J. J. and Godfrey, D. A. (1973). Stimulus coding at caudal levels of the cat's auditory nervous system: II. Patterns of synaptic organization. In *Basic Mechanisms in Hearing* (ed. A. Møller), pp. 479–504. Academic Press, New York and London.

Morrison, D., Schindler, R. A. and Wersäll, J. (1975). A quantitative analysis of the afferent innervation of the organ of Corti in guinea pig. *Acta Otolaryng.* **79**, 11–23.

Mountain, D. C. (1980). Changes in endolymphatic potential and crossed olivo-cochlear bundle stimulation alter cochlear mechanics. *Science* **210**, 71–72.

Mountcastle, V. B. (1957). Modality and topographic properties of single neurons of cat's somatic sensory cortex. *J. Neurophysiol.* **20**, 408–434.

Moushegian, G., Rupert, A. L. and Gidda, J. S. (1975). Functional characteristics of superior olivary neurones to binaural stimuli. *J. Neurophysiol.* **38**, 1037–1048.

Nedzelnitsky, V. (1980). Sound pressures in the basal turn of the cat cochlea. *J. Acoust. Soc. Am.* **68**, 1676–1689.

Neff, W. D. (1960). Role of the auditory cortex in sound discrimination. In *Neural Mechanisms of the Auditory and Vestibular Systems* (eds G. L. Rasmussen and W. F. Windle), pp. 211–216. Thomas, Springfield.

Neff, W. D. (1961). Neural mechanisms of auditory discrimination. In *Sensory Communication* (ed. W. A. Rosenblith), pp. 259–278. Wiley, New York.

Neff, W. D. (1968). Localization and lateralization of sound in space. In *Hearing Mechanisms in Vertebrates* (eds A. V. S. de Reuck and J. Knight), pp. 207–231. CIBA Foundation Symposium. Churchill, London.

Neff, W. D., Diamond, I. T. and Casseday, J. H. (1975). Behavioral studies of auditory discrimination. In *Handbook of Sensory Physiology* Vol. 5/2 (eds W. D. Keidel and W. D. Neff), pp. 307–400. Springer, Berlin.

Nelson, D. A. and Turner, C. W. (1980). Decay of masking and frequency resolution in sensorineural hearing-impaired listeners. In *Psychophysical, Physiological and Behavioural Studies in Hearing* (G. van den Brink and F. A. Bilsen, eds), pp. 175–182. Delft University Press, Delft.

Nelson, P. G. and Erulkar, S. D. (1963). Synaptic mechanisms of excitation and inhibition in the central auditory pathway. *J. Neurophysiol.* **26**, 908–923.

Nelson, P. G. and Evans, E. F. (1971). Relationship between dorsal and ventral cochlear nuclei. In *Physiology of the Auditory System* (ed. M. B. Sachs), pp. 169–174. National Educational Consultants Inc, Baltimore.

Nelson, P. G., Erulkar, S. D. and Bryan, J. S. (1966). Responses of units of the inferior colliculus to time-varying acoustic stimuli. *J. Neurophysiol.* **29**, 834–860.

Newman, J. D. and Wollberg, Z. (1973). Multiple coding of species-specific vocalizations in the auditory cortex of squirrel monkeys. *Brain Res.* **54**, 287–304.

Niimi, K. and Matsuoka, H. (1979). Thalamocortical organization of the auditory system in the cat studied by retrograde axonal transport of horseradish peroxidase. *Adv. Anat. Embryol. Cell. Biol.* **57**, 1–56.

Nomoto, M., Suga, N. and Katsuki, Y. (1964). Discharge pattern and inhibition of primary auditory nerve fibers in the monkey. *J. Neurophysiol.* **27**, 768–787.

Nordmark, J. O. (1970). Time and frequency analysis. In *Foundations of Modern Auditory Theory*, Vol. 1 (ed. J. V. Tobias), pp. 57–83. Academic Press, New York and London.

Oakley, D. A. and Russell, I. S. (1977). Subcortical storage of Pavolvian conditioning in the rabbit. *Physiol. Beh.* **18**, 931–937.

Oatman, L. C. (1976). Effects of visual attention on the intensity of auditory evoked potentials. *Exp. Neurol.* **51**, 41–53.

Oesterreich, R. E., Strominger, N. L. and Neff, W. D. (1971). Neural structures mediating sound intensity discrimination in the cat. *Brain Res.* **27**, 251–270.

Oonishi, S. and Katsuki, Y. (1965). Functional organization and integrative mechanism on the auditory cortex of the cat. *Jap. J. Physiol.* **15**, 342–365.

Osen, K. K. (1969). Cytoarchitecture of the cochlear nuclei in the cat. *J. Comp. Neurol.* **136**, 453–483.

Osen, K. K. and Roth, K. (1969). Histochemical localization of cholinesterases in the cochlear nuclei of the cat, with notes on the origin of acetylcholinesterase-positive afferents and the superior olive. *Brain Res.* **16**, 165–185.

Palmer, A. R. and Evans, E. F. (1980). Cochlear fibre rate-intensity functions: no evidence for basilar membrane nonlinearities. *Hearing Res.* **2**, 319–326.

Papçun, G., Krashen, S., Terbeek, D., Remington, R. and Harshman, R. (1974). Is the left hemisphere specialised for speech, language, and/or something else? *J. Acoust. Soc. Am.* **55**, 319–327.

Patterson, R. D. (1976). Auditory filter shapes derived with noise stimuli. *J. Acoust. Soc. Am.* **59**, 640–654.

Peake, W. T., Sohmer, H. S. and Weiss, T. F. (1969). Microelectrode recordings of intracochlear potentials. In *Quarterly Progress Report, M.I.T. Research Laboratory of Electronics* **94**, 293–304.

Peterson, L. C. and Bogert, B. P. (1950). A dynamical theory of the cochlea. *J. Acoust. Soc. Am.* **22**, 369–381.

Pfeiffer, R. R. (1966a). Classification of response patterns of spike discharges for units in the cochlear nucleus: tone-burst stimulation. *Exp. Brain Res.* **1**, 220–235.

Pfeiffer, R. R. (1966b). Anteroventral cochlear nucleus: wave forms of extracellularly recorded spike potentials. *Science* **154**, 667–668.

Pfeiffer, R. R. (1970). A model for two-tone inhibition of single cochlear nerve fibers. *J. Acoust. Soc. Am.* **48**, 1373–1378.

Pfeiffer, R. R. and Kim, D. O. (1973). Considerations of nonlinear response properties of single cochlear nerve fibers. In *Basic Mechanisms in Hearing* (ed. A. Møller), pp. 555–587. Academic Press, New York and London.

Pfingst, B. E., O'Connor, T. A. and Miller, J. M. (1977). Response plasticity of neurons in auditory cortex of the rhesus monkey. *Exp. Brain Res.* **29**, 393–404.

Pick, G. F., Evans, E. F. and Wilson, J. P. (1977). Frequency resolution in patients with hearing loss of cochlear origin. In *Psychophysics and Physiology of Hearing* (eds E. F. Evans and J. P. Wilson), pp. 273–281. Academic Press, London and New York.

Pickles, J. O. (1975). Normal critical bands in the cat. *Acta Otolar.* **80**, 245–254.

Pickles, J. O. (1976a). Role of centrifugal pathways to cochlear nucleus in determination of critical bandwidth. *J. Neurophysiol.* **39**, 394–400.

Pickles, J. O. (1976b). The noradrenaline-containing innervation of the cochlear nucleus and the detection of signals in noise. *Brain Res.* **105**, 591–596.

Pickles, J. O. (1979a). Psychophysical frequency resolution in the cat as determined by simultaneous masking and its relation to auditory-nerve resolution. *J. Acoust. Soc. Am.* **66**, 1725–1732.

Pickles, J. O. (1979b). An investigation of sympathetic effects on hearing. *Acta Otolar.* **87**, 69–71.

Pickles, J. O. (1980). Psychophysical frequency resolution in the cat studied with forward masking. In *Psychophysical, Physiological and Behavioural Studies in Hearing* (eds G. van den Brink and F. A. Bilsen), pp. 118–126. Delft University Press, Delft.

Pickles, J. O. and Comis, S. D. (1973). Role of centrifugal pathways to cochlear nucleus in detection of signals in noise. *J. Neurophysiol.* **36**, 1131–1137.

Pickles, J. O. and Comis, S. D. (1976). Auditory-nerve fiber bandwidths and critical bandwidths in the cat. *J. Acoust. Soc. Am.* **60**, 1151–1156.

Pierson, M. and Møller, A. R. (1980). Effect of modulation of basilar membrane position on the cochlear microphonic. *Hearing Res.* **2**, 151–162.

Plomp, R. (1967). Pitch of complex tones. *J. Acoust. Soc. Am.* **41**, 1526–1533.

Plomp, R. (1976). *Aspects of Tone Sensation.* Academic Press, London and New York.

Ranke, O. F. von. (1950). Hydrodynamik der Schneckenflüssigkeit. *Zeits. f. Biol.* **103**, 409–434.

Rasmussen, G. L. (1946). The olivary peduncle and other fiber projections to the superior olivary complex. *J. Comp. Neurol.* **84**, 141–220.

Rasmussen, G. L. (1960). Efferent fibers of the cochlear nerve and cochlear nucleus. In *Neural Mechanisms of the Auditory and Vestibular Systems* (eds G. L. Rasmussen and W. F. Windle), pp. 105–115. Thomas, Springfield.

Rasmussen, G. L. (1964). Anatomic relationships of the ascending and descending auditory systems. In *Neurological Aspects of Auditory and Vestibular Disorders.* (eds W. S. Fields and B. R. Alford), pp. 1–19. Thomas, Springfield.

Rassmusen, G. L. (1965). Efferent connections of the cochlear nucleus. In *Sensori-neural Hearing Processes and Disorder* (ed. A. B. Graham), pp. 61–75. Little Brown, Boston.

Ravizza, R. J. and Belmore, S. M. (1978) Auditory forebrain: evidence from anatomical and behavioral experiments involving human and animal subjects. In *Handbook of Behavioral Neurobiology* (ed. R. B. Masterton), pp. 459–501. Plenum Press, New York.

Ravizza, R. J. and Masterton, R. B. (1972). Contribution of neocortex to sound localization in opossum (*Didelphis Virginiana*). *J. Neurophysiol.* **35**, 344–356.

Reale, R. A. and Imig, T. J. (1980). Tonotopic organization in auditory cortex of the cat. *J. Comp. Neurol.* **192**, 265–291.

Rhode, W. S. (1971). Observations of the vibration of the basilar membrane in squirrel monkeys using the Mössbauer technique. *J. Acoust. Soc. Am.* **49**, 1218–1231.

Rhode, W. S. (1977). Some observations on two-tone interaction measured with the Mössbauer effect. In *Psychophysics and Physiology of Hearing* (eds E. F. Evans and J. P. Wison), pp. 27–38. Academic Press, London and New York.

Rhode, W. S. (1978). Some observations on cochlear mechanics. *J. Acoust. Soc. Am.* **64**, 158–176.

Rhode, W. S. (1980). Cochlear partition vibration — recent views. *J. Acoust. Soc. Am.* **67**, 1696–1703.

Rhode, W. S., Geisler, C. D. and Kennedy, D. T. (1978). Auditory nerve fiber responses to wide-band noise and tone combinations. *J. Neurophysiol.* **41**, 692–704.

Ritsma, R. J. (1967). Frequencies dominant in the perception of the pitch of complex sounds. *J. Acoust. Soc. Am.* **42**, 191–198.

Robards, M. J. (1979). Somatic neurons in the brain-stem and neocortex projecting to the external nucleus of the inferior colliculus: an anatomical study in the opossum. *J. Comp. Neurol.* **184**, 547–566.

Robards, M. J., Watkins, D. W. and Masterton, R. B. (1976). An anatomical study of some somesthetic afferents to the intercollicular terminal zone of the midbrain of the opossum. *J. Comp. Neurol.* **170**, 499–524.

Robertson, D. and Johnstone, B. M. (1979). Aberrant tonotopic organization in the inner ear damaged by kanamycin. *J. Acoust. Soc. Am.* **66**, 466–469.

Robles, L., Rhode, W. S. and Geisler, C. D. (1976). Transient response of the basilar membrane measured in squirrel monkeys using the Mössbauer effect. *J. Acoust. Soc. Am.* **59**, 926–939.

Rockel, A. J. and Jones, E. G. (1973a). The neuronal organization of the inferior colliculus of the adult cat. I. The central nucleus. *J. Comp. Neurol.* **147**, 11–60.

Rockel, A. J. and Jones, E. G. (1973b). The neuronal organization of the inferior colliculus of the adult cat. II. The pericentral nucleus. *J. Comp. Neurol.* **149**, 301–334.

Rose, J. E. (1949). The cellular structure of the auditory region of the cat. *J. Comp. Neurol.* **91**, 409–439.

Rose. J. E. and Woolsey, C. N. (1958). Cortical connections and functional organization of the thalamic auditory system of the cat. In *Biological and Biochemical Bases of Behavior* (eds H. F. Harlow and C. N. Woolsey), pp. 127–150. University of Wisconsin Press, Madison.

Rose, J. E., Galambos, R. and Hughes, J. R. (1959). Microelectrode studies of the cochlear nuclei of the cat. *Bull. Johns Hopkins Hosp.* **104**, 211–251.

Rose. J. E., Galambos, R. and Hughes, J. (1960). Organization of frequency sensitive neurons in the cochlear nuclear complex of the cat. In *Neural Mechanisms of the Auditory and Vestibular Systems* (eds G. L. Rasmussen and W. F. Windle), pp. 116–136. Thomas, Springfield.

Rose, J. E., Greenwood, D. D., Goldberg, J. M. and Hind, J. E. (1963). Some discharge characteristics of single neurons in the inferior colliculus of the cat. I. Tonotopic organization, relation of spike counts to tone intensity, and firing patterns of single elements. *J. Neurophysiol.* **26**, 294–320.

Rose, J. E., Gross, N. B., Geisler, C. D. and Hind, J. E. (1966). Some neural mechanisms in the inferior colliculus of the cat which may be relevant to the localization of a sound source. *J. Neurophysiol.* **29**, 288–314.

Rose, J. E., Hind, J. E., Anderson, D. J. and Brugge, J. F. (1971). Some effects of stimulus intensity on response of auditory nerve fibers in the squirrel monkey. *J. Neurophysiol.* **34**, 685–699.

Roth, G. L., Aitkin, L. M., Andersen, R. A. and Merzenich, M. M. (1978). Some features of the spatial organization of the central nucleus of the inferior colliculus of the cat. *J. Comp. Neurol.* **182**, 661–680.

Russell, I. J. and Roberts, B. L. (1974). Active reduction of lateral-line sensitivity in swimming dogfish. *J. Comp. Physiol.* **94**, 7–15.

Russell, I. J. and Sellick, P. M. (1978). Intracellular studies of hair cells in the mammalian cochlea. *J. Physiol. (Lond.)* **284**, 261–290.

Rutherford, W. (1886). A new theory of hearing. *J. Anat. Physiol.* **21**, 166–168.

Ryan, A. and Miller, J. (1977). Effects of behavioral performance on single-unit firing patterns in inferior colliculus of rhesus monkey. *J. Neurophysiol.* **40**, 943–956.

Ryan, A. and Miller, J. (1978). Single unit responses in the inferior colliculus of the awake and performing rhesus monkey. *Exp. Brain Res.* **32**, 389–407.

Ryan, A. F., Wickham, G. M. and Bone, R. C. (1980). Studies of ion distribution in the inner ear: scanning electron microscopy and X-ray microanalysis of freeze-dried cochlear specimens. *Hearing Res.* **2**, 1–20.

Ryugo, D. K. and Weinberger, N. M. (1976). Corticofugal modulation of the medial geniculate body. *Exp. Neurol.* **51**, 377–391.

Ryugo, D. K. and Weinberger, N. M. (1978). Differential plasticity of morphologically distinct neuron populations in the medial geniculate body of the cat during classical conditioning. *Behav. Biol.* **22**, 275–301.

Sachs, M. B. and Abbas, P. J. (1974). Rate versus level functions for auditory-nerve fibers in cats: tone-burst stimuli. *J. Acoust. Soc. Am.* **56**, 1835–1847.

Sachs, M. B. and Kiang, N. Y.-S. (1968). Two-tone inhibition in auditory nerve fibers. *J. Acoust. Soc. Am.* **43**, 1120–1128.

Sachs, M. B. and Young, E. D. (1979). Encoding of steady-state vowels in the auditory nerve: representation in terms of discharge rate. *J. Acoust. Soc. Am.* **66**, 470–479.

Sachs, M. B. and Young, E. D. (1980). Effects of nonlinearities of speech encoding in the auditory nerve. *J. Acoust. Soc. Am.* **68**, 858–875.

Sachs, M. B., Young, E. D., Schalk, T. B. and Bernardin, C. P. (1980). Suppression effects in the responses of auditory-nerve fibers to broadband stimuli. In *Psychophysical, Physiological and Behavioural Studies in Hearing* (eds G. van den Brink and F. A. Bilsen), pp. 284–291. Delft University Press, Delft.

Saunders, J. C., Bock, G. R., James, R. and Chen, C. S. (1972). Effects of priming for audiogenic seizure on auditory evoked responses in the cochlear nucleus and inferior colliculus of BALB/C mice. *Exp. Neurol.* **37**, 388–394.

Schankweiler, D. and Studdert-Kennedy, M. (1967). Identification of consonants presented to left and right ears. *Quart. J. Exp. Psychol.* **19**, 59–63.

Scharf, B. (1970). Critical bands. In *Foundations of Modern Auditory Theory*, Vol. 1 (ed. J. V. Tobias), pp. 159–202. Academic Press, New York and London.

Scharf, B. and Meiselman, C. H. (1977). Critical bandwidth at high intensities. In *Psychophysics and Physiology of Hearing* (eds E. F. Evans and J. P. Wilson), pp. 221–232. Academic Press, London and New York.

Scharlock, D. P., Neff, W. D. and Strominger, N. L. (1965). Discrimination of tone duration after bilateral ablation of cortical auditory areas. *J. Neurophysiol.* **28**, 673–681.

Scheibel, M. E. and Scheibel, A. B. (1974). Neuropil organization in the superior olive of the cat. *Exp. Neurol.* **43**, 339–348.

Schindler, R. A., Merzenich, M. M., White, M. W. and Bjorkroth, B. (1977). Multielectrode cochlear implants: nerve survival and stimulation patterns. *Archs. Otolar.* **103**, 691–699.

Schouten, M. E. H. (1980). The case against a speech mode of perception. *Acta Psychologica* **44**, 71–98.

Schroeder, M. R. (1975). Models of hearing. *Proc. I.E.E.E.* **63**, 1332–1350.

Schubert, D. (1978). History of research on hearing. In *Handbook of Perception* Vol. 4 (eds E. C. Carterette and M. P. Friedman), pp. 41–80. Academic Press, New York and London.

Schuknecht, H. F. (1960). Neuroanatomical correlates of auditory sensitivity and pitch discrimination in the cat. In *Neural Mechanisms of the Auditory and Vestibular Systems* (eds G. L. Rasmussen and W. F. Windle), pp. 76–90. Thomas, Springfield.

Sellick, P. M. (1979). Recordings from single receptor cells in the mammalian cochlea. *Trends in Neuroscience* **2**, 114–116.

Sellick, P. M. and Russell, I. J. (1979). Two-tone suppression in cochlear hair cells. *Hearing Res.* 1, 227–236.

Sellick, P. M. and Russell, I. J. (1980). The responses of inner hair cells to basilar membrane velocity during low-frequency auditory stimulation in the guinea pig. *Hearing Res.* 2, 439–445.

Semple, M. N. and Aitkin, L. M. (1979). Representation of sound frequency and laterality by units in central nucleus of cat inferior colliculus. *J. Neurophysiol.* 42, 1626–1639.

Shaw, E. A. G. (1974). The external ear. In *Handbook of Sensory Physiology*, Vol. 5/1 (eds W. D. Keidel and W. D. Neff), pp. 455–490. Springer, Berlin.

Simmons, F. B. (1964). Perceptual theories of middle ear muscle function. *Ann. Otol. Rhinol. Laryngol.* 73, 724–740.

Simmons, F. B., Matthews, R. G., Walker, M. G. and White, R. L. (1979). A functioning multichannel auditory nerve stimulator. *Acta Otolar.* 87, 170–175.

Smith, C. A. (1961). Innervation pattern of the cochlea. The inner hair cell. *Ann. Otol. Rhinol. Laryngol.* 70, 504–527.

Smith, C. A. (1968). Ultrastructure of the organ of Corti. *Advan. Sci.* 24, 419–433.

Smith, C. A. (1975). The inner ear: its embryological development and microstructure. In *The Nervous System* Vol. 3 (ed. D. B. Tower), pp. 1–18. Raven Press, New York.

Smith, C. A. (1978). Structure of the cochlear duct. In *Evoked Electrical Activity in the Auditory Nervous System* (eds R. F. Naunton and C. Fernandez), pp. 3–19. Academic Press, New York and London.

Smith, C. A., Lowry, O. H. and Wu, M. L. (1954). The electrolytes of the labyrinthine fluids. *Laryngoscope* 64, 141–153.

Smith, D. E. and Moskowitz, N. (1979). Ultrastructure of layer IV of the primary auditory cortex of the squirrel monkey. *Neuroscience* 4, 349–359.

Smith, R. L. (1979). Adaptation, saturation and physiological masking in single auditory-nerve fibers. *J. Acoust. Soc. Am.* 65, 166–178.

Smolders, J. W. T., Aertsen, A. M. H. J. and Johannesma, P. I. M. (1979). Neural representation of the acoustic biotope: a comparison of the response of auditory neurons to tonal and natural stimuli in the cat. *Biol. Cybern.* 35, 11–20.

Smoorenberg, G. F. (1972). Combination tones and their origin. *J. Acoust. Soc. Am.* 52, 615–632.

Sohmer, H. (1966). A comparison of the efferent effects of the homolateral and contralateral olivo-cochlear bundles. *Acta Otolar.* 62, 74–87.

Sokolich, W. G., Hamernik, R. P., Zwislocki, J. J. and Schmiedt, R. A. (1976). Inferred response polarities of cochlear hair cells. *J. Acoust. Soc. Am.* 59, 963–974.

Sousa-Pinto, A. (1973). The structure of the first auditory cortex in the cat. I. Light microscopic observations on its organization. *Arch. Ital. Biol.* 111, 112–137.

Sovijärvi, A. R. A. (1975). Detection of natural complex sounds in the primary auditory cortex of the cat. *Acta Physiol. Scand.* 93, 318–335.

Sovijärvi, A. R. A. and Hyvärinen, J. (1974). Auditory cortical neurons in the cat sensitive to the direction of sound source movement. *Brain Res.* 73, 455–471.

Spoendlin, H. (1966). The organization of the cochlear receptor. *Adv. in Otolaryngol.* 13, 1–227. Karger, Basel.

Spoendlin, H. (1972). Innervation densities of the cochlea. *Acta Otolar.* 73, 235–248.

Spoendlin, H. (1978). The afferent innervation of the cochlea. In *Evoked Electrical Activity in the Auditory Nervous System* (eds R. F. Naunton and C. Fernandez), pp. 21–39. Academic Press, New York and London.

Spoendlin, H. and Lichtensteiger, W. (1966) The adrenergic innervation of the labyrinth. *Acta Otolar.* **61**, 423–434.

Springer, S. P. (1979). Speech perception and the biology of language. In *Handbook of Behavioral Neurobiology*, Vol 2 (ed. M. S. Gazzaniga), pp. 153–177. Academic Press, New York and London.

Starr, A. and Wernick, J. S. (1968). Olivocochlear bundle stimulation: effects on spontaneous and tone-evoked activities of single units in cat cochlear nucleus. *J. Neurophysiol.* **31**, 549–564.

Steele, C. R. (1976). Cochlear mechanics. In *Handbook of Sensory Physiology* Vol. 5/3 (eds W. D. Keidel and W. D. Neff), pp. 443–478. Springer, Berlin.

Stepien, L. S., Cordeau, J. P. and Rasmussen, T. (1960). The effect of temporal lobe and hippocampal lesions on auditory and visual recent memory. *Brain* **83**, 470–489.

Stillman, R. D. (1971). Characteristic delay neurons in the inferior colliculus of the kangaroo rat. *Exp. Neurol.* **32**, 404–412.

Strelioff, D., Haas, G. and Honrubia, S. (1972). Sound-induced electrical impedance changes in the guinea pig cochlea. *J. Acoust. Soc. Am.* **51**, 617–620.

Strominger, N. L. (1969). Localization of sound in space after unilateral and bilateral ablation of auditory cortex. *Exp. Neurol.* **25**, 521–533.

Swanson, L. W. and Hartman, B. K. (1975). The central adrenergic system. An immunofluorescence study of the location of cell bodies and their efferent connections in the rat utilizing dopamine-β-hydroxylase as a marker. *J. Comp. Neurol.* **163**, 467–506.

Tanaka, Y., Anasuma, A. and Yanagisawa, K. (1980). Potentials of outer hair cells and their membrane properties in cationic environments. *Hearing Res.* **2**, 431–438.

Tasaki, I. (1954). Nerve impulses in individual auditory nerve fibers of guinea pig. *J. Neurophysiol.* **17**, 97–122.

Tasaki, I. (1960). Afferent impulses in auditory nerve fibers and the mechanisms of impulse initiation in the cochlea. In *Neural Mechanisms of the Auditory and Vestibular Systems* (eds G. L. Rasmussen and W. F. Windle), pp. 40–47. Thomas, Springfield.

Tasaki, I. and Fernandez, C. (1952). Modification of cochlear microphonics and action potentials by KCl solution and by direct currents. *J. Neurophysiol.* **15**, 497–512.

Tasaki, I. and Spyropoulos, C. S. (1959). Stria vascularis as a source of endocochlear potential. *J. Neurophysiol.* **22**, 149–155.

Tasaki, I., Davis, H. and Eldredge, D. H. (1954). Exploration of cochlear potentials in guinea pig with a microelectrode. *J. Acoust. Soc. Am.* **26**, 765–773.

Thompson, G. C. and Masterton, R. B. (1978). Brain stem auditory pathways involved in reflexive head orientation to sound. *J. Neurophysiol.* **41**, 1183–1202.

Thompson, R. F. (1960). Function of auditory cortex of cat in frequency discrimination. *J. Neurophysiol.* **23**, 321–334.

Tilney, L. G., DeRosier, D. J. and Mulroy, M. J. (1980). The organization of actin filaments in the stereocilia of cochlear hair cells. *J. Cell Biol.* **86**, 244–259.

Tobias, J. V. (1970). *Foundations of Modern Auditory Theory*, Vol. 1. Academic Press, New York and London.

Tobias, J. V. (1972). *Foundations of Modern Auditory Theory*, Vol. 2. Academic Press, New York and London.

Tonndorf, J. (1973). Cochlear nonlinearities. In *Basic Mechanisms in Hearing* (ed A. Møller), pp. 11–44. Academic Press, New York and London.

Trahiotis, C. and Elliott, D. N. (1970). Behavioral investigation of some possible effects of sectioning the crossed olivocochlear bundle. *J. Acoust. Soc. Am.* **47**, 592–596.

Tsuchitani, C. (1977). Functional organization of lateral cell groups of cat superior olivary complex. *J. Neurophysiol.* **40**, 296–318.

Tsuchitani, C. and Boudreau, J. C. (1966). Single unit analysis of cat superior olive S-segment with tonal stimuli. *J. Neurophysiol.* **29**, 684–697.

Tunturi, A. R. (1952). A difference in the representation of auditory signals for the left and right ears in the iso-frequency contours of the right middle ectosylvian auditory cortex of the dog. *Am. J. Physiol.* **168**, 712–727.

Vinnikov, Ya. A. (1974). Sensory reception. *Molecular Biology, Biochemistry and Biophysics.* **17**, 1–392.

Voigt, H. F. and Young, E. D. (1980). Evidence for inhibitory interactions between neurons in dorsal cochlear nucleus. *J. Neurophysiol.* **44**, 76–96.

Vries, H. de. (1948). Die Reichswelle der Sinnesorgane als physiologisches Problem. *Experientia* **4**, 205–240.

Walsh, S. M., Merzenich, M. M., Schindler, R. A. and Leake-Jones, P. A. (1980). Some practical considerations in development of multichannel scala tympani prostheses. *Audiology* **19**, 164–175.

Warr, W. B. (1975). Olivocochlear and vestibular efferent neurons of the feline brain-stem: their location, morphology and number determined by retrograde axonal transport and acetylcholinesterase histochemistry. *J. Comp. Neurol.* **161**, 159–182.

Warr, W. B. (1978). The olivocochlear bundle: its origins and terminations in the cat. In *Evoked Electrical Activity in the Auditory Nervous System* (eds R. F. Naunton and C. Fernandez), pp. 43–63. Academic Press, New York and London.

Warr, W. B. and Guinan, J. J. (1979). Efferent innervation of the organ of Corti: two separate systems. *Brain Res.* **173**, 152–155.

Watanabe, T., Yanagisawa, K., Kanzaki, J. and Katsuki, Y. (1966). Cortical efferent flow influencing unit responses of medial geniculate body to sound stimulation. *Exp. Brain Res.* **2**, 302–317.

Webster, W. R. and Aitkin, L. M. (1975). Central auditory processing. In *Handbook of Psychobiology* (eds M. S. Gazzaniga and C. Blakemore), pp. 325–364. Academic Press, New York and London.

Wegener, J. G. (1973). The sound localizing behavior of normal and brain-damaged monkeys. *J. Aud. Res.* **13**, 191–219.

Weiskrantz, L. and Mishkin, M. (1958). Effects of temporal and frontal lesions on auditory discrimination in monkeys. *Brain* **81**, 406–414.

Weiss, T. F., Mulroy, M. J. and Altman, D. W. (1974). Intracellular responses to acoustic clicks in the inner ear of the alligator lizard. *J. Acoust. Soc. Am.* **55**, 606–619.

Wever, E. G. (1949). *Theory of Hearing.* Wiley, New York.

Wever, E. G. and Bray, C. W. (1930). Action currents in the auditory nerve in response to acoustical stimulation. *Proc. Nat. Acad. Sci. USA.* **16**, 344–350.

Wever, E. G. and Lawrence, M. *Physiological Acoustics.* Princeton University Press, Princeton.

Wever, E. G. and Vernon, J. A. (1955). The effects of the tympanic muscle reflexes upon sound transmission. *Acta Otolar.* **45**, 433–439.

Whitfield, I. C. (1979). The object of the auditory cortex. *Brain Behav. Evol.* **16**, 129–154.

Whitfield, I. C. and Evans, E. F. (1965). Responses of auditory cortical neurons to stimuli of changing frequency. *J. Neurophysiol.* **28**, 655–672.

Whitfield, I. C. and Purser, D. (1972). Microelectrode study of the medial geniculate body in unanaesthetised, free-moving cats. *Brain Behav. Evol.* **6**, 311–322.

Whitfield, I. C. and Ross, H. F. (1965). Cochlear-microphonic and summating potentials and the outputs of individual hair cell generators. *J. Acoust. Soc. Am.* **38**, 126–131.

Whitfield, I. C., Cranford, J., Ravizza, R. and Diamond, I. T. (1972). Effects of unilateral ablation of auditory cortex in cat on complex sound localization. *J. Neurophysiol.* **35**, 718–731.

Wiederhold, M. L. (1970). Variations in the effects of electric stimulation of the crossed olivocochlear bundle of cat single auditory-nerve-fiber responses to tone bursts. *J. Acoust. Soc. Am.* **48**, 966–977.

Wiederhold, M. L. (1976). Mechanosensory transduction in 'sensory' and 'motile' cilia. *Ann. Rev. Biophys. Bioeng.* **5**, 39–62.

Wiener, F. M. and Ross, D. A. (1946). The pressure distribution in the auditory canal in a progressive sound field. *J. Acoust. Soc. Am.* **18**, 401–408.

Wightman, F., McGee, T. and Kramer, M. (1977). Factors influencing frequency selectivity in normal and hearing-impaired listeners. In *Psychophysics and Physiology of Hearing* (eds E. F. Evans and J. P. Wilson), pp. 295–306. Academic Press, London and New York.

Willott, J. F., Shnerson, A. and Urban, G. P. (1979). Sensitivity of the acoustic startle response and neurons in subnuclei of the mouse inferior colliculus to stimulus parameters. *Exp. Neurol.* **65**, 625–644.

Wilson, J. P. (1974). Basilar membrane vibration data and their relation to theories of frequency analysis. In *Facts and Models in Hearing* (eds E. Zwicker and E. Terhardt), pp. 56–63. Springer, Berlin.

Wilson, J. P. (1980a). Subthreshold mechanical activity within the cochlea. *J. Physiol.* **298**, 32–33P.

Wilson, J. P. (1980b). Evidence for a cochlear origin for acoustic re-emissions, threshold fine structure and tonal tinnitus. *Hearing Res.* **2**, 233–252.

Wilson, J. P. (1980c). Model for cochlear echoes and tinnitus based on an observed electrical correlate. *Hearing Res.* **2**, 527–532.

Wilson, J. P. and Johnstone, J. R. (1975). Basilar membrane and middle ear vibration in guinea pig measured by capacitive probe. *J. Acoust. Soc. Am.* **57**, 705–723.

Winer, J. A., Diamond, I. T. and Raczkowski, D. (1977). Subdivisions of the auditory cortex of the cat: the retrograde transport of horseradish peroxidase to the medical geniculate and posterior thalamic nuclei. *J. Comp. Neurol.* **176**, 387–417.

Woolsey, C. N. (1960). Organization of cortical auditory system: a review and a synthesis. In *Neural Mechanisms of the Auditory and Vestibular Systems* (eds G. L. Rasmussen and W. F. Windle), pp. 165–180. Thomas, Springfield.

Worden, F. G. and Marsh, J. T. (1963). Amplitude changes of auditory potentials evoked at cochlear nucleus during acoustic habituation. *Electroenceph. Clin. Neurophysiol.* **15**, 866–881.

Wright, C. G. and Barnes, C. D. (1972). Audio-spinal reflex responses in decerebrate and chloralose-anaesthetised cats. *Brain Res.* **36**, 307–331.

Young, E. D. and Brownell, W. E. (1976). Responses to tones and noise of single cells in dorsal cochlear nucleus of unanesthetized cats. *J. Neurophysiol.* **39**, 282–300.

Zakrisson, J.-E. and Borg, E. (1974). Stapedius reflex and auditory fatigue. *Audiology* **13**, 231–235.

Zwicker, E. (1954). Die Verdeckung von Schmalbandgeräuschen durch Sinustöne. *Acustica* **4**, 415–420.

Zwicker, E. (1970). Masking and psychological exciation as consequences of the ear's frequency analysis. In *Frequency Analysis and Periodicity Detection in Hearing* (eds R. Plomp and G. F. Smoorenberg), pp. 376–394. Sijthoff, Leiden.

Zwicker, E. (1974). On a psychoacoustical equivalent of tuning curves. In *Facts and Models in Hearing* (eds E. Zwicker and E. Terhardt), pp. 132–141. Springer, Berlin.

Zwicker, E., Flottorp, G. and Stevens, S. S. (1957). Critical band-width in loudness summation. *J. Acoust. Soc. Am.* **29**, 548–557.

Zwislocki, J. J. (1965). Analysis of some auditory characteristics. In *Handbook of Mathematical Psychology* Vol. 3 (eds R. Luce, R. Bush and E. Galanter), pp. 1–97. Wiley, New York.

Zwislocki, J. J. (1975). The role of the external and middle ear in sound transmission. In *The Nervous System*, Vol. 3 (ed. D. B. Tower), pp. 45–55. Raven Press, New York.

Zwislocki, J. J. (1980) Five decades of research on cochlear mechanics. *J. Acoust. Soc. Am.* **67**, 1679–1685.

Zwislocki, J. J. and Kletsky, E. J. (1980). Micromechanics in the theory of cochlear mechanics. *Hearing Res.* **2**, 505–512.

Index

O

P